THE PROBIOTIC DIET

JORDAN RUBIN & DR. JOSH AXE
WITH JOSEPH BRASCO M.D.

THE PROBIOTIC DIET

IMPROVE DIGESTION, BOOST YOUR BRAIN HEALTH,
AND SUPERCHARGE YOUR IMMUNE SYSTEM

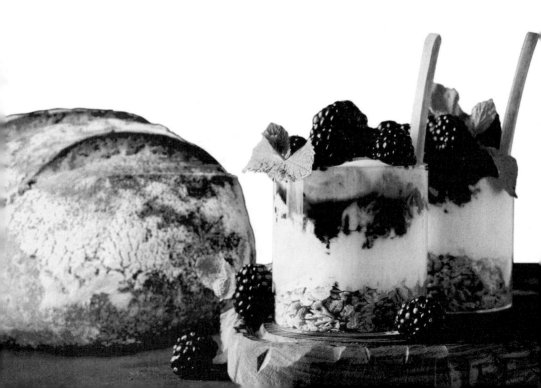

DESTINY IMAGE® PUBLISHERS, INC.
P.O. Box 310, Shippensburg, PA 17257-0310
"Publishing cutting-edge prophetic resources to supernaturally empower the body of Christ"

This book and all other Destiny Image and Destiny Image Fiction books are available at Christian bookstores and distributors worldwide.

For more information on foreign distributors, call 717-532-3040.

Reach us on the Internet: www.destinyimage.com.

ISBN 13 TP: 978-0-7684-7222-6

ISBN 13 eBook: 978-0-7684-7223-3

ISBN 13 HC: 978-0-7684-7225-7

ISBN 13 LP: 978-0-7684-7224-0

For Worldwide Distribution, Printed in the U.S.A.

2 3 4 5 6 7 8 / 27 26 25 24 23

CONTENTS

1

FREE PROBIOTICS

"Pro-by-*what?*"
—Oprah Winfrey, after hearing Mehmet Oz, M.D.,
mention the word "probiotics"

A few years ago, my wife, Nicki, and I drove to Nashville, Tennessee, for two incredibly good reasons. First, to visit Samuel, a two-month-old infant boy we were planning to adopt as we hurdled over the paperwork logjam. And second, to meet with Joe Brasco, M.D. and board-certified gastroenterologist, to discuss an idea—a book about probiotics. Dr. Joe lived 90 minutes southwest of Nashville in Huntsville, Alabama, so it was convenient for him to drive up and discuss.

I felt in my gut—pun intended—that it was time to figure out how to put together a book like *The Probiotic Diet*. For years, I'd been studying how probiotics had gone AWOL in the modern American diet, and their absence meant that the body's "terrain"—or internal environment—was more susceptible to digestive problems such as ulcers, constipation, irritable bowel syndrome, GERD or chronic heartburn, gastritis, inflammatory bowel disease, bacterial diseases like salmonella, and a group of viruses called calicivirus, also known as the Norwalk virus.

I had a soft spot in my heart for probiotics ever since they were instrumental in my recovery from a two-year battle against a variety of digestive diseases that nearly killed me when I was

19 years old. I felt that a lifestyle built around intentionally adding probiotics to your daily eating plan was sorely needed in our disease-stricken nation today.

After Joe and I made great headway that afternoon, we made plans to meet for dinner at the Cheesecake Factory in Brentwood, a leafy suburb of Nashville. Joe's wife, Christi, and their two children would be joining us. On our way to Brentwood, Nicki and I stopped at a Publix supermarket to pick up a few things. Just before stepping inside the gleaming spic-and-span store, I spotted a colorful green poster affixed next to the entrance.

"Free Antibiotics!" blared the headline. The tagline was obviously meant to stop shoppers in their tracks because everyone loves getting something for nothing. Publix, like any commercial enterprise, was not in the business of giving something away unless it drives more business their way. Curious what the fine print would say—since Joe and I had been talking about *probiotics* an hour earlier—I peered for a closer look. The small print at the bottom of the poster provided the details: "Just bring in your prescription for one of the oral antibiotics listed below to your neighborhood Publix pharmacy, and receive it FREE, up to a 14-day supply."

Then the poster listed the common antibiotics that it would honor with a free prescription:

- Amoxicillin
- Lephalexin
- Sulfamethoxazole/Trimethoprim (Sm2-TMP)
- Penicillin VK
- Ampicillin
- Erythromycin

I knew that many of these antibiotics were oral medicines that physicians routinely prescribe to treat children's ear infections, help adults fight off sinus problems, or combat sexually transmitted diseases. These antibiotics either annihilate bacteria in the body or weaken them so the immune system can deliver the *coup de grace*. All this makes sense since antibiotics, which comes from the Greek words *anti* (meaning "against") and *bios* (meaning "life") are chemical compounds known for killing or inhibiting the growth of infectious organisms.

Antibiotics are ineffective, however, against infections caused by viruses, such as colds, the flu, COVID-19, and most coughs and sore throats. This information doesn't stop some parents—especially working moms and dads who can't afford to stay home with a sick child—from viewing antibiotics as "cure-alls" for any sort of ailment. They'll drag their sick children to the doctor's office and practically demand that they walk out with an antibiotic prescription in hand, even though first-year interns could tell them that most cold and flu bugs naturally run their course with bed

GROWING UP WITH ANTIBIOTICS

Did my mother rush me to the doctor whenever I had an earache as a kid?

Actually, I didn't have ear infections growing up, but I did come down with sinusitis on occasion, which is pain and pressure in the face along with a stuffy or runny nose. Doctors say that symptoms indicate a bacterial infection, so the default treatment is antibiotics.

Dad and Mom were wary of antibiotics, but since I didn't come down with sinusitis very often—perhaps every couple of years—they followed our family doctor's advice and got me an antibiotic prescription.

rest and plenty of liquids. So the harried family physician relents and writes the prescription, an action that happens millions of times each year.

"That's exactly the problem with antibiotics," railed talk-show host John Kobylt of the "John and Ken Show" on KFI radio in Los Angeles. "Too many dopey moms not understanding science are giving their kids antibiotics when they have a three-day virus." All these antibiotics are creating antibiotic-resistant "super bugs," ranted the talk-show host, "and it's all because of the excessive prescriptions of antibiotics that doctors are bullied [into giving] by the mothers who doctor-shop until they find one who will prescribe the antibiotics."[1]

You could say the overprescription of antibiotics was inevitable given that these medicines were called "miracle drugs" when they were first introduced over a hundred years ago. German physician and chemist Paul Ehrlich is credited with discovering the world's first modern antibiotic in 1909 when he successfully synthesized organic compounds that would selectively attack an infecting organism without harming the host. His development of salvarsan, a synthetic compound that exhibited selection action against spirochetes—the bacteria that caused syphilis—was hailed as a major advancement in medicine.

Ehrlich's discovery blazed a trail for British bacteriologist Sir Alexander Fleming, whose experiments with the mold *Penicillium notatum* led to the discovery of penicillin, the archetype of antibiotics, in 1928. Penicillin is credited with saving the lives of hundreds of thousands of American GIs during World War II—as well as the baseball career of one of my baseball heroes, New York Yankee centerfielder Mickey Mantle. When Mantle was playing high school football in the late 1940s, he was kicked hard in his right shin. His ankle swelled to twice its normal size at the same time a 104° fever hit. Doctors diagnosed him with a bone infection called osteomyelitis, and they thought the only thing that could be done was to amputate his leg. Mickey's mother would have none of that, so she took her son to another hospital for a second opinion, where doctors treated him with penicillin—and saved a Hall of Fame baseball career.

Feel-good stories about penicillin can be repeated in millions of households, and there's no doubt that human history would have to be rewritten if antibiotics had never been discovered. The number of diseases that have been controlled or cured because of antibiotics would fill a couple of pages of this book. Wounds, gashes, and even simple infections—like an ingrown toenail that can turn septic—are no longer deadly, and pregnant women no longer have to fear dying from an infection after childbirth. Infants and toddlers screaming for relief from ear infections can be healed by the right antibiotic.

For all the good that these wonder drugs do, however, there's a downside to antibiotics that must be reckoned with. Antibiotics can be called molecules of biological warfare, destroying or compromising *all* bacteria, including the good. Often, this action can leave the body temporarily without defenses, especially in the digestive tract. That's why certain antibiotics are known for a high incidence of side effects, such as upset stomach, diarrhea, and vaginal yeast infections.

The dark cloud hanging above the sunny landscape of good health is that various bacteria in our bodies can become resistant to the antibiotic trying to kill it. Antibiotic-resistant pathogens are emerging at an alarming rate, meaning the antibiotic that worked last year could be ineffective today. The body's growing resistance to various antibiotics has been growing for the last 20 or 30 years and is increasing among viruses, bacteria, fungi, and parasites.

The U.S. Food and Drug Administration says that disease-causing microbes that have become resistant to drug therapy are an increasing public health problem. Tuberculosis, gonorrhea, malaria, and childhood ear infections are just a few of the diseases that have become harder to treat with antibiotic drugs. For instance, the incidence of penicillin resistance for patients suffering from a strain of pneumonia—*Streptococcus pneumoniae*—now tops 35 percent, and 70 percent of bacteria that cause infections in hospitals are resistant to at least one of the drugs commonly used to fight infections.[2] In 2009, a striking 20-year-old Brazilian fashion model and beauty queen, Mariana Bridi, had her hands and feet amputated—then died a week later after the bacteria *Pseudomonas aeruginosa* successfully resisted multiple kinds of antibiotics. Mariana was originally treated for a urinary tract infection.[3]

The unseen picture is that you're taking in antibiotics all the time—and don't even know it. Antibiotics are used as a growth stimulant for livestock, and food-producing animals are routinely given antibiotic drugs, through their feed or by injection, for disease prevention. When you eat a juicy steak or spaghetti and meatballs from conventionally raised cattle, you're consuming antibiotics. That's why I will eat only beef and other red meat that's been raised in pastures and grass-fed. You've heard that you are what you eat, but when it comes to eating meat, you are what *they* ate!

Dairy products, too. If you're drinking commercial milk—or even spooning popular brands of yogurt with labels crowing "Probiotics Inside!"—you're consuming more antibiotics. Dairy cows are fed a constant supply of antibiotics from birth because of crowded living conditions, which contributes to their sickly nature. Every sip of commercial milk gives you the residue of up to 80 different antibiotics![4]

I share this information not to write a manifesto declaring that antibiotics are no good and should be abandoned. There's a time and a place for antibiotics. My point—and it's the point of this book—is, we need to look for ways to add *probiotics* to our diets, which can counterweight the antibiotics we're receiving either through medical treatment or through the foods and dairy products we routinely eat. Intentionally looking for ways to promote the growth of beneficial microorganisms in the human body is what *The Probiotic Diet* is all about. Some 400 species of microorganisms are said to live inside your body's terrain, so when those living organisms aren't circulating in your blood and your gut in the numbers they should, then you're setting yourself up for even *worse* health problems.

This is where following the Probiotic Diet comes in. In the following pages, you'll learn:

- how good germs can create great health
- how to raise your metabolism and balance your terrain
- how transforming your terrain will transform your life and provide the best defense for a host of health ailments

We have a lot of ground to cover, but by the time you're done reading *The Probiotic Diet*, you'll understand why the pendulum needs to swing away from antibiotics and more toward a probiotic culture. That's why I wasn't surprised to hear that Swedish researchers discovered that "good" germs may work as well as antiseptics in protecting hospital patients from dangerous infections. In this study, patients swabbed with probiotic bacteria called *Lactobacillus plantarum* escaped infection as well as those who cleaned up using the antiseptic chlorhexidine.[5]

Lactobacillus plantarum is a probiotic bacteria found in fermented foods such as sauerkraut. I'll be talking a lot more about particular probiotics in coming chapters, but keep in mind that when you see the words *lactobacillus* or *bacillus* written in italics, that represents a family of probiotic microorganisms that are beneficial for your health and your longevity.

NATURE'S ANTIBIOTIC: CHICKEN SOUP FOR THE SOUL

I was rarely sick growing up, but on the few occasions when I caught a cold, had a fever, or didn't feel well, Mom didn't bundle me up, rush me to the family doctor, and then dash into the pharmacy to fill a prescription for an antibiotic.

Instead, she kept me home and served up a heaping helping of "Jewish penicillin," otherwise known as homemade chicken soup. (I was raised in a Messianic Jewish home, but with a last name of Rubin, perhaps you figured that out.) There's something about slurping a zesty soup made from scratch with fiber-rich vegetables such as celery, carrots, onion, and zucchini that's mmm-mmm good for you.

For our family, chicken soup was nature's antibiotic—and good for the soul.

If You've Got Digestive Problems...

I understand that a certain percentage of readers will be picking up *The Probiotic Diet* because of their digestive troubles. Whenever I speak in public, I can't tell you how many hurting folks pull me aside to describe how their rampant diarrhea or constant gut pain have made their lives miserable. Quite frankly, I've learned more about other people's bowel habits than most would care to know, but that's fine with me because I view helping others as my purpose in life.

If you're coping with constipation, got gas, are bloated as a Goodyear blimp, or are dealing with diarrhea, then count yourself among the estimated 30 million men, women, and children in this country—10 percent of the U.S. population—plagued by persistent "gut" issues that disrupt life throughout the daylight hours and often through the night. The pain in your gut takes on many manifestations: constant or intermittent; stabbing like a knife or mildly uncomfortable; debilitating or manageable. Whether your digestive distress is piercing or pedestrian, it's no fun going through life hobbled by pain or feeling lousy.

The cause of your alimentary agitation may be from the microorganisms living in your intestinal tract—more than 100 trillion, according to scientists who've wet a finger in the wind and made an educated guess. Most of these microorganisms are benign or "friendly," and they assist the body in the digestive process, synthesizing valuable nutrients from the foods you eat and the liquids you drink. Other microorganisms, however, have minds of their own: waging skirmishes to gain territory in your digestive tract, a turf war where there are no victors and just one loser—you.

You can turn the battle in your favor by adopting the Probiotic Diet. I've also teamed up with my great friend and fellow co-founder of Ancient Nutrition, Dr. Joshua Axe, to ensure that this book is filled with life-changing and gut-transforming information. Dr. Axe, Dr. Brasco, and I are confident that this groundbreaking nutrition and lifestyle program will improve your digestive health naturally. We believe the Probiotic Diet can help you deal with:

- inflammatory bowel disease (Crohn's disease and ulcerative colitis)
- irritable bowel syndrome
- heartburn and GERD
- Candida
- parasites
- constipation
- ulcers
- gas and bloating
- food allergies
- system problems

- skin conditions (acne, eczema, and psoriasis)
- urinary tract infections
- frequent colds and flus
- dental problems (teeth and gums, including bad breath)
- overweight and obesity

The protocols in this book have gone through years of rigorous testing. Back in 2008, Dr. Brasco started testing *The Probiotic Diet* with his patients at the Center for Colon & Digestive Disease in Huntsville—patients who had resigned themselves to a lifetime of digestive distress and inflammatory bowel disease symptoms. The results were phenomenal, and while they were anecdotal, you'll see how these courageous folks were handed the tools to transform their digestive terrains and live in ways they never thought possible.

You can have access to those same tools as well. If you're ready to add probiotic foods and nutritional supplements to your diet, you could dramatically improve your health in the next few months, whether your health is "normal" or you're besieged by intestinal distress. *The Probiotic Diet* can help you experience an amazing transformation in your ability to fight off various bugs and improve your gut health, and you do that by following our three-phase, 12-week program that provides:

- a comprehensive eating plan containing an abundance of probiotic-rich foods
- a targeted nutritional supplement protocol
- probiotic beverages
- a thorough cleansing of the digestive system
- specific regimens designed for specific digestive issues

I wish I had access to a plan like the Probiotic Diet back when I was 19 years old. I had just finished a six-week summer semester at Florida State University in Tallahassee following my freshman year of college. My hometown was Palm Beach Gardens, Florida, a palm-swept city of wide boulevards and 35,000 residents along South Florida's Treasure Coast. Dad was a naturopathic physician and a chiropractor, and my mother was a wonderful homemaker for my younger sister, Jenna, and me.

I had accepted the typical summer job for a college student: working as a camp counselor at Lake Swan near Gainesville, located in central Florida a couple of hours from home. Camp Swan, as it was called, was sponsored every summer by my home church, First Baptist Church of West Palm Beach.

I knew Camp Swan wasn't just another sports camp since I had gone there as a camper during my high school years. Sure, we did rope courses, waterskiing, and tubing behind a speedboat during the day, but the evenings were reserved for listening to an inspirational speaker, clapping to energetic worship music, and participating in skits and drama presentations.

In the summer of 1993, I was looking forward to my first Camp Swan as a counselor. It's funny how you can look back and remember certain things like yesterday, and for me, it was viewing a new film, *Forrest Gump*, after our orientation with the other rookie counselors. Although *Forrest Gump* could never be confused with a biblical movie, Tom Hanks's character resonated with me. Here was someone—okay, Forrest Gump was a simpleton—who had the right motives and wanted to change people's lives for the better. The other overriding message was the importance of being in the right place at the right time.

Voiceover by Forrest Gump: "Lieutenant Dan got me invested in some kind of fruit company. So then I got a call from him, saying we don't have to worry about money no more. And I said, 'That's good!' One less thing."

Of course, the "fruit company" turned out to be Apple Computers during their start-up days in the mid-1970s, and Forrest Gump made millions. I came out of the theater that night motivated about life.

Even though Florida's summer heat is oppressive, I enjoyed being outdoors and impacting young teens' lives. The biggest excitement during the first couple of days was when some high-school kid on water skis ran over an alligator. That shook everyone up.

Then it was *my* turn to get shook up. One afternoon after lunch, my stomach felt like it was doing a break dance. I tried to blame my digestive distress on something I ate—after all, camp chow was often a mix of mystery meat and runny sauces—but suddenly, I had a gigantic urge to go. After excusing myself to the other counselors, I walked *very quickly*—running was out of the question—to the nearest toilet, which was one of those hole-in-the-floor jobs.

The relief didn't last long. An hour or two later while out on the ropes course, I had to make the same "penguin walk" for the primitive toilets. Thus began around-the-clock nausea, constant stomach cramps, horrible digestive problems, and a fiery fever. My energy was sapped by the relentless diarrhea, causing me to lose 20 pounds in just six days. Unable to perform my duties, I was one sick puppy and asked to leave camp.

I felt a little better when I got home, but the rest of the summer was a blur of doctor visits and lying low. My family doctor performed the requisite tests, and in an effort to leave no stone unturned, he even tested me for the HIV virus. None of the test results discovered a reason for what ailed me. My sudden digestive stress remained a medical mystery. All my doctor could do was write me a prescription for antibiotics, which, looking back, may have exacerbated my problems.

I was determined to return to Florida State that fall, where I moved into a six-bedroom house with seven other guys. Thank goodness I had my own bedroom. A month into the fall semester, my health nosedived when the diarrhea returned with a vengeance. I'll never forget the time when I got lost driving around Tallahassee. I never had a good sense of direction anyway, but on this one occasion, I got lost in a hilly area when I *really had to go*. To make matters worse, I was driving a stick shift, which I wasn't good at, and I kept stalling at every stop. I panicked that day and barely made it home.

My diarrhea got so bad that it was foolhardy to venture outside. I probably visited the toilet one to two dozen times a day, and most of my stools were bloody. Nighttime was the worst: I rarely slept more than 45 minutes to an hour before I had to get to the bathroom lickety-split.

Let me tell you: it was no fun making a mad dash for the porcelain throne, and you can only imagine how unsanitary conditions were inside the "Animal House" I was renting with my college buddies. The pounds melted off my robust 19-year-old frame like a snowman in the Sahara Desert. I persevered as long as I could until my body completely rebelled and broke down. I had to drop out of Florida State—and take Incompletes in my Biology Lab, Non-Verbal Communications, Nutrition 201, Public Speaking, Early Church History, and Intro to Guitar classes. I flew back home to South Florida to a mother and father very concerned about my failing health.

That was the start of a two-year health odyssey that resulted in numerous hospitalizations, dozens of doctor visits, and long-shot trips to Mexico and Germany in search of an elusive cure. I reached bottom during one of my periodic stays at a hospital in West Palm Beach. On this occasion, fever spikes tormented me, and my heart beat like a Florida State drum major—more than 200 beats per minute. I had lost more than 80 pounds and wasn't much more than a 104-pound stick-and-bones figure who resembled a Nazi death camp survivor. My medical team prepared my parents for the news that I might not make it.

I'll never forget the night in my hospital room when I made peace with God and accepted whatever He had planned for me—including my imminent death. That evening, I asked the Lord not to give up on me. If He would heal me and help me get out of that hospital, I promised that I would make it my life's mission to help others lead healthy lives.

That very night, my health rallied like Mickey Mantle delivering a game-winning double in the bottom of the ninth inning. Even though I still had some distance to make up, I eventually made a full recovery employing many of the principles that comprise *The Probiotic Diet*. Today, God has blessed me with excellent health and incredible energy, and those debilitating digestive and immune system problems are in my rearview mirror. You wouldn't recognize me these days, all these years after my brush with death, and I give a lot of the credit to probiotics.

I'll describe later what precise probiotics I took, but I can assure you that I wouldn't be alive without probiotics.

Along Came Nicki

Two years after I recovered from my severe digestive problems, I was introduced to a wonderful young woman named Nicki at my singles group—called Souled Out Singles—that met on Monday nights at Christ Fellowship Church in Palm Beach Gardens.

The week before, I had shared my health journey—the one I just described—and one of the other guys in the singles group told me that I had to show Nicki the snapshot of me when I weighed 111 pounds.

"This can't be you!" she exclaimed as she held the photo of a gangly college kid with pipestem legs in boxer shorts. You could count every rib on my upper torso.

"That's me," I replied, but I wasn't thinking about those lonely days and interminable nights. Nicki was a beautiful young woman, and I couldn't take my eyes off her. You could say that she set off my attraction bells.

Soon, I began looking forward to every Monday night when I could sit next to Nicki and get to know her better. We remained "good friends" for six months before I finally worked up the courage to ask her out. We dated for a year, had a seven-month engagement, and were married on September 5, 1999.

Like many newly married couples in our mid-twenties, our future looked limitless in the afterglow of the honeymoon. Long before GPS systems became standard equipment in today's nicer cars, we saw a roadmap that stretched as far as the eyes could see from our modest one-bedroom apartment in Palm Beach Gardens.

I had founded a health and wellness company called Garden of Life a year earlier, and our stratospheric growth was like hanging onto a Delta V rocket launched at nearby Cape Canaveral. Nicki, a certified public accountant, kept her fingers busy punching a numeric keypad; she was being handed more and more responsibility with a major East Coast accounting firm.

We worked insane hours those first couple of years of marriage, driven to make our mark in the corporate world before we'd "settle down" and start a family. Then Garden of Life *really* took off, and I needed Nicki's savvy business acumen as well as her CPA skills to help manage our skyrocketing sales in the early '00s. We didn't mind working until eight or nine o'clock in the evening because we were striding toward a common goal and experiencing unexpected success.

Nicki and I began trying in earnest to bring an offspring into the world. Remember, we had life all mapped out. Once Nicki became pregnant, she would deliver a strapping son. (Hey, all dads say that!) As for Nicki, she wanted to be a stay-at-home mom while keeping a part-time hand in our health and wellness company.

But as José, the unassuming chef in the movie *Bella*, says, "If you want to make God laugh, just tell Him your plans."

First of all, Nicki wasn't becoming pregnant. Despite taking all the right steps, we battled infertility for more than two years. The situation became serious enough for us to schedule a series of appointments with a fertility specialist. I checked out fine, but as for Nicki, the doctor suspected endometriosis, a condition in which endometrial tissue—the lining inside the uterus—grows *outside* the womb and attaches to other organs, such as the ovaries and fallopian tubes. Tiny islands of endometrium, or cells, can block important pathways in and around the uterus.

Our infertility difficulties came to a head in the summer of 2003, when Nicki was 33 years old. She was four-and-a-half years older than me, surely not too old to become pregnant, but at an age when conception becomes more difficult. The doctor hemmed and hawed before recommending a laparoscopy to remove any ovarian cysts or adhesions in Nicki's pelvic cavity. We didn't like the surgical option, but if that's what it took for Nicki to become pregnant, then that's what we would do.

Meanwhile, I was busy writing *The Maker's Diet* that summer as well as running Garden of Life, so I had a lot on my plate as well. At the end of my manuscript, I devised a 40-day "health experience" section with a comprehensive meal plan. I felt that I should personally test the 40-day health plan as a matter of accountability, but it didn't make much sense if I were the only one in our household following a fairly strict diet for breakfast, lunch, and dinner.

I asked Nicki to undergo the 40-day health plan with me, but deep down, an ulterior motive was in play: I believed the Maker's Diet could help Nicki become pregnant because her diet could use some cleaning up. You see, my lovely wife had a love affair with Starbucks and their Caramel Macchiatos—extra caramel, and extra whip. Cherry-flavored Twizzlers were another weakness.

I believed Nicki's occasional forays into the world of junk food could have been impacting her ability to get pregnant since I had come across research showing that consuming too many carbohydrates, particularly sugar and starches, could raise a woman's insulin levels and produce a hormonal imbalance impeding the ovulation process. I had a gut feeling that if she stuck with the Maker's Diet for 40 days, then her womb would be more predisposed, as it were, to becoming pregnant.

At first, Nicki resisted my suggestion to join me on the Maker's Diet, but she eventually came around because she didn't want to submit to invasive surgery any more than I wanted her to. She was desperate enough to try anything—even a regimented diet that included goat's milk yogurt and cultured vegetables and a "partial fast" every Thursday (no breakfast or lunch). The result was a miracle in more ways than one: Nicki and I are *sure* that she became pregnant on the fortieth and final day of the Maker's Diet while on a trip to Springfield, Missouri! I'm convinced that Nicki's consumption of probiotic-rich foods and supplements helped her digestion and led to her conceiving.

Around nine months later on May 29, 2004, our hopes and dreams were realized when Joshua Michael Rubin entered this world with a set of healthy lungs. We certainly wanted our little guy to have a brother or sister. Because Nicki had so much difficulty, however, becoming pregnant and breastfeeding—she suffered from engorgement, blocked ducts, and mastitis—she broached the idea of adopting a child from a foreign country. We decided that we would see where God would lead us.

An Unexpected Detour

In the spring of 2007, I happened to fly to Nashville at the request of Mercy Ministries (now called Mercy Multiplied), a non-profit Christian organization for young women facing life-controlling issues such as eating disorders, substance addiction, and the residue of sexual and emotional abuse. Some of the young women—who are in their teens and early twenties—arrive at Mercy dealing with a crisis pregnancy, and the compassionate counselors are there to present alternatives to abortion, such as placing their child for adoption.

The founder of Mercy Multiplied, Nancy Alcorn, asked me to speak to the girls for a couple of days on various health and well-ness topics, walking them through a list of practical steps that they could take to change their lives for the better. Many of the girls had lived for years by skipping breakfast and subsisting on fast-food fare—burger-and-fries and pepperoni pizza—for their nutritional needs. Others thought they were getting their "fruit" when they ordered a raspberry-topped sundae at Dairy Queen.

I urged them to eat only foods that God created, which meant choosing foods as close to the natural source as possible to give them the healthiest lives possible. In practical terms, this meant seeking out organically grown meat, fruits, and vegetables, as well as pasture-raised dairy products high in omega-3s, unpro-cessed grains, and various nuts and seeds. Because many of the Mercy girls had digestive issues due to the years of disordered eating, getting probiotics into their diets was a must.

The young women responded well, and the staff thanked me for carving out several days from my busy schedule. As I was leaving the group home that afternoon, I happened to get into a conversation with a Mercy Multiplied counselor about their adoption services. I asked some leading questions, but I never indicated that Nicki and I were leaning toward the adoption

option. I did, however, pick up a packet of information upon my departure. Back home, Nicki and I didn't feel any compunction to fill out the application to be considered adoptive parents, however.

Two months later, I received a phone call from someone at Mercy Multiplied who remembered that I had taken an adoption packet. What she said stunned me.

"Jordan, we have a situation with one of the birthmothers," she began, "and she wrote down the characteristics she would like to see in the child she's placing for adoption. We think you and Nicki have a lot of those characteristics. Would you and your wife be interested in adopting?"

Would we? This time around, Nicki and I talked more seriously about the opportunity, certainly prayed about it, and then we gave our enthusiastic yes. We filled out all the necessary paper-work and flew to Nashville two days after the baby was born on August 6, 2007. The birthmother had named her son Samuel because she was devoting him to God, much like how Hannah in the Old Testament (see 1 Samuel) named her son Samuel and gave him to be in service to the Lord.

Unfortunately, the courts and paperwork barred us from immediately bringing Samuel home with us where we lived at the time in Palm Beach Gardens, which is why we found ourselves in Nashville on that Labor Day weekend. Meanwhile, Samuel was looked after by a wonderful foster mom. While all of this was happening, suddenly, and I mean out of nowhere, a friend who ran the Place of Hope children's home founded by our former church in Palm Beach Gardens mentioned that one of their residents had an unplanned pregnancy and was looking to place the child in an adoptive home. Would we be interested? This happened in mid-October.

Once again, Nicki and I thought about it and prayed about it, and once again, we said yes. On October 29, 2007, Alexis was

OUR PROBIOTIC INFANT FORMULA

Following Joshua's birth in 2004, he was a wonderful, normal boy, but he was also colicky and prone to screaming to the high heavens when hungry. Nicki was committed to breastfeeding our son because we both believed that nothing could match the high-quality nutrients found in breast milk or replace God's perfect design for breastfeeding.

Poor Nicki. She never slept more than three or four hours a night the first few months. She was continually exhausted, and while I tried to be supportive when our son wailed from his crib at half-past-two in the morning, we both knew there wasn't much I could do: Nicki was the sole provider for his sustenance.

When Nicki began running into problems related to breastfeeding (engorgement, blocked

born, and she became a permanent part of our family just two days later. But baby Samuel was still in Nashville, and we wanted very much for him to join our family. Finally, on February 26, 2008, the paperwork got resolved, and Nicki and I held him as we experienced an awesome adoption placement ceremony at the Mercy Multiplied headquarters.

Meet Dr. Joe Brasco

I already mentioned that during our Labor Day weekend trip to visit Samuel, Dr. Joe Brasco and I laid down the foundation for *The Probiotic Diet* book. Now that you've gotten to know me and my background, it's time I introduce my co-author.

I knew that Dr. Joe would be a great resource to collaborate with on *The Probiotic Diet*. We met in 1999—shortly after my engagement to Nicki—when I spoke at a seminar on clinical nutrition about my digestive tract problems and how I overcame them. Sitting in the front row that afternoon was Dr. Brasco.

After my talk, Joe introduced himself, sensing that he had found a kindred spirit in a more natural approach to digestive health. We remained in contact, and our friendship blossomed. In 2002, we joined forces to write my first book, *Restoring Your Digestive Health*, and we later collaborated on another dozen books in the *Great Physician's Rx* series on topics ranging from irritable bowel syndrome to high cholesterol.

Joe has quite an interesting story himself. Growing up in an Italian immigrant family on Staten Island—one of New York City's five boroughs—he was like any other kid in the neighborhood who loved baseball and the Bronx Bombers—the New York Yankees. Every afternoon after school and on Saturday mornings in the 1960s, Joe and his friends played energetic pick-up games until the sun set over Upper New York Bay. Number 7 in pinstripes, Mickey Mantle, was his baseball idol, too.

Following Mass on Sunday, Joe and the extended family gathered around an oversized dining room table at tow o'clock to savor a Sunday afternoon dinner straight out of the film *The Godfather*. A dozen or so family members—representing three generations—passed oversized platters of antipasti, chicken

ducts, and mastitis), it wasn't long before her run-down body couldn't produce enough milk for our hungry boy. We knew the last thing we wanted to feed Joshua was pasteurized cow's milk or commercial formula because homogenization of the milk alters the fats and makes them more likely to damage arteries and potentially harm the body.

Necessity being the mother of invention—since Nicki and I were determined to find an alternative to commercial formula—I devised a homemade infant formula that was rich in probiotics and closely matched the high-quality nutrients found in breast milk.

The major ingredient, I decided, would be raw goat's milk because it was unpasteurized and delivered an easily digestible protein that did not contain the same complex proteins found in cow's milk. Goat's milk has higher amounts of medium-chain fatty acids

(MCFAs) than any other milk and 7 percent less lactose than cow's milk. Furthermore, raw or cultured goat's milk fully digests in a baby's stomach in 20 minutes, while pasteurized cow's milk takes eight hours because of the difference in the goat milk's structure: its fats and protein molecules are tiny in size, which is the key to rapid absorption in the digestive tract.

When Alexis and Samuel joined our family a couple of years later, I made huge batches of my homemade infant formula every Sunday that would last us the week. Poor Samuel. After bringing him home with us, the little guy's body was covered from head to foot with eczema. His skin had turned red and itchy and resembled pimply acne. He also suffered from constipation.

The probiotic ingredients in his infant formula cleared up his eczema in a jiffy and put a smile on his face, happy that he no longer had to strain to poop into his diaper.

cacciatore, pasta Milanese, and marinated vegetables and ate for hours until their stomachs burst. But the younger ones always left room for homemade dessert: mascarpone-rich tiramisu, cream-filled cannoli, and lemony vanilla gelato.

Although Joe could eat all afternoon—and get hungry enough to raid the refrigerator at seven o'clock—he didn't grow to a strapping six-footer but leveled out at five-feet, five inches during adolescence. "I didn't become the Italian Stallion like Sylvester Stallone," he jokes. "More like the Italian Pony."

Of greater concern than his slight stature was persistent acne, for which he sought treatment from a dermatologist. On top of that, during his freshman year of high school Joe began experiencing a run-down feeling—low energy and listlessness. His mom, worried that something might be drastically wrong, felt the back of his head for any lumps but didn't find any sign of a tumor.

When Joe's energy continued to ebb, she made an appointment to see the family doctor. After listening to Joe describe the symptoms, the doctor poked and prodded a bit before opining that Joe must have some type of virus—probably mononucleosis. He counseled bed rest and wrote him a prescription.

While on bed rest for a couple of weeks—and missing his sandlot baseball games—Joe passed the time by reading books about his health condition. Something in his heart told him that prescription drugs weren't a magic panacea—that he would be better off gravitating toward a more natural way of getting better.

So, at the age of 14, Joe took the train to the nearest health food store, which in those days—1974—was located in the New Dorp neighborhood of Staten Island. There he purchased books by health pioneers Adele Davis and Paul Bragg, who pointed out that the standard American diet—tasteless white bread baked from nutrient-stripped refined flour, deep-fried chicken and greasy hamburgers served up in fast-food restaurants, single-skillet meals made out of a box, and mass-produced "treats" high in refined sugar, artificial flavoring, and preservatives—provided woefully inadequate nutrition.

As he read more about the ingredients of good health, the Staten Island teenager dropped junk food and stopped consuming nutritionally bankrupt products like soda pop, white bread, and—*Mama mia!*—pasta made from enriched flour. "I told Mom that I didn't want to eat any more of those things," Joe said, "so she let me go to the health food store and shop for better foods and products to eat."

With Mom's spending money in his pocket, he filled his satchel with whole wheat pasta, raw milk cheese, yogurt made from organic milk, juicy organic apples, and nutritional supplements like brewer's yeast. For his complexion, Joe purchased a box of Swiss Kriss, a mixture of powdered herbs and flowers that was administered via a facial steam bath.

Joe's quest for a non-traditional approach to what ailed him resulted in greater energy and an eventual clearing up of his skin. As he continued to have his consciousness raised—to use a '70s term—Joe thought about what he wanted to do with his life. During high school, he entertained thoughts about becoming a medical doctor, but he didn't tell his parents or three younger brothers about his secret ambition.

Following graduation from an all-boys Catholic high school, Joe quietly took the prerequisite pre-med courses at Rutgers University in nearby New Brunswick, New Jersey: biology, organic chemistry, and math. After earning excellent grades, he applied to three medical schools, telling his family that he didn't want to become a doctor just so he could write "M.D." behind his name. "I wanted to become a doctor with a cause," he said, "and my cause was that I would try to revolutionize medicine and show people that they can recapture their health without relying on drugs and surgery, that good health could be obtained through natural means."

To do so, however, meant working *within* the system, or as Joe put it: "I needed the credentials of orthodoxy if I wanted to enact changes in the way we treat people." With acceptances from three medical schools in his hip pocket, Joe chose the Medical College of Wisconsin in Milwaukee with a vague idea of pursuing something to do with nutrition. When he had to declare a direction in his third year, Joe chose internal medicine. "I knew family practice was too general for what I wanted to do, and internal medicine would be a tighter focus, the better route to go."

Following graduation from medical school and residency, Joe was assigned to the University of Illinois campus for his internship. He hasn't forgotten a pivotal conversation that occurred during his first week—one that would change the course of his life. It was a Saturday, 12:30 p.m., and Joe was in a care room off the ICU kibitzing with Dr. Lou Agnone, the senior resident and gastroenterologist appointed to work with him. Dr. Agnone had taken an interest in the young doctor, so he asked him, "Tell me, Joe, what are you going to specialize in?"

"Well, I want to go into nutrition," Dr. Brasco replied.

"What are you going to do with nutrition?" queried Dr. Agnone, clearly unimpressed.

"I do believe you can really improve people's health that way."

"Are you going to do a fellowship in nutrition? You could do a fellowship in nutrition, but that's not going to take you anywhere," the experienced doctor declared. Dr. Agnone paused for a moment before plunging ahead. "Here's what you ought to do," he began. "You have a medical education to pay for, so you need to make a living. You said you wanted to pursue something in nutrition. What's nutrition? Answer: it's the GI tract. So if you really want to do nutrition, you need to become a gastroenterologist."

"I don't know about that," Dr. Brasco replied hesitantly.

"No, you need to think this through like I have. Gastroenterology is where you want to specialize."

So that's what Joe did. After four years of medical school, three years of residency, and two years of fellowship, Joe joined a gastroenterology practice in Indianapolis, Indiana, and began seeing dozens of patients each day seeking relief for their digestive ailments. "I was thrust into the real world," Joe said. "The real world is that most people don't want to put in the work to get better. They don't believe they can feel as bad as they do just from their diet. They don't believe that a simple thing like changing what they eat could help them. Patients placate you and make some changes for a day or two, but they never fully heed your advice to drink more water for their constipation or stop eating fried jalapenos for their acid reflux. I would say that 95 percent never stick with the program for longer than 24 hours. Sometimes I wonder what I have to say to convince them to change."

But the 5 percent who follow his advice—advice that's part of the Probiotic Diet—experience a renaissance in their digestive health.

Presently, Dr. Brasco is practicing at the Center for Colon & Digestive Disease in Huntsville, where he skillfully combines diet, supplementation, and judicious use of medications to provide a comprehensive treatment program for his patients. "My goal is to help patients realize that a good diet is essential to good health," Dr. Brasco explained. "However, most people are still new to the idea of probiotics. One of the mantras of my profession is that depending on the health of the GI tract, so goes the rest of the body."

The license plate on his car says it all: GI JOE. You have to love that, especially if you're a patient of Dr. Brasco.

Meet Dr. Joshua Axe

Long before Josh and I partnered together to form Ancient Nutrition, he was paving the way for gut health. When he started his website, DrAxe.com, in 2006, there wasn't much out there in terms of probiotic or gut information. That didn't stop Josh. He was on a mission from the day he got a call from his mom, Winona, when he was just 24 years old.

Josh was in school training to become a doctor and working as a clinical nutritionist just outside of Orlando, Florida, when he received a phone call from home. His mother was on the line, and she sounded upset.

"What's wrong, Mom?" Josh asked.

"The cancer has come back," she said through tears.

His heart sank, and he was immediately transported back to his seventh-grade year, when his mom was told that she had stage-4 breast cancer that had spread to her lymph nodes. At the time, Winona was 41 years old; she was a gym teacher and a swim instructor. Everyone thought she was the picture of fitness and health.

Soon after her diagnosis, Winona underwent a total mastectomy of her left breast and started the first of what would be four cycles of chemotherapy that left her too weak to get out of bed in the days that followed. It was painful for Josh to see how sick she got on chemo.

Thankfully, months later she was declared cancer-free, but her health continued to spiral downward. Even after bouncing back from chemotherapy and returning to her job, she felt lousy. Every day, she would get home at 3:30 p.m. and nap until dinner time. When she told her doctor that she couldn't cope with being a wife, mother, and schoolteacher, she prescribed an antidepressant.

Depressed and exhausted: this was the mother Josh knew throughout his teenage years. She lived in fear that the cancer would return.

And now, ten years later, it had.

Her distressed voice shook Josh back to the present. "My oncologist told me they found a tumor on my lungs that was 2.5 centimeters," she said. "He wants to do surgery and start radiation and chemotherapy right away."

Josh tried to be as encouraging as possible. "Mom, please don't worry. Your body has the ability to heal. We just need to stop feeding the cancer cells and get to the root cause of the disease." He was confident her health could be restored—but, in order to do that, they'd need to take care of her whole body.

The next day, he flew home to help her lay out a health program. Josh asked Winona to tell him about any symptoms she had been experiencing in the time leading up to her diagnosis.

She sighed. "Well, I'm still struggling with depression," she said. "And even if I get a good night's sleep, I'm always tired the next day." She described symptoms that indicated she had multiple food sensitivities. She also revealed that she'd been diagnosed with hypothyroidism.

All of this was quite troubling—but it was her last symptom that shocked Josh. When he asked about her digestive habits, she revealed that she'd had an average of one to two bowel movements a week, for the last ten years.

"Wow, Mom," Josh said, stunned. "Why didn't you talk to your doctor about this earlier?"

"I thought it was normal," she said. Her face crumpled.

"Mom," Josh said, "this is actually good news. We can definitely do something about your digestion, and that alone will make a big difference in how you're feeling." And hopefully will help stop the cancer, too, he thought.

That's when Josh told his mother about leaky gut syndrome—a condition in which the intestinal wall breaks down, allowing microbes and food particles to leak out of the digestive tract, triggering an inflammatory immune response—and how dangerous it was. Josh believed it was the cause of her constipation and several other health problems, and that they needed to address it immediately. "We can do this, Mom."

Josh proceeded into his mom's kitchen and grabbed a black garbage bag and opened kitchen cupboards. "We're starting all over," he announced. "From now on, you're not eating anything that comes out of a box."

Together, they threw out every processed food they could find:

- boxed cereals like Honey Nut Cheerios and Honey Bunches of Oats (she thought these cereals were healthy)

- plastic bottles of Juicy Juice billed as "90 percent real fruit juice" but made with apple juice concentrate and "natural" flavors that weren't natural at all
- chips and crackers made with MSG and genetically modified corn
- cereal bars made with high fructose corn syrup, artificial colors, and soy protein
- salad dressings with artificial thickeners, emulsifiers, and hydrogenated oils
- bags of highly refined white sugar and white flour

All of these processed foods create an imbalance of the good bacteria in the gut. This imbalance leads to a cascade of problems, including leaky gut.

Then they drove to a local health food store, where Josh walked his mother through the aisles and talked her through the types of foods she should be eating and the probiotic-rich food that would help support her body in its fight to kill the cancer cells.

At that time, the mainstream antibacterial craze was at its height, and almost every product in conventional grocery stores—from floor cleaner to toothpaste to number-two pencils—seemed to have added antibacterial ingredients. Scientists had started to sound the alarm about the overprescription of antibiotics causing resistance to some strains of illnesses, and the danger of overly sterile environments to our immune systems, but their research wasn't trickling down to most neighborhoods just yet. The evidence of these issues was showing up every day in Josh's natural medicine practice, though. For several years he'd seen the collateral damage these antibacterials and other supposedly "sanitary" chemicals were causing.

If part of the problem centered on being too clean, he felt certain the solution must be the opposite—to get dirty. To consciously create repeated "micro-exposures" to dirt that held long-lost bacteria, viruses, and other microbes that could function as nature's immunizations. To fortify and replenish the beneficial bacteria our bodies lost during the onslaught of antibacterial products in our environment. To completely reeducate the immune system so it could once again learn how to defend itself without going overboard. To not be afraid of a little dirt here and there, but instead, more consciously follow the rhythms of nature and embrace the healing power that surrounds us every day.

And so, to start his mother's healing program, he went straight for the dirt. In his years of medical research, Josh developed a special interest in probiotics. One of the most novel and interesting threads of research he found centered on microorganisms in soil, which possesses many vital microbes often missing in the human body. Right away, he started Winona on a probiotic supplement with soil-based organisms (SBOs) believed to improve the absorption of nutrients, eliminate yeast overgrowth, and improve bowel function.

In her kitchen, Josh taught his mom how to make green drinks with servings of spinach, celery, cucumber, cilantro, lime, green apple, and stevia. She consumed a daily regimen of supplements, high-quality extracts derived from medicinal plants. She downed many cups of bone broth soup, the healing elixir made from the bones and innards of chicken, beef, lamb, or fish—animal parts previously considered dirty waste, now known to be an excellent source of collagen, glutamine, and other nutrients that help "heal and seal" the lining of the gut. She spent time outside in her garden every day, digging in the flower beds, or simply being still and giving thanks.

Josh's mom was a model patient—she followed his diet and lifestyle advice very closely. Over the next several months, she saw many positive changes in her health: her constipation problems resolved, and she began having one bowel movement every day. She noticed a major upswing in her energy. Her thyroid issues disappeared. She lost 22 pounds, and she no longer felt depressed. She reported feeling more joy than she had ever experienced.

When Josh's mom went in four months later for a CT scan, her surgeons were mystified by the results. Not only was her blood work normal, but her cancer markers had also dropped dramatically.

"What's happened is very unusual," the oncologist said, with obvious surprise. "We don't see cancer shrink very often." Her largest tumor had shrunk by 52 percent. The oncologist encouraged her to keep doing what she was doing, "because whatever it is, it's working." Her medical team decided to hold off on surgery. Winona was greatly relieved to avoid going under the knife again.

Now, Josh would never claim that his protocols "cured" his mom's cancer. Many factors come into play with an outcome like hers, and Winona was very diligent about following the guidance and directions of her other doctors. But where her doctors' instructions left off, her diet and lifestyle changes began. And Josh and I believe it is due to the integration of all of these factors and an emphasis on gut health that today—more than 20 years after she first learned she had breast cancer, and a decade after this second diagnosis—his mother is healthy and enjoying the fruits of her lifestyle changes.

Since then, Dr. Axe has written scores of articles on gut health, leaky gut, and probiotics, as well as programs and books like *Eat Dirt*. The protocol that his mother followed forms the backbone of the Eat Dirt program. For more information on Josh's books as well as thousands of health articles and scores of healthy recipes, visit www.DrAxe.com.

Where We Go Next

I'm thrilled to introduce you to *The Probiotic Diet*. I know this is a timely book with a timely message because the overprescription of antibiotics and overconsumption of antibiotic-laden and generally unhealthy foods means that millions of Americans and people worldwide go through life not feeling well.

That can all change if you adopt the principles behind *The Probiotic Diet,* but you'll have to be open because there's a good chance that everything you think you know about good health is about to change. The first area we'll explore is germs, and who better to start with than the famous 19th century French scientist Louis Pasteur, the founder of microbiology and father of "germ theory."

2

"IT'S THE TERRAIN"

As a rule, I don't shop at supermarkets very often since I prefer to purchase my groceries and meats at natural health food stores, which offer a better selection of organic fruits and vegetables as well as wild-caught fish and grass-fed meats like buffalo and bison. Nutrition S'Mart and Whole Foods are where we do our shopping in Palm Beach Gardens.

The large supermarket chains are getting the message that there's a growing market for organic foods, however. In the last few years, Safeway, Vons, Kroger's, Fred Meyer, Ralphs, Winn-Dixie, and Albertsons have dedicated entire aisles to organic foods. Publix is another mainstream chain offering organic eggs, milk, fruit, and vegetables. I've forgotten why Nicki and I stepped into the Nashville Publix that Labor Day weekend—it was probably to pick up some toiletries—but perhaps I wanted a couple of organic apples for the hotel room.

Since I'm not a regular customer of these grocery emporiums, I've noticed how supermarkets don't leave anything to chance. The "end caps" feature alluring displays of barbecue chips or stacks of soft drinks, and their aisles are wide enough for two carts to pass each other, but not too wide: grocers want you to easily pick things off both shelves as you pass. You can choose from 147 kinds of breakfast cereal, 22 brands and types of peanut butter, and 25 brands of chocolate chip cookies. An abundance of cheery signs guides you along, and in the produce department, the track lighting illuminating the fresh fruits and vegetables dazzles the eyes.

Have you noticed how supermarkets purposely place the produce section on one end of their humongous building and the milk and other dairy products way on the other side? If you're dropping in for a head of lettuce and a gallon of milk, you better have your walking shoes on. The idea is to make you pass by a *lot* of tempting treats on your way to the high-traffic staples. The hope, of course, is that you'll fill up your cart with foods fresh on your mind but not on your shopping list.

If Nicki sent me to the supermarket to pick up a head of Romaine and a gallon of whole milk, I would probably return home empty-handed. That's because organic lettuce can be hit-or-miss in supermarkets, but commercial milk—even if it's organic—presents a problem, and that's because of pasteurization.

I describe why I'm sour on pasteurized milk in a sidebar on page 44, but there's fascinating information about the man behind the word we find on every label of milk and juice in America. Louis Pasteur—the 19th century French scientist for whom pasteurization was named—discovered a process that relates directly to the premise of the Probiotic Diet.

But first, you need the backstory.

The period between 1775 and 1875 was marked by the phenomenal changes throughout the Western world as scientific discoveries, labor-saving inventions, and technological innovations opened the door to the Industrial Age. This pivotal era was also marked by social upheaval: the 13 original American colonies declared their independence from England and formed the United States, followed by the violent French Revolution and its Reign of Terror, which lopped off the heads of the monarchy and noble class and sent shivers through palace walls from London to Vienna.

France fell under the dictatorship of a victorious general, Napoleon Bonaparte, who enacted a uniform and modern administrative system, gave land tenure to the peasant proprietors, and left the bourgeoisie—the middle or merchant class—a political heritage that they claimed during the 19th century.

I relate this history lesson to help you understand why France, from its Napoleonic height in 1812 to its stunning defeat in the Franco-Prussian War of 1870-71, exerted a powerful diplomatic influence in the civilized world, shaped Western thought, and pioneered significant scientific advancements throughout much of the 19th century. "France led Europe in theoretical and industrial chemistry, and her self-sufficiency during the Revolutionary and Napoleonic Wars was in no small part the result of her scientific superiority," wrote author René Dubos.[1]

Many of the scientific discoveries that impact our health today came from the fertile minds of three 19th century French scientists: Louis Pasteur, Claude Bernard, and Antoine Béchamp. It turned out that Pasteur gained immortality while Bernard and Béchamp became historical footnotes, which is a shame. As you'll soon learn, Louis Pasteur—for all the fame he received—promulgated a huge mistake nearly 150 years ago, and the repercussions are being felt by millions of people today.

Louis Pasteur: The Road to Immortality

If Louis Pasteur, dressed in a dark waistcoat with a white turnover collar and wide tie, were to stroll through a Publix supermarket today, I think he would be rather bemused that a variation of his name—pasteurization—is prominently lettered on milk cartons, yogurt containers, boxes of fruit juice, and even bottles of beer. It's the old-school equivalent of having your jersey number retired in every stadium in the world, I guess.

The French scientist is credited with numerous and wondrous scientific advancements: laying the foundation for the science of microbiology, solving the mystery of rabies and silkworm diseases, and contributing to the development of the first vaccines. His most famous discovery relates to the causes of fermentation, which opened the door to the eponymous pasteurization process.

Born in 1822, the son of a tanner, and a star pupil at the École normale supérieure, the young Pasteur initially turned his attention to studying the difference between quartz crystals and salts, a problem baffling scientists because of their different properties. Through a series of experiments—with primitive laboratory instruments that he constructed himself—Pasteur proved that each isomer had different qualities because they were optical in nature, meaning some were left-handed and some were right-handed.

This might not seem like a big deal today, but in the 1840s, Pasteur's observations and ability to survey all the known data and link strands of information into a coherent hypothesis quickly won him superstar status among scientists in France and abroad. He was quickly inducted into the French Legion of Honor, and England presented him with the Copley Medal. Pasteur developed such a sterling reputation that in 1854, at just 32 years of age, he was appointed Dean of the Faculty of Science at the University of Lille.

Lille happened to be the center of France's winemaking industry, an integral cog of the French economy and linchpin of French *gastronomie*. In the summer of 1856, *le grand professeur* received a visit from a Monsieur Bigot, whose son attended Pasteur's classes. After describing his son's enthusiastic tales of

THE PROBIOTIC DIET

Pasteur's lectures and experiments, Monsieur Bigot wondered if the new dean could solve *un petit problème*. It seemed that Monsieur Bigot owned a distillery that manufactured alcohol through a fermentation process that began with adding yeast to sugar beets in large vats. The problem was that many of the fermentations were turning sour—and Monsieur Bigot had no idea why. Tired of dumping tons of sour alcohol down the drain and losing money, the factory owner asked Pasteur to investigate why this was happening.

How fermentation was initiated was a mystery in the mid-19th century. Most chemists of the day understood that the process entailed the chemical breakdown of sugar into alcohol and carbon dioxide, but what caused fermentation was essentially unknown. Yeast cells were found in fermenting vats of wine, but these living organisms were believed to be the product, not the cause, of fermentation. The scientific establishment shrugged their shoulders and attributed the chemical changes occurring during fermentation to mysterious life forces. This attitude didn't help contemporary winemakers, who never knew when their wine might turn sour or taste like vinegar. Monsieur Bigot faced the same problem with producing alcohol from sugar beets.

Pasteur's first step was using a microscope to analyze samples from the vats of alcohol. He found thousands of tiny microorganisms, asymmetrical in structure, and since they possessed this structure, he concluded that the living cells—in this case, the yeasts—were responsible for breaking down the sugar into alcohol. What turned the alcohol sour, he believed, were various undesirable microbes contaminating the alcohol during fermentation.

The 64,000-franc question was this: Where did the yeasts come from? Well, Pasteur felt he couldn't blame "spontaneous generation," a moldy-oldy theory dating from ancient times that postulated that life could arise spontaneously in organic materials.

YOU WANT THAT MILK PASTEURIZED?

As you'll find out in the Probiotic Diet program on page 237, pasteurized dairy products are generally off the menu. I won't drink pasteurized and homogenized milk, and I won't let my children swallow any type of commercially produced milk either. I prefer raw, unpasteurized milk, cheese, and yogurts produced from sustainable farms in the family refrigerator.

I've got nothing against Louis Pasteur, and Lord knows he only meant well, but pasteurization kills probiotics, zaps most of the enzymes, and alters the protein and fat in milk. "In spite of modern techniques of pasteurization, pasteurized milk is dead milk that will rot on standing," contends William Campbell Douglass II, M.D. and author of *The Milk Book*:

Pasteur conducted a series of experiments that destroyed every argument supporting spontaneous generation. In his mind, he was sure that the yeasts and other microorganisms found during fermentation entered from *outside* the vat. To prevent the fermentation from turning sour, Pasteur suggested heating the alcohol slightly to kill the contaminating organisms *after* the fermentation was complete.

This process of eradicating undesirable microorganisms through heating eventually became known as *pasteurization*. Today, pasteurization is most often associated with dairy products and bottled or packaged juices, although it wasn't until the 1920s that the process of quickly raising the temperature of milk to 161 degrees Fahrenheit and keeping it there for at least 15 seconds to kill off bacteria and pathogenic microorganisms was uniformly adopted throughout the United States.

Public health drove the need for pasteurization in the early decades of the 20th century. Before pasteurization, you literally put your life—or your children's lives—at risk when you served industrially produced milk. As city populations on both sides of the Atlantic skyrocketed in the early 1900s, green pasture-land for cows became scarce in urban areas. To make up for the loss, "swill dairies" began feeding their cows a mixture of waste grain from distilleries. The cows became diseased and emaciated, and coupled with poor sanitation and zero refrigeration, commercial milk killed thousands of adults, youngsters, and babies each year. Pasteurization was viewed as the solution to the growing "milk problem."

The commercial rise of pasteurization in Europe and America happened after Pasteur's death in 1895. While the French chemist was still alive, though, another beehive of scientific inquiry in the last half of the 19th century was the subject of germs. It was Pasteur's "germ theory" that inadvertently paved the way for the Probiotic Diet.

Pasteur's Germ Theory

The hospital was the last place you wanted to go when you were sick in the 19th century. You went to the hospital to die, not to be cured. If leeches, bloodletting, tortuous surgery without anesthesia, or benign

The Milk of Human Kindness Is Not Pasteurized.

Although Pasteur is generally given credit for coming up with the idea of parboiling milk, the record shows that Pasteur never pasteurized milk himself. "I doubt he ever drank it either," Dr. Douglass added. It was a German chemist, Franz Ritter von Soxhlet, who first proposed that pasteurization be applied to milk in 1886. Yet in one of the more ironic twists in history, it is Pasteur's name that's forevermore associated with a process that doesn't produce the healthiest dairy products.

While pasteurization is not intended to kill all pathogenic microorganisms in the milk—just reduce those likely to cause disease—the process destroys the beneficial bacteria available in milk. Fifty percent of milk's calcium cannot be assimilated by the body after pasteurization. Furthermore, pasteurization turns the milk sugar lactose into beta-lactose, which is more rapidly absorbed into the bloodstream and raises blood sugar levels. "The sudden rise in blood sugar is followed by a fall leading to low blood sugar, hypoglycemia, which induces hunger," wrote Dr. Douglass. "The end result is obesity. Obesity has become one of the most common diseases of childhood. Pasteurized milk makes you fat; raw milk does not."[2]

Homogenization is a non-starter for me, too. Auguste Gaulin—another Frenchman—patented a nifty machine in 1899 that shoots milk through a fine nozzle to break up fat globules so that butterfat will not rise to the top. In the old days when cow's milk was bottled and put on store shelves, globules of butterfat separated from the milk and floated to the top of the bottle. That's why we have the expression, "The cream always rises to the top."

neglect didn't kill you, then infectious germs would hasten your ultimate demise.

Physicians and scientists still had no idea what germs were in the mid-19th century, but they were getting warm. The first breakthrough came from Dr. Ignaz Semmelweis, a Hungarian physician posted at the Vienna General Hospital, site of the world's largest maternity clinic, in the 1850s. Most women still gave birth at home back then, attended by a midwife, but "problem pregnancies" ended up at Vienna General. The problem is that too many mothers and too many children were leaving in pine boxes because mortality rates were ten, 20 times higher inside the maternity ward than at home. No one knew why the mortality rate was so high. Doctors rubbed their Van Dyke beards and blamed poor ventilation or crowded conditions in the maternity ward.

Dr. Semmelweis noticed something about his colleagues at Vienna General: doctors left the dissection room with their hands bloodied from working on cadavers and didn't do much more than give their hands a cursory wipe on a towel before reporting to the delivery room, where they assisted in bringing a newborn into the world. No scrubbing or plastic gloves in those days!

On a hunch, Dr. Semmelweis established a new policy: from now on, doctors had to scrub their hands in chlorinated water after working on cadavers. (Dr. Joseph Lister of Scotland wouldn't discover how to kill germs with heat and antiseptics for another 18 years.) Within a month, the mortality rate in the maternity ward dropped six-fold to 2 percent! He wrote a book about his discovery, which was released in 1861, a year before Pasteur and Claude Bernard completed their first pasteurization test on April 20, 1862.

I'm sure a copy of Dr. Semmelweis's book was circulated in Pasteur's vicinity, and this is where Pasteur's story takes a detour—a fascinating turn. A rising body of academic thought believes that Louis Pasteur "borrowed" reams of research from other scientists, passed it off as his own, and capitalized on being "first." Remember, he apparently didn't mind the prestigious awards, audiences with royalty, or respect in the most prestigious academic settings.

The problem is that the homogenization process creates an enzyme called xanthine oxidase, or "XO," which contributes to heart disease by damaging the arteries and building up arterial plaque. The milk industry says that pasteurization kills XO, which is highly debatable, but pasteurization also alters vital amino acids, which reduces our ability to access the proteins, fats, vitamins, and minerals in milk.

I read Dr. Douglass's book in the mid-1990s when I was recovering from my gastrointestinal diseases, and he made me a believer in raw milk and the beneficial probiotics it contained. The problem was that I couldn't buy raw milk in Florida at the time. (Selling raw milk is illegal in 24 states as of the time of publishing this book.) So I got creative and found a woman, Joanne Nightingale, who nursed me back to health by providing me with raw goat's milk from her backyard herd.

As you will see in the Probiotic Diet, I recommend cultured and fermented dairy products from cows, goats, and sheep, and these are best if they come from raw dairy sources.

FOOD IRRADIATION— THE SAME AS PASTEURIZATION

Most people associate "pasteurization" with milk, yogurt, and other dairy products. But there's another process that's just as capable of damaging or killing microorganisms— including probiotics—and that's called irradiation.

Irradiation is a process that uses light, infrared heat— the same kind of radiant energy found in household microwave ovens—to kill off microorganisms that contaminate food or

Not that Pasteur wasn't deserving of accolades, because he harbored a brilliant mind, but during the middle of the 19th century, two other scientists—Antoine Béchamp and Robert Koch, a German—were also conducting pioneering experiments in chemistry, particularly in the areas of fermentation, yeast, and the new discovery of little organisms called bacteria. "All three were involved in similar research, but there was much competition and 'borrowing' of discoveries, always with the undercurrent of politics and influence," wrote Tim O'Shea, author of *The Sanctity of Human Blood: Vaccination Is Not Immunization*. "These individuals were not colleagues but worked independently. Each one was onto a whole new area of human discovery, and the race was on to influence the medical world."[3]

Some believe that Pasteur's greatest influence on the medical world was *not* his discovery of heating microbes to kill them—what later came to be known as pasteurization—but his dissemination of his "germ theory," which has huge ramifications on our health today and creates the need for the Probiotic Diet.

For several years, Pasteur worked with curved neck flasks that allowed contact with air but inhibited movement of non-gaseous particles. From these experiments, Pasteur demonstrated that microorganisms were present in the air but not created by air, which was critical for the refutation of spontaneous generation (as mentioned before), as well as the development of his "monomorphic germ theory" of disease.

In 1862, Pasteur theorized that:

- germs, or microbes, caused disease
- germs invade the body from the outside
- human blood is sterile and can only be infected by outside microbes
- germs are monomorphic, meaning they are non-changeable and have only one form and can be identified by species
- the shapes and colors of microorganisms are constant
- every disease is associated with a particular microorganism
- germs should be killed by drugs[4]

cause food spoilage and deterioration.

Since 1986, all irradiated products must carry an international symbol called a radura, which resembles a stylized flower. The U.S. Food and Drug Administration has approved irradiation for wheat, potatoes, flour, spices, fruits, vegetables, and nuts. If there has been a salmonella outbreak, then irradiation is mandatory.

That's been the case with domestic almonds, which must be irradiated (or pasteurized) following two isolated cases of salmonella in 2004 that were traced to raw almonds. Yet cooking almonds to 200 degrees to kill supposed pathogens also destroys the delicious smell, taste, and texture of raw almonds, as well as the enzymes and probiotics that are part of the skin.

I've been forced to purchase foreign almonds that have not been irradiated so that I can continue to receive the probiotics from the skin of the almonds.

FOOD FOR THOUGHT

Have you ever wondered why there's an expiration date for sour cream?

GET THEE BEHIND ME, MR. PEANUT!

Have you noticed the growing number of parents *sure* that their children are allergic to peanuts—like peanuts have germs and should be avoided at all costs? These days, it's not unusual for schools to ban peanut-butter-and-jelly sandwiches, and some airlines have replaced the tiny bag of honey-roasted peanuts with pretzels, lest some passengers complain about being "exposed" to peanut particles at 35,000 feet.

The so-called "allergy craze" has gotten so out of hand that 25 percent of parents

In other words, since germs cause disease, it was medicine's challenge to find the right drug or vaccine to kill the nasty bug without killing the patient. This theory hardened into a scientific dogma that is considered conventional wisdom in the halls of medicine today. Pasteur's germ theory is widely hailed as the single most important contribution by the science of microbiology for the general welfare of the world's people. Furthermore, you could say that the paradigm of modern medical treatment—diagnose the germ or bacteria causing the ill health and then prescribe something to destroy it or make the patient feel better—is based on Pasteur's germ theory of disease.

Yet two contemporaries of Louis Pasteur—Claude Bernard and Antoine Béchamp—were shuffled to history's side rail because they had different ideas about germs and microorganisms. Nearly 150 years after the fact, however, Bernard and Béchamp are getting a second look after the overprescription of antibiotics has swung the pendulum *way* toward killing every germ in sight instead of realizing that life is a process, not a fixed state.

Claude Bernard, even though he counted Pasteur as a friend, didn't completely agree with his colleague's germ theory. He believed germs and microorganisms were constantly changing within the body's internal environment, or what he called in French, the body's *milieu* or *milieu interieur*. Bernard's research convinced him that the body is constantly striving to maintain a stable, well-balanced environment, one that is not overly affected by outside influences, which is the same theory from which we created the Probiotic Diet.

Claude Bernard: It's All About the Terrain

Claude Bernard never set out to become a doctor or physiologist. Born in 1813 as the son of poor vineyard workers living in Saint-Julien, France, the young Bernard was educated in a simple village school and dreamed of becoming a writer. He composed a vaudeville comedy, *La Rose du Rhône*, that met with some local success. That prompted the young playwright to draft a prose drama in five acts called *Arthur de*

believe their kids have allergies when research shows that only 4 percent of boys and girls are actually allergic to something like nuts and peanuts.[5] That's why we read news reports about teachers confiscating school lunches with nut products or school buses that had to be steam-cleaned after a stray peanut hit the floor.

Harvard doctor and social scientist Nicholas Christakis thinks these stories are ridiculous. In an essay published in the *British Medical Journal*, Dr. Christakis wrote that about as many people die from lightning strikes as they do from food allergies, and parents gone wild about peanuts and the like "bear many of the hallmarks of mass psychogenic illness." Of the roughly 3.3 million Americans with nut allergies, about 150 people die from allergy-related causes each year, he noted. I did the math: that's a miniscule .000045 percent chance.

Christakis also wrote that the "wholesale avoidance of nuts contribute to the problem because children who lack exposure become more sensitized to them." Perhaps you've never thought about food allergies in those terms before, but as it relates to the Probiotic Diet, it's almost always *good* for kids to come into contact with more "germs" that are "supposedly" dangerous to their health.

Not that peanuts always have germs on them, but you get my point.

Bretagne. With his play in hand, Bernard set off for Paris at the age of 21. A well-known critic, Saint-Marc Girardin, gave his writings the once-over and imperiously announced that young Bernard may want to do something else with his life than pen stage plays.

Bernard accepted the critic's rebuke and applied to medical school in Paris. Despite finishing at the bottom of his class, Bernard passed his *études* and obtained his medical degree, where he gravitated toward experiments centering on the digestive process. He read about a U.S. Army surgeon named William Beaumont, who became known as the "father of gastric physiology" after he devoted several years peering into the digestive tract of a patient who was shot in the stomach. Beaumont's patient had survived the shooting, but a hole—or fistula—in his stomach never healed, which allowed the American doctor to observe the digestion process with his very own eyes.

Beaumont performed this research by tying a piece of food to a string and dropping it through the hole in the patient's stomach. Every few hours, the American physician would slowly reel in the string and observe how well the food had been digested. This novel research led to the important discovery that digestion was a chemical process, not a mechanical one. Stomach acids, or gastric acids, digested foods into nutrients the body could use.

Claude Bernard decided to create artificial fistulas, or openings, in live animals such as horses. What the Frenchman discovered is that the stomach was not the sole digestive organ; much more digestion took place in the small intestine. He also demonstrated the importance of the pancreas, whose secretions broke down fat molecules.

Bernard also discovered a starch-like substance in horses's livers, which he named glycogen. Then he turned his attention to the portion of the nervous system that governed blood circulation and how the blood's red corpuscles carry oxygen from the lungs to body tissues. Each of his findings convinced Bernard that the body's *milieu interieur* was continually striving to maintain a stable, well-balanced state. Disease, therefore, was caused by variations in the body's internal environment or terrain, to which the microbes responded by changing form to survive.

"The living body, though it has need of the surrounding environment, is nevertheless relatively independent of it," he wrote. "This independence, which the organism has of its external environment, derives from the fact that in the living being, the tissues are, in fact, withdrawn from direct external influences and are protected by a veritable internal *milieu,* which is constituted, in particular, by the fluids circulating in the body."[6]

By virtue of his discoveries and influence in French medical and biological sciences, Bernard was accorded many honors like Louis Pasteur. In fact, Bernard became the first French scientist to be given a national funeral in 1878, an honor usually reserved for political and military heroes. (In case you're wondering, Pasteur was also accorded a state funeral at the Cathedral de Nôtre

Dame following his death in 1895, and his body was placed in a permanent crypt at the Louis Pasteur Institute in Paris.)

Bernard's legacy, as it relates to the Probiotic Diet, was that "the terrain is everything." Bernard hypothesized that germs could not make a person sick unless the person's internal environment—or terrain—supported illness. He literally put his theory where his mouth was. Bernard drank a glass of water infected with cholera but didn't get sick! He took the risk, he said, because he knew he was healthy, had a strong immune system, and didn't believe he had any reason to get sick. When Pasteur heard about Bernard's crazy self-experiment, he called him "lucky."

But think about the millions of doctors, nurses, and health workers who are around sick people all day long, breathing in their germs and coming into physical contact with conta-gions. Yet they don't get sick (for the most part). Why does that happen?

It's because the body's terrain is armed with the proper micro-organisms—microorganisms that form the essential message of the Probiotic Diet.

Antoine Béchamp: Overlooked But Not Forgotten

I purchased an important book as I did my probiotic research called *Béchamp or Pasteur? A Lost Chapter in the History of Biology*, written by E. Douglas Hume in 1923.

Now, with a name like "E. Douglas Hume," you picture a pipe-smoking academic in a tweed jacket toiling away in a musty university library. And with a niche book like *Béchamp or Pasteur?*, you figure that this volume has been gathering dust in those same musty university libraries for the last 85 years.

Well, let me burst two bubbles. E. Douglas Hume is actually Ethel Douglas Hume, and her book *Béchamp or Pasteur?* is getting a second look after nine decades of academic neglect. I'm figuring that Ethel went with "E. Douglas" because a woman wasn't expected to write a serious tome declaring that the "germ theory" of the esteemed Louis Pasteur had more holes than a slice of Swiss cheese. Pasteurized, of course.

The author sought to show that Pasteur, the hero of traditional medicine, was a "chemist who, without ever being a doctor, dared nothing less than to profess to revolutionize medicine" with his declarations that every disease could be tied to a particular microorganism, and it was medicine's job to figure out the right drug to kill those germs.

She contrasted Pasteur's goal of personal success and honors with a rival named Antoine Béchamp, who had a different theory: germs were the *consequence* of disease, not the cause.

After reading up on Béchamp, I now regard him as one of the foremost pioneers of science of his generation, and his discoveries could have saved humanity immense misery and suffering. Béchamp, who lived from 1816-1908, was one of France's most prominent researchers and biologists. He earned degrees in biology, chemistry, physics, pharmacy, and medicine, and he practiced, researched, and taught in all those disciplines—up until the day he died at the age of 91.

The reason why you've never heard of Béchamp is because he called Pasteur's theory that infectious and contagious disorders were caused by germs "the greatest scientific silliness of the age." Béchamp's voice was ignored by the elites guarding the gates of traditional medicine in the latter half of the 19th century. As Pasteur's germ theory became set in clinics and the classroom, that laid the foundation for modern medicine's view that doctors should diagnose the disease and then write the proper prescription for "treating" the illness. Today's medicine is practiced that

ANOTHER PERSPECTIVE ON PASTEUR'S DEATHBED CONFESSION

Michael A. Schmidt, Lendon H. Smith, and Keith W. Sehnert, authors of *Beyond Antibiotics*, had this to say about Louis Pasteur's deathbed realization that his theories about germs were erroneous:

> Pasteur recognized that it was not the bacteria that were responsible for disease, but the "terrain" (the surrounding land), the inability of the host to combat them. If the host was "strong" (i.e., the immune system was active), the organisms could not get a foothold. If the host was weak, the organisms could "settle in" and "overcome." Pasteur had come to the conclusion that myriad factors, including diet, nutrition, stress, heredity,

way: you describe your symptoms to the doctor, he or she diagnoses what ails you, and you walk out with a prescription—usually for an antibiotic.

Béchamp's contrarian view stated that it was not the bug that caused disease but rather the condition in which the bugs lived in the *milieu interieur,* or internal terrain. Disease happened when an imbalance in the body's terrain caused the bad or pathogenic microbes, including bacteria, to take over. Béchamp discovered that tiny organisms, which he named "microzymas," were present in all things—animal, vegetable, and mineral, whether living or dead. Microzymas means "tiny fermenters."

"Depending on the host, these microzymas could assume various forms," said Dr. Tim O'Shea. "Bad bacteria and viruses were simply the forms assumed by the microzymas when there was a condition of disease. In a diseased body, the microzymas became pathological bacteria and viruses. In a healthy body, microzymas formed healthy cells."[7]

Béchamp called his theory "pleomorphism" and stated that

microorganisms can travel through different stages of development and evolve into various growth forms. According to the French professeur, disease came from inside the body when microzymas—the particles in blood—reacted to changes in the body's terrain.

Pleomorphism maintains that germs occur in many forms, and what starts as a virus can change into bacteria, which can change into a fungus. Any of these forms—viral, bacterial, or fungal—can and eventually do break apart and start all over again. That's the nature of life, according to Béchamp's pleomorphism theory.

Béchamp, as well as Claude Bernard, kept insisting that the germ was not what was important, but rather what should be studied was the body's terrain, where germs and microbes end up. "Bernard argued that it was the state of the host organism that largely determined its own fate and that of the germ," wrote Jane G. Goldberg, author of *Deceits of the Mind and Their Effects on the Body.* "Germs—bacteria and viruses—do, after all, surround us all the time; yet only some of us 'catch' them, and only some of the time. So, Bernard maintained, it cannot be environment and state of mind, had a profound effect on resistance to microbes.

The view of infectious disease was divided into two camps: those who adhered to Pasteur's original germ theory and those who believed the health of the host was more important. The discovery of sulfa drugs and penicillin in the 1930s and 1940s launched medicine fully into the chemotherapeutic approach to infection and all but laid to waste the notion of host resistance. Thus was born the Antibiotic Age.[8]

HOW HISTORY HAS TREATED PASTEUR, BERNARD, AND BÉCHAMP

Louis Pasteur has been cared for kindly by history with honorifics and respect. While he was still alive, the Pasteur Institute opened its doors in Paris in 1888, and the Institute has been responsible for breakthrough discoveries that have enabled medical science to control such virulent diseases as tetanus, tuberculosis, and yellow fever. The biomedical research organization was the first to isolate HIV, the virus that causes AIDS. In many ways, the Pasteur legacy is alive and well in the 21st century.

Claude Bernard didn't fare as well, but he has not been forgotten. As mentioned earlier, he was given a national funeral upon his death, and a statue of Bernard was erected in his honor at his birthplace,

the entry of the germ into the system that produces disease. It must be the state of the ground on which it falls—the host organism—that determines whether the germ damages us, or we damage the germ, or we and the germ live in peaceful coexistence."[9]

So, two completely different viewpoints or worldviews: Pasteur certain that germs caused disease, while Béchamp argued that disease causes or allows germs to flourish in the body. One was lauded as the "father of modern medicine," the other man was forgotten by history.

Here's where their stories get really interesting. There's strong evidence that Louis Pasteur, at the end of his life, recognized that his lifelong preoccupation with his "germ theory" had been misdirected all along. On this deathbed, he reportedly whispered: *Bernard avait raison. Le germe n'est rien; c'est le terrain qui est tout.*[10]

Translation: "Bernard was right. The germ is nothing; it's the terrain that's everything."

From all the reading and studying I've done, I agree completely with Bernard, Béchamp, and (hopefully) Pasteur: the terrain *is* everything, and that's why following the Probiotic Diet and introducing the right microorganisms into your body creates an impenetrable *milieu interieur*—or terrain—that will keep you healthier and feeling better. For too long, we've been led down a primrose path that all you needed to recover from an illness was to find the right medicine, the right antibiotic, the right vaccine.

By now, I hope you're waking up to the fact that taking steps to improve your body's terrain by following an internal health program such as the Probiotic Diet will do more to protect you from disease and ill health—or improve the symptoms that ail you—than practically anything else you can do. Since the Probiotic Diet is all about creating a healthy internal environment or terrain within your body, which encompasses the digestive system, parts of your lymphatic system, and the immune system located in the gastrointestinal tract, we'll focus on this area of your body in our next chapter.

So read on, if you've got the "guts."

Saint-Julien. If you travel to Paris, you can even book a room at the Hotel Claude Bernard, a three-star establishment located on the Left Bank near the Sorbonne.

Antoine Béchamp has been swept aside since his death a century ago because his findings challenged the foundation of modern medicine. Thanks to the Internet and a revival of Ethel Douglas Hume's book *Béchamp or Pasteur?*, however, his research about how disease causes germs—not the other way around—has received a renaissance. I'm pleased to help get the word out about this respected scientist whose thoughts and discoveries were overlooked for too long.

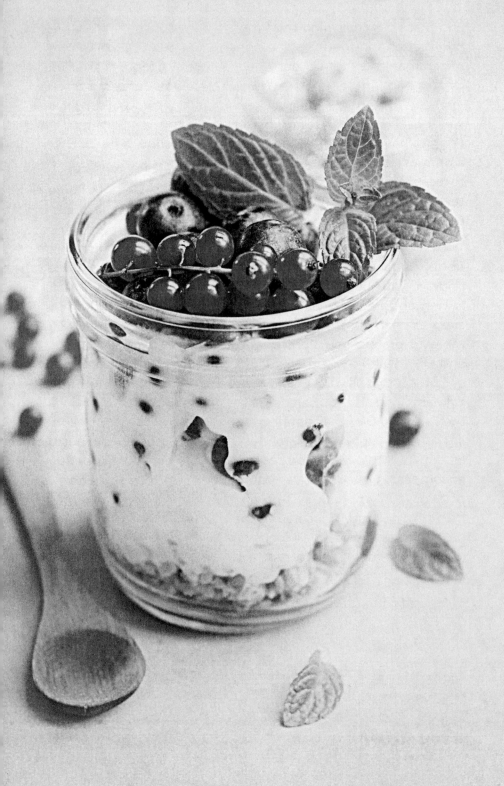

3

THE GUTS OF THE MATTER

When I was 19 years old, on summer break from college and hanging out with my friends, I never thought diddly squat—in a manner of speaking—about my digestive system.

Of course, that all changed at Camp Swan, when my stomach churned like an overloaded washing machine and my bowels needed instant relief. Up until that time, though, I was like 90 percent of Americans who wake up in the morning and never give their digestive systems a second thought. I figured you eat what you enjoy eating, you wash it down with your favorite beverage, and 24 hours later, you take care of business. Like a German intercity train, everything rolls out of the station on time.

In principle, that's how our digestive systems should work, but if the thousands of e-mails I receive each month are any indication, it's apparent that far too many people live with far too much digestive distress these days. Dealing with gas, bloating, constipation, debilitating pain, and nausea isn't fun, and it's not a topic you typically share with neighbors or loved ones. Discussing your bathroom habits and "BMs"—bowel movements—does not make for palatable dinner table conversation.

CHEW ON THIS FOR A WHILE

If friends or family members have teased you about "inhaling" your food, take that as a gracious reminder to chew your food better. Chewing food well does a body good, and I cannot emphasize enough how critical it is to become a good chewer when you embark on the Probiotic Diet.

I wish I had listened to my mother back in my teenage years. Before I went off to college, I wolfed down food like I was competing in the Nathan's Famous Hot Dog Eating Contest held every Fourth of July at Coney Island. I can still hear Mom's voice admonishing me: "Jordan, quit eating so fast. You're swallowing your food whole!"

In high school, I needed only four or five bites to finish a "gut-bomb" burrito or monster sandwich. When I didn't take my time to

Listen, I understand. Many find it embarrassing to bring up "bathroom talk." When Sandra Benitez, author of *Bag Lady: A Memoir*, was a young American girl growing up in El Salvador, she began experiencing symptoms of ulcerative colitis at the age of five and suffered in silence for nearly 50 years until she underwent life-changing ileostomy surgery. "As a young girl, I suffered mostly from constipation," she said. "There was a lot of bleeding and mucous. I would spend long hours every day, sitting and straining on the toilet, yet in spite of my efforts, I would frequently go days without a bowel movement."

Rather than inform her mother, young Sandra didn't say a word because of the embarrassment. In retrospect, she finds this self-imposed reticence incomprehensible. "It's amazing how people don't like to talk about this subject," she said. "I mean, think about it. Everyone has to poop! If we don't, we'll die! But to talk about it is a no-no."

These days, Sandra has no problems using words that cause most people to blush. "When you're not feeling good from something that has to do with sitting on the toilet, nobody wants to discuss this.

People don't like talking about bodily functions and are repulsed by anything that has to do with feces or the anus or the rectum. They'll talk about anything else, but those words are taboo."[1]

We're going to discuss some of those taboo words because it's necessary to have a good understanding about the physiological side of digestion. So consider this chapter a primer on your gut, which, in our opinion, is the key to good health. Pay close attention because this information builds on the foundation of the Probiotic Diet. As Michael Gershon, M.D., author of *The Second Brain*, once said, "Take care of your gut, and your gut will take care of you."

Where It All Begins

By definition, digestion is a process by which food is broken down into smaller pieces so that the body can use these nutrients to build and nourish cells, which provides energy. As William Beaumont and Claude Bernard first discovered 150 years ago, digestion involves a chemical breakdown of the macronutrients

chew properly, I sent chunks of partially undigested food down my gullet. My saliva never got a chance to do its job, which was to start the breakdown of carbohydrates.

Undigested carbohydrates in the gut are a strong source of intestinal ailments and the reason why so many need to follow the Probiotic Diet, but more on that subject later. Chewing your food properly—by that, I mean carefully chewing each morsel of food 25 to 50 times before swallowing—ensures that plenty of digestive juices are added to the food before it begins to wind through the digestive tract. Well-chewed food should be almost in a liquid form before you swallow because the length of time your food spends in the esophagus before reaching the stomach depends on how well it was chewed.

Food that has been chewed 25 times or *more* usually makes the trip through the esophagus in seven seconds, but "inhaled" food can get stuck in the ten-inch tube between the throat and the stomach for up to a minute. Sometimes longer. Dr. Brasco said that he can't tell you how many times he's been called out in the middle of the night to dislodge food—with an endoscope—that's stuck in a patient's esophagus.

I'm beyond the age where Mom reminds me to chew my food well, but she wouldn't have to bite her lip, so to speak, after watching me eat today. I'm a careful chewer who takes "mastication" seriously. I can raise my right hand and solemnly state that I eat my food *real* slow.

(protein, carbohydrates, and fats) in foods and beverages into smaller and smaller nutrients that the body can absorb, assimilate, and utilize.

The digestive system is made up of the digestive tract, which consists of a long tube of organs that runs from the mouth to the anus—there's the A word again—and includes the esophagus, stomach, small intestine, and large intestine. While we're talking about what's inside the gut, we might as well add the liver, gall bladder, and pancreas, which produce important secretions for digestion that drain into the small intestine. The digestive tract in an adult is about 30 feet long, or the length of a ten-yard sideline marker used on the gridiron. Think about how long your intestine is the next time you watch an NFL umpire stretch the "chains" to see if the team on offense gained enough yardage to earn another first down.

Digestion begins the instant you take a bite of an apple or lift a forkful of food into your mouth, even though digestive secretions can begin when you smell dinner being prepared in the kitchen. Like the choreographed chaos that ensues after a quarterback yells "Hut" to start a play, all sorts of physiological things happen when you begin chewing on food. Saliva, or spit, charges out of its three-point stance and floods the mouth when the salivary glands (located under the tongue and near the lower jaw) begin producing saliva. Saliva moistens food so that it will be easier to swallow and contains a digestive enzyme called ptylin, which is a salivary amylase. Ptylin gets to work breaking down the carbohydrates, or starches and sugars, in each bite of food.

One of the important functions of the mouth is chewing because chewing mashes the food into a soft mass that can be swallowed into the esophagus and travel on to the stomach. Movements by the tongue and mouth push the food to the back of the throat, where a flexible flap called the epiglottis closes over the trachea to ensure the food enters the esophagus and not the windpipe to prevent choking. As you can see, just the act of chewing and swallowing a bite of food is an amazing physiological process.

Down Time

Once chewed food enters the esophagus, wavelike contractions known as *peristalsis* push the food down through the esophagus to the stomach. A muscular ring called the lower esophageal sphincter allows food to enter the stomach. Then the lower esophageal sphincter squeezes shut to prevent food and fluid from going back up into the esophagus.

With age, stress, or poor physical condition, however, the lower esophageal sphincter can weaken, allowing food and acid to back up the hatch. Result: heartburn and acid reflux. Left untreated, acid reflux can lead to ulcers and bleeding of the esophagus as well as increase the risk of developing cancer of the esophagus.

This juncture where the esophagus and the stomach meet is where digestive distress usually rears its ugly head. Heartburn and acid reflux are quintessential American digestive disorders that have made over-the-counter antacid products like Tums, Rolaids, Pepto-Bismol, and Alka-Seltzer into household names and cloying jingles like "plop, plop, fizz, fizz, oh what a relief it is" impossible to get out of our cluttered minds. According to the latest government statistics, 25 million suffer from heartburn daily, while more than 60 million American adults endure occasional occurrences of heartburn. Men and women are affected equally, but the incidence of heartburn increases after age 40.[2]

That's not good news for a nation that loves to celebrate every occasion with food—and lots of it. From football weekends to festive, holiday dinners, we commemorate life's richest moments—and even life's worst times—with the mouth, tongue, and stomach. The problem is that we are indulging rich, processed, fatty foods six days a week and twice on Sunday while washing everything down with generous amounts of soda, caffeine, and alcohol. Maybe a glass of pasteurized milk and chocolate chip cookies for dessert, for all I know.

If the lower esophageal sphincter weakens for some reason, as it sometimes does with those who overeat, ferocious stomach acids can rise into the esophagus, resulting in a burning sensation behind the breastbone lasting from a few minutes to several hours. That's why heartburn has nothing to do with the heart, even though many experience a quite-noticeable burning sensation in the cardiovascular area. The inflammation or irritation can feel like dancing flames in the upper chest. Some say that when they lie down it feels like lava is eroding their tonsils.

For those fortunate enough not to deal with heartburn or acid reflux, let's continue to follow the food as the softened mass reaches the stomach, the J-shaped organ that has three functions. The stomach has three tasks:

- store the swallowed food and liquids
- mix the food and liquids with digestive juices produced by the stomach
- and slowly empty its contents into the small intestine

A normal stomach can hold three pints of food or 24 ounces of food, which is a large plate of food. Only a few substances, like water and alcohol, can be absorbed directly by the stomach; the rest must undergo the "wash-and-spin" cycle that the stomach's known for. The stomach's strong muscular walls chum the food with acids and enzymes, breaking it into smaller pieces and eventually a semi-liquid form called chyme. About four hours after eating a meal, the chyme is released a little bit at a time through the pyloric sphincter, a thickened muscular ring between the stomach and the small intestine.

More digestion and absorption of food happens in the small intestine, which extends to about 20 feet of length, or two-thirds of the entire digestive system. The small intestine's twisting tubes occupy most of the lower abdomen between the stomach and the beginning of the large intestine.

You'd think that the heavy lifting in digestion happens in the large intestine, but that's not the case. Glands in the small intestine's walls secrete enzymes to finish the breakdown of carbohydrates, fats, and proteins. Any undigested material—like fiber from fruits and vegetables—travels next to the large intestine.

The large intestine forms an upside-down U over the coiled small intestine. With a length of five to six feet—the length of your body!—the large intestine is comprised of three parts: the cecum, the colon, and the rectum. The cecum is a pouch at the beginning of the large intestine that allows food to pass from the small intestine to the large intestine. The middle part, the colon, is where fluids and salts are absorbed as the waste material

THE NITTY GRITTY

The topic on the table is stools, and I'm not talking about the kind that you sit on next to a kitchen counter. You can choose to skip this sidebar, but there's some good information ahead.

Stools should be the color of walnut brown, although there could be a greenish hue if you're eating a lot of salad and green vegetables. Stools should have a firm but soft consistency and come out about the length of a banana. If you're producing the human version of "rabbit pellets" or small balls, then you're probably not drinking enough water.

You should have at least one good bowel movement a day, but two or even three are ideal. A normal stool should leave the body easily, settle in the toilet water, and gently submerge. If there is not enough fiber in the diet, the stool will sink to the bottom of a toilet like a

makes its final journey to the rectum, and it's also where the feces is stored before being expelled from the body through the anus as a bowel movement.

The storage of feces inside the body—or I should say, the *excess* storage—is half the reason why *The Probiotic Diet* needs to be read and followed. When transit time for feces slows to a snail's pace, your body's waste stays in the colon longer, where it putrefies and results in toxins entering the bloodstream through the intestinal wall. This can lead to a condition called autointoxification, which can cause everything from headaches to autoimmune disorders.

I've long felt that autointoxication is a form of self-poisoning that results in bloating, indigestion, gas, body odor, and a lengthy list of maladies. Colon cancer, the second leading cause of death in the United States, could result from years of autointoxication. Even the traditional medical community recognizes the connection between constipation and serious disease. *The Lancet*, a prestigious British medical journal, reported that women who are constipated are four times more likely to develop breast cancer.[3]

When the eliminative system of the human body is not in top-notch working order, sluggish and clogged as a kitchen sink full of oatmeal, the digestive tract cannot properly process and eliminate food wastes and toxins.

This virtually guarantees toxic build-up in the colon, which, over time, results in serious illness or chronic degenerative disease. Health statistics show that more North Americans are hospitalized due to intestinal tract illnesses than for any other group of disorders. The medical costs of these diseases are estimated to be $20 billion or more per year, and the bloated market for laxatives, antacids, and antihemorrhoidals tops $2 billion each year.[4]

The idea that putrefaction of the stools causes diseases such as intestinal autointoxication originated with physicians in ancient Egypt, according to a National Institutes of Health study. The ancient Egyptians believed that a putrefactive principle associated with feces was absorbed into the general circulation, where it acted to produce fever and pus. "The ancient Greeks extended the concept of putrefaction to involve not only the submarine submerging on a dive mission.

I believe there are four causes of constipation, or, if you choose to look at the bright side, four things you can do to reverse the condition:

1. Increase your water intake.

Constipation is often caused by dehydration. Drink a minimum of eight glasses of water a day, or better yet, a half-ounce of water per pound of body weight. If you weigh 150 pounds, that will mean 75 ounces of water, close to ten glasses a day. For those weighing 200 pounds, that means 100 ounces, or 12 glasses of water. Great hydration can jump-start the peristaltic action of a sluggish colon. If you enjoy sparkling water, don't choose brands with added carbonation, such as Perrier.

2. Practice de-lipidation, which means improving fat deficiency.

You need to consume healthy fats and oils every day. Some of the healthiest fats to improve elimination are extra-virgin coconut oil and extra-virgin olive oil. Consume 2 to 4 tablespoons of healthy fats and oils per day in smoothies and on salads to eliminate constipation.

3. Increase the consumption of probiotics in the form of foods and supplements.

Much more on this later, but contrary to popular belief, most of the weight of a bowel movement comes not from fiber but from trillions of microorganisms. Probiotic consumption can greatly increase elimination and over time "eliminate" stubborn constipation.

residues of food, but also those of bile, phlegm, and blood, incorporating it into their humoral theory of disease," the NIH study declared.[5]

Many factors lead to a constipated colon, including a glaring lack of probiotics, which we'll get into shortly. But let's face it: autointoxication occurs because Americans have a love affair with *crap,* as signified by this acronym:

- **C**offee and cruddy foods
- **R**efined sugar and starches
- **A**lcohol
- **P**rocessed foods

Autointoxication symptoms can also be extenuated by a lack of exercise, which cuts off lymphatic flow. A good workout has a way of stimulating a good bowel movement, although, in my experience, jumping on a mini-trampoline or rebounder for ten to 20 minutes is the best form of exercise to improve lymphatic flow and speed elimination. A brisk morning walk can also do the trick. President Harry Truman was famous for his "morning constitutional" walks around Lafayette Park next to the White House, accompanied by a single Secret

Service agent. (Those simple days are long gone, of course.)

These days, many medications, especially antibiotics, cause constipation. Changing your routine—like traveling to San Francisco from the East Coast—can disrupt normal bowel habits. Not giving the body enough time to let peristalsis work—that series of organized muscle contractions that often occur after eating—is a common route to autointoxication. In the morning, too many people rush out the front door after grabbing a bowl of cereal, topped with pasteurized and homogenized milk. As they start up the car, they feel a slight urge to eliminate, but since they're running late, they're too busy to act upon that inclination. And so the seeds of constipation are sown.

We're Talking Trillions

I hope you were taking notes during Human Digestion 101. Now that you have the basics of digestion down, let me add some technical information that will help you understand better why you need to intentionally

4. Consume at least 25 grams of fiber per day to ensure healthy elimination.

If you're going to try to eliminate twice a day—or at least get up to once a day—it's important to eat plenty of fiber. Fiber is the indigestible remnants of plant cells found in vegetables, fruits, whole grains, nuts, seeds, and beans. Fiber-rich foods take longer to break down and are partially indigestible, which means that as these foods work their way through the digestive tract, they absorb water and increase the elimination of fecal waste in the large intestine.

Good sources of fiber are berries, fruits with edible skins (apples, pears, and grapes), citrus fruits, whole non-gluten grains (quinoa, millet, amaranth, and buckwheat), green peas, carrots, cucumbers, zucchini, and tomatoes. Green leafy vegetables such as spinach are also fiber rich. Sprouted, soaked, or sour-leavened whole grain products are high in fiber as well.

A sure way to live a constipated life is to ignore and suppress your gastro-colic reflex. This is the sensation you feel in your colon shortly after a meal to evacuate the bowels. As mentioned earlier, due to our hectic schedules and busy lives, we ignore this urge, and eventually that urge is severely lessened.

add probiotic foods and supplements to your terrain.

Inside your digestive tract, you have trillions of microorganisms swimming around, colonizing every nook and cranny, every millimeter of surface space, from the tip of your tongue to your... well, you know what end I'm talking about. You've been living with these microorganisms ever since you were born. "You may have been a sterile, singular being in the womb, but once you entered the birth canal and then the world of nipples and hands and bed sheets, you picked up an ark of microbial handmaidens," said Jennifer Ackerman, author of *Sex Sleep Eat Drink Dream*. "Soon the little buggers were everywhere, like words filling a page, in folds of skin, in orifices of nose and ears, and especially in the warm, cozy tunnels of your digestive tract, from mouth to anus."[6] Breastfed infants have significantly higher amounts of beneficial microbes in their guts than do formula fed infants. This is most likely due to a combination of contact with the mother's skin and the contents of the breast milk itself.

Our son Samuel didn't receive the beneficial bacteria that come from intimate contact with the mother and consistent breastfeeding. I mentioned in Chapter 1 that Samuel had developed a nasty case of eczema by the time we were able to complete the formal adoption arrangements, and his skin didn't get better until I put him on a probiotic-rich infant formula. Samuel is not alone with his eczema problem: a study at Lund University in Sweden showed that children with only a limited variety of bacteria in their feces after birth often develop eczema by the age of the 18 months.[7]

We know that when Samuel grows up big and strong, his body will consist of 10 trillion cells. To help you put a trillion in perspective—timely, since the politicians in Washington, DC, have no problem running a trillion-dollar deficit these days—here's a good analogy: you could spend $1 million a day—every day—since the day Jesus Christ was born up to today and still not reach a trillion dollars. (The actual total is $734 billion, give or take a few billion.)

Yes, 10 trillion is an astronomical number, but your gut has *ten times* the number of microorganisms circulating in your terrain. We call these digestive tract microorganisms

ELIMINATION ROUND

When you're dealing with autointoxification or stubborn constipation, you park yourself on the chamber throne a great deal. Sitting on a Western-style toilet may not be the best way to eliminate your colon, however.

For centuries, people dug themselves a latrine trench or found a secluded spot behind a tree and squatted to relieve themselves. Anatomically speaking, squatting works because at the end of the rectum, there's a 90-degree bend known as the anorectal angle that's designed to prevent incontinence. When you squat, that 90-degree bend straightens out and elimination is more complete.

Hundreds of millions of people still squat 'n' go around the world today— even in Western Europe. I'll never forget traveling to Italy the first time and stepping into a bathroom stall where there was a porcelain hole in the floor flanked by two ceramic footpads. In a rank-smelling Italian public restroom, I admit that you better have strong thighs to squat 'n' go without holding on to something.

Bending at the waist while sitting on a toilet strains your colon, however, and straining is what causes tubes of Preparation H to fly off the shelves. If you've been pushing too hard, you don't have to get rid of your Western toilet and replace it with a Turkish footpad model. Instead, consider using an "elimination bench" that you place in front of your toilet. When you sit down and set your feet on the bench, it places your body in a more anatomically correct squatting position. You could also raise your feet by placing a few large books on the floor.

I have an elimination bench at home and highly recommend its use.

"intestinal flora." Even though flora refers to plants, this term seems to have stuck for these microbial cells inhabiting the gut. Of these trillions and trillions of intestinal "bugs," it's been estimated that about 500 different bacterial species are swimming around in your abdominal area. These bacteria make up most of the flora in the colon and 60 percent of the dry mass of feces.[8] Taken together en masse, the total weight of this microbial zoo is between two and three pounds.

These tiny microorganisms are your friends—or at least, most of them should be. "Your intestinal tract is surprisingly smart, versatile, and brain-like," said author Jennifer Ackerman. "Your resident bacteria play a far larger role in digestion than ever imagined."[9]

Intestinal flora perform a host of useful functions, such as helping you digest and absorb your food, shore up your immune system, detoxify noxious compounds, and even contribute to the manufacture of essential vitamins that your body needs. All your intestinal flora need is a hospitable environment, where they can flourish, help with digestion, and deal with rogue bacteria roaming around your terrain.

Inside your terrain, however, billions of unfriendly intestinal flora lurk, like bandits crouched behind rocks, waiting to surprise the next pioneer wagon train coming around the bend. These impaired or imbalanced flora can take the form of bacteria, viruses, fungi, and protozoans, and their fingerprints are all over heart disease, allergies and asthma, skin disorders, obesity, irritable bowel syndrome, urinary tract infections—a whole host of acute conditions and chronic diseases. An imbalance of intestinal flora crops up after antibiotic treatments or when a powerful flu bug makes the rounds, resulting in constipation or diarrhea.

This Wild, Wild West scene is apropos to what's happening in your terrain. At this moment, while you're reading these words, there's a white-hat-versus-black-hat standoff on Main Street in Dodge City. Over at the Crystal Palace Saloon, the good, bad, and indifferent bacteria are duking it out like one of those old-time Westerns where wingback chairs are tossed about, bottles of whiskey crash against heads, and haymaker punches are landed.

That's a good description of the tussle going on every second of

WE NEED HEALTHY SKIN, TOO

Did you know that we have trillions of natural flora on our skin as well as in our gut? That's why I shake my head every time I see a soap commercial touting its ability to "fight bacteria while keeping your skin clean and sparkling."

As we discussed in the introduction to my friend Dr. Axe in Chapter 1, antibacterial soaps are not the answer because they kill the beneficial bacteria on your skin as well as any lurking germs. They also destroy the healthy oils present on your skin, which create an acid mantle of protection to stop bad germs from entering your body. A common ingredient of commercial antibacterial soaps is triclosan, a chlorinated aromatic chemical that destroys bacteria and microbes on contact.

We *need* beneficial bacteria on our skin to fight off the critters hibernating under and around our fingernails and folds of the skin. But I'm not proposing that we don't wash our hands or practice good hygiene. In fact, I take good hygiene very seriously, especially washing the hands, because the hands are one of the five main areas where germs enter the body—the bad germs that assault the body's immune system. (About 80 percent of your immune system lives in your gastrointestinal tract.)

That's why each morning and evening, I plunge my fingernails into a tub of special semisoft hand soap and work the creamy material around the tips of my fingers, cuticles, and fingernails for 15 or 20 seconds, knowing I'm applying a soap that is rich in essential oils and *not* antibacterial. This creamy soap does not disrupt the delicate balance of microflora necessary for healthy skin.

your life inside your terrain. Friendly bacteria in your gut are doing their darnedest to keep the bad bacteria in check as each side seeks an upper hand. When the good guys are winning, you should have a balance of 85 percent "white hat" intestinal flora and 15 percent "black hat" organisms in the intestinal tract.

The problem is that our modern lifestyle, with its heavy reliance on antibiotics, consumption of too much sugary foods, drinking too much alcohol and soft drinks, and cavalier attitude about chemical food additives kills off zillions of beneficial bacteria. I wouldn't be surprised if you could flip that 85:15 ratio on its head for all the millions of Americans experiencing auto-intoxication or chronic digestive problems like irritable bowel syndrome or Crohn's disease.

Following the Probiotic Diet will introduce live bacteria cultures into your gut and be a preventive and therapeutic measure to help you keep the balance of intestinal flora in your terrain tipped toward the positive side.

The Second Brain

I was nine years old when Mom heard that the Village Players theater in nearby Palm Beach was putting on the popular musical *Oliver!* based on the classic Charles Dickens book *Oliver Twist*. Like plenty of other mothers in South Florida, she thought I was the perfect kid to play the lead role of Oliver Twist. I knew all the songs by heart because Mom used to play a 33-rpm record—those were the days—of the *Oliver!* soundtrack during naptime. I loved singing, *Food, glorious food... hot sausage and mustard... while we're in the mood... cold jelly and custard...*

Even though I had never acted professionally before, that didn't deter Mom from escorting me to an open casting call with dozens of stage moms and their young sons in tow. Knowing all the lines and all the songs by heart impressed the director, and it didn't hurt that I had the right street urchin look.

I got the part. The troupe rehearsed for well over three months, and then Opening Night arrived. Let me tell you: after winning this key role for a major musical in South Florida, boy, was I nervous! I still haven't forgotten the butterflies that fluttered around my stomach whenever the orchestra warmed up just before the rise of the curtain.

I don't recall running to the bathroom before an *Oliver!* performance, but it's a physiological fact that when people get nervous, they often have to have a bowel movement because the sphincter loosens its grip. There's a strong link between the emotions and gut health, and when you're under stress, the body's response sometimes causes the large intestine to move spontaneously, which results in rapid evacuation. On the other hand, stress can prompt a decrease in motility in the small intestines, which leads to constipation.

Michael Gershon, M.D., a neurobiologist at New York City's Columbia-Presbyterian Medical Center, has devoted his career to studying the human bowel—the stomach, esophagus, small intestine, and colon. His 30 years of research have led to an electrifying discovery: we have two brains—the one inside our craniums and a hidden but powerful brain in the gut known as the enteric nervous system. The presence of a "second brain" is why we feel queasy when called to speak in public—or sing "Food, Glorious Food" before 800 patrons in a crowded auditorium.

What happens is that the nervous system in your gut, which contains an independent network of over half of the body's nerve cells, can sense nutrients, measure acids, and trigger peristaltic waves that propel food along the digestive tract. "The brain is not the only place in the body that's full of neurotransmitters," Dr. Gershon explained. "One hundred million neurotransmitters line the length of the gut—approximately the same number found in the brain." These neurotransmitters coordinate with the immune system to defend your terrain from invaders.

So, if you've ever had butterflies in your stomach, then the "second brain" in your gut is producing emotion-based feelings. Your two brains communicate back and forth by way of a nerve trunk extending from the base of the brain all the way down to your abdomen. When one brain is upset, the other knows about it right away.

The brain, the terrain, and the bugs make for a fascinating triangle, and beneficial bacteria, digestion, and nutrition make for a dynamic partnership. Good intestinal flora can prevent bloating, gas, and unfriendly yeast overgrowth by controlling the pH level of the intestines through the production of lactic acid. (The pH level refers to the level of acidity versus alkalinity.) In addition, probiotics have been found in a Canadian medical study to influence the brain-gut axis, especially in the areas of stress management.[10]

Where We Go Next

I mentioned earlier that around 500 different types of bacteria—good and bad—live in the colon and the lower portion of the small intestine. Your head may be spinning, wondering why you're not sick all the time, but only 20 species make up 75 percent of that number. The most prominent bacterial species are *Bacteroides, Bifidobacteria, Pepto streptococcus, Fusobacteria, Rheumanococcus, Lactobacillus, Clostridia,* and *Escherichia coli,* better known as *E. coli.*

I'm figuring that every Latin name is unknown to you—as well as unpronounceable—except for the last one, *E. coli.* Most *E. coli* strains are harmless, but a serotype 0157:H7 can cause serious food poisoning, which is why you occasionally see *E. coli* in the news after people get sick after eating at a fast-food chain where ground beef tainted by *Escherichia coli* bacteria has been served. This will gross you out, but the way E. coli is spread from person to person is by what infectious scientists call the "fecal-oral" route. That's a nice way of saying that a restaurant employee who went No. 2 failed to wash his hands after cleaning his tush, and then he spread the bacteria on the foods he was preparing.

Excuse me for the digression, but all these bacterial species are examples of microbes, but not all are probiotics. Most are good, some are indifferent, and a few are bad bugs. When your body receives probiotics through foods and supplementation, they work to colonize the intestinal tract with beneficial flora while crowding out the disease-causing bacteria, viruses, and yeasts.

But like a baseball scorecard, you need to know "who's who" in the probiotic world. You'll start learning how to tell one probiotic from another in our next chapter.

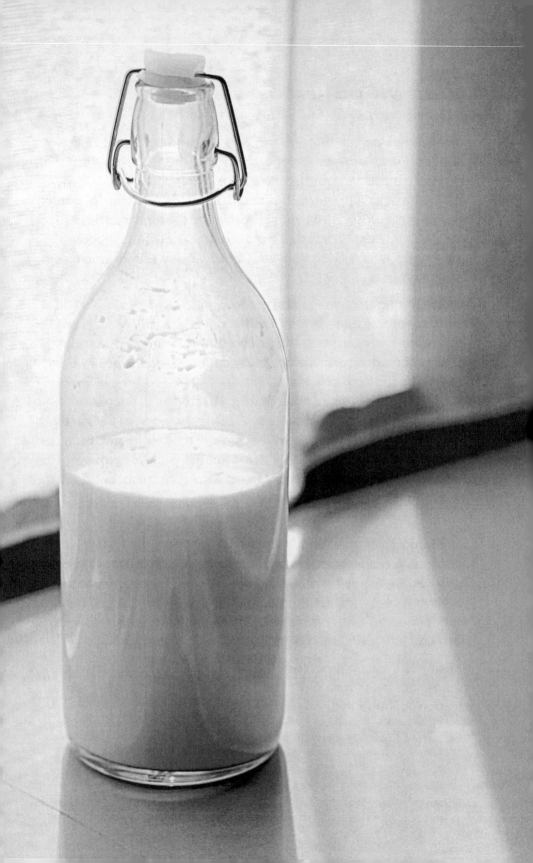

4

PROBIOTICS: THE GOOD GERMS

I had a special relationship with my Grandma Rose.

I lost three grandparents before I turned ten years old, but Grandma Rose was always there for me—right up until her death in 2005 at the age of 82. When I was confined to a bed for months at a time during my life-and-death struggles with Crohn's disease back in the mid-1990s, she spelled my parents whenever they needed a break from their caregiver duties. I'll never forget the tender way my gentle grandmother carried steaming bowls of her homemade chicken soup to my bedroom, pressed a cool cloth to my feverish forehead, and cleaned up after me without complaint.

What a remarkable woman! Grandma Rose grew up in another era, a time that seems far away from 21st century America. Born in 1922 in a small Polish village that could have doubled as the set of *Fiddler on the Roof*, Rose was the youngest of seven children to Gidalia and Simma Catz. Her relatives were persecuted Russian Jews who sought sanctuary in places like Hungary, Czechoslovakia, and Poland. On their small family farm 60 kilometers west of Warsaw, her father operated a mill that pressed poppy seeds and flaxseeds into oil. A big taste treat in those days was to take the pressed seeds and patty them into hard cakes, which were dipped into schmaltz, or the rendered fat from chicken soup.

Grandma Rose used to tell me stories about how their family—poor but not destitute—bartered eggs for milk from the village dairyman. She would lug the tin pail of fresh cow's milk home to the family cellar and leave it there. Remember, this was raw, unpasteurized, and unhomogenized milk—the real deal—and did not have to be refrigerated. (Even if the Catz family could have afforded a refrigerator, they didn't have electricity anyway.)

After two or three days in the cellar (one day in warm weather or two to three days in cooler weather), the raw milk would culture and thicken, and Rose and her siblings fought over who would get to taste the tangy cream that formed at the top of the pail. If you've ever enjoyed crème fraîche, then you know what I'm talking about.

What remained in the pail was a type of fermented dairy called "clabbered cream" or "clabbered milk." The explanation for the culturing process in the cellar is that the bacteria in the milk began the process of converting lactose—a sugar, so therefore sweet—into lactic acid, which, being an acid, is tart or sour. In addition to changing the taste, this fermentation caused a slight curdling, which thickened the milk as it rose toward the top as cream. The clabbered cream skimmed off the top tasted delicious.

The clabbered milk left behind had a sour, tangy taste from the slight curdling that had occurred. Clabbered milk was still quite drinkable and could be made into curds to form a soft cheese.

The reason why the Catz family could leave raw dairy out for a number of days, either at room temperature or below, was because the natural probiotics in the raw milk would culture it. When you leave pasteurized milk out overnight *without* refrigeration, however, the milk putrefies because all the good probiotic organisms were zapped when the milk was heated to 161 degrees Fahrenheit during the pasteurization process.

This story about Grandma Rose growing up in Poland and consuming crème fraîche and clabbered milk is a great segue to the story of a Russian biologist named Élie Metchnikoff, who first recognized the health benefits of probiotics in the early 1900s. It was Metchnikoff who discovered that Bulgarian peasants consuming large quantities of sour milk containing fermenting bacteria—much like Grandma Rose did as a young girl—appeared to enjoy extraordinarily good health and, for those days, an extraordinarily long life.

Born in 1845 in the Ukraine, Ilya Ilyich Metchnikoff, nicknamed Élie, was the son of an officer of the Imperial Guard who was a landowner in the Ukraine steppes. His mother was Jewish.

As a young boy, Élie was fascinated by natural history and loved to give lectures to his smaller brothers and other children in his village of Kharkoff. He studied natural sciences at the nearby University of Kharkoff and showed that he was an academic prodigy by completing four years of university in just two years. After graduation, he studied intracellular digestion in flatworms at the University of Giessen in Germany, an observation that portended his future interest in human digestion and how that impacted health.[1]

At age 32, Metchnikoff returned to Russia and the University of St. Petersburg, where he became a professor of zoology. Not much is written about Metchnikoff's private life, but he must have been a tortured soul as he reached his mid-thirties. He was not married, but that changed when he fell in love with Ludmilla Feodorovitch, who suffered from such a severe case of tuberculosis that she had to be carried down the aisle in a chair for the wedding. For five years, Metchnikoff tended to her care and did all he could to save the life of the woman he loved, but Ludmilla died in 1873, and with her death, the light in Metchnikoff's life dimmed. Devastated by the loss, troubled by weak eyesight and heart troubles, and tired of how he was being treated at the university, Metchnikoff attempted to take his own life by swallowing a dose of opium.

Fortunately for us—and this book—the opium dose was not fatal.

Metchnikoff seemed to rebound two years later when he met and married his second wife, Olga, but then she was struck by a severe attack of typhoid fever. Although she survived, her illness threw Metchnikoff into another mental tailspin. He attempted suicide a second time by inoculating himself with relapsing fever, but his hopes to kill himself were dashed when the attack of relapsing fever, while severe, wasn't potent enough to kill him.

It was at this juncture that life turned brighter. Olga came into an inheritance, which freed him from financial concerns. Feeling renewed, he returned to his laboratory, where he developed the theory of phagocytosis, which stated that various amoeboid cells—notably white blood cells—were able to engulf and destroy harmful substances such as toxins and bacteria.

Crossing Paths

Metchnikoff's paper on phagocytosis made the rounds and raised his profile in the scientific world. His spirits were lifted further in 1886 when he was appointed director of an institute established at the University of Odessa to carry out Louis Pasteur's research on a vaccine treatment for rabies. Some of his Odessa colleagues raised a stink about Metchnikoff's involvement, however, saying that he was unqualified since he did not have a medical degree. Humiliated, Metchnikoff fled Odessa and traveled to Paris, where he met with Louis Pasteur and asked the *éminence grise* (French for "gray eminence") for his advice on what to do next.

In what has to be one of the probiotical ironies of the late 19th century, the future "father of probiotics" was asked by the "father of modern medicine" to stay and work for the Louis Pasteur Institute. Pasteur gave him an appointment and a laboratory, and Metchnikoff remained in Paris for the rest of his life. For his work on immunity from infectious diseases, Metchnikoff was awarded, together with Paul Ehrlich, the Nobel Prize for Physiology and Medicine in 1908.

It was during his tenure at the Pasteur Institute—again, the irony is delicious—that Metchnikoff followed a different muse. As he was getting along in years (the Russian microbiologist was in his late fifties at the time), he began to study longevity. "Metchnikoff came to view the aging process as largely abnormal in modern man," said John G. Simmons, author of *Doctors and Discoveries*. "He suggested the possibility of a normal life expectancy of about 120 years."[2]

Metchnikoff speculated that senility might be due to chronic autointoxication caused by intestinal bacteria, which, in turn, were caused by toxins present in the diet. The Russian researcher laid all the blame on the large intestine, which was "the reservoir of the waste of the digestive processes, and the waste stagnating long enough to putrefy. The products of putrefaction are harmful."[3] This thinking fit in with the mindset of the late 19th century that constipation was the bane of mankind. In Jewish folklore, the call of nature could not be delayed a minute longer than necessary, lest the bowels release more toxins into the bloodstream.

For a while, Metchnikoff was attracted to the theories of English surgeon Sir W. Arbuthnot Lane, who introduced the surgical removal of the colon as a cure for "autointoxication diseases." An estimated 1,000 patients submitted to this dubious procedure. Metchnikoff eventually rejected Lane's extreme surgical method and decided to pursue a different approach to autointoxication: improving the bacterial population of the intestines by adding beneficial bacteria, said Peter Cartwright, author of *Probiotics for Crohn's & Colitis.*

As Metchnikoff poked around, he heard about Bulgarian peasants living in the Caucasus Mountains who had an average lifespan of 87 years, exceptional for the early 1900s when the average life expectancy was in the mid-forties. During that era, the *New York Times* printed a picture taken in a small Bulgarian village of Baba Vasilka, who was described as the "oldest woman in the world" at age 126, and her son, Tudor, a youth of 101 years, who was portrayed as still active and vigorous.

The Bulgarian diets, Metchnikoff learned, contained large amounts of fermented dairy—just like the crème fraîche and clabbered milk that Grandma Rose consumed as a girl growing up in Poland. According to Metchnikoff's empirical observations, eating bowl after bowl of cultured dairy—what we could call Crème Bulgare today—caused the Bulgarian bowels to become acidic and form an inhospitable environment for the unfriendly bacteria, yeasts, viruses, and parasites that would otherwise produce toxins.[4]

Arguing that the bacteria in the Bulgarian cultured dairy kept putrefactive bacteria in check, Metchnikoff set off to find which bacterium in the fermented dairy improved the intestinal flora. The Russian researcher hypothesized that replacing or diminishing the number of putrefactive bacteria in the gut with lactic acid bacteria, or LABs, would bring about normal bowel health and prolong life. He successfully isolated a bacterium in the peasants' cultured dairy and named it *Lactobacillus bulgaricus* (pronounced just the way it looks: *lack-toh-bah-sill-us bull-gare-i-cus*) in honor of the Bulgarians. The *Lactobacillus bulgaricus* chased out the "wild, putrefying *bacilli* in our large intestine," he claimed.[5] *Bacilli* are Latin for bacteria.

To prove his hypothesis that toxins in the bowel could be the root cause of serious disease, Metchnikoff orally and rectally implanted the bacteria in the gastrointestinal tract of volunteer subjects to scientifically determine if a substantial positive effect on health could be measured after consuming *Lactobacillus bulgaricus*.

Unfortunately, the *Lactobacillus bulgaricus* could not survive the passage through the gastrointestinal tract, but when the cultured yogurt-type dairy was consumed intact with its naturally occurring friendly microorganisms, the test volunteers were as fit as a fiddle. This supports a major tenet of the Probiotic Diet: that an excellent way to enhance the health of the gastrointestinal tract is to consume lacto-fermented foods and not merely *Lactobacillus*-based probiotics.

The Father of Probiotics

Metchnikoff explained his scientific rationale for the health benefits of lactic acid bacteria in his book *The Prolongation of Life*, which was published in 1907. Remember: Metchnikoff, in a way, was searching for a fountain of youth, and for him, that fountain was filled with fermented milk. "The dependence of intestinal microbes on the food makes it possible to adopt measures to modify the flora in our bodies and to replace the harmful microbes with useful microbes," he wrote as his thesis statement.[6]

As one of the first scientists to propose a link between disease and harmful bacteria in the terrain, Metchnikoff's theories received extensive attention and were responsible for a surge in the consumption of fermented milk and cultured dairy products in the decade leading up to the Roaring Twenties. It's said that Metchnikoff drank copious amounts of sour milk—the Crème Bulgare—to test his hypothesis that consuming lactic acid bacteria would reap wonderful health benefits and extend his life.

Unfortunately, consuming a couple of liters of cultured dairy every single day could not overcome a balky heart, and Metchnikoff died of cardiac arrest at the age of 71 in 1916. Even though he lived well beyond the average life expectancy of his time, the Russian failed to last as long as his Bulgarian compatriots, which dampened enthusiasm for his theories. His remains were buried at the Pasteur Institute in Paris, presumably not far from the plot containing the bones of Louis Pasteur.

Today, Metchnikoff's legacy lives on. His idea that certain lactic acid bacteria acidify the gut and keep putrefying bacteria in check earned him the title "The Father of Probiotics," apropos since he is also credited with coining the term "probiotics," which, according to its Latin roots, means "for life." His research into the potential life-lengthening properties of lactic acid bacteria inspired other scientists to study the relationship between bacteria and good intestinal health as well as the idea that "beneficial" bacteria could be used medically to combat deleterious bacteria.

Following his death, however, Metchnikoff's ideas lost traction in research labs on the European continent. Reason? The "germ theory" of his mentor, Louis Pasteur—which held that germs caused disease and it was up to modern medicine to find the right drugs to kill those germs—still held sway. When antibiotics came along in the 1930s and received wider use during World War II to treat wounded soldiers, the wondrous "miracle drug" known as penicillin became the preferred method of anti-microbial therapy, and Metchnikoff's research was largely forgotten.

"There is little evidence to indicate that Metchnikoff's concept [regarding the benefits of lactic acid bacteria] was taken seriously," wrote Canadian researchers Kingsley C. Anukum, Ph.D., and Gregor Reid, Ph.D. "Indeed, between 1908 and 1964, little or nothing was heard of microbial therapy in Western countries."[7]

The Power of Harmful Bacteria

Élie Metchnikoff was on to something, though, during an exciting time when knowledge about human physiology was exploding in the early 20th century. The pH scale, the standard measurement of acidity, was developed in 1909 by Soren Sorensen, a Danish biochemist who performed pioneering research into proteins, amino acids, and enzymes—the basis of today's protein chemistry.

Basically meaning the "power of hydrogen," the pH scale helped researchers measure the level of acidity in the intestines. On a logarithmic scale from 0 to 14, the lower the number, the more acidic the terrain. The higher the number, the more alkaline. Ideally, the large intestine should have a low pH since harmful bacteria thrive in an alkaline environment, not in an acidic one.

Besides acidifying the colon, scientists learned that friendly bacteria assisted the immune system by preventing infection, manufacturing important B-complex vitamins, and increasing the absorption of the proteins found in the foods you eat. Friendly microorganisms improved the absorption of minerals such as calcium, copper, iron, magnesium, and manganese and stiffened the body's resistance to food poisoning.

The early 20th century was also the era when biochemists were having success isolating bacterial strains. Among the first to be identified were friendly bacteria from the *Lactobacillus* or *Bifidobacterium* genera. (*Bifidobacterium* is also pronounced as how it looks: bif-i-doh-bact-tear-i-um.) Lactobacillus converts lactose and other sugars to lactic acid and are present in the gastrointestinal tract as well as the vaginas of women. *Lacto* is a Latin prefix for "milk," while *bifido* means "forked" or "split into two parts" because under a microscope, *Bifidobacterium* appear to have branches. The bacteria in the bifidobacteria genus are found mostly in the colon, where, like the lactobacillus bacteria, they are good at adhering to the intestinal walls and crowding out harmful bacteria.

Let's take a closer look at some of the members in these two families of friendly bacteria:

Lactobacillus plantarum

This lactic acid-producing bacteria is commonly found in fermented vegetables that have been pickled in vinegar. Sauerkraut, pickles, brined olives, and Korean *kimchi* are examples. This probiotic helps ensure that vitamins and minerals reach your cells.

Lactobacillus casei

This lactic acid-producing bacteria found in the human intestine and mouth has been found to assist in the growth of other desirable bacteria in your terrain.

Lactobacillus acidophilus

This lactic acid-producing bacteria gets its name from *lacto-* (meaning milk), *-bacillus* (meaning rod-like in shape), and *acidophilus* (meaning acid-loving). In the last ten years, the sale of milk cartons festooned with *lactobacillus acidophilus* has exploded as word has gotten out that this probiotic can guard the health of your entire digestive tract. *Lactobacillus acidophilus* is effective against chronic diarrhea because it inhibits the growth of many kinds of harmful bacteria.

Lactobacillus bulgaricus

You already know about this probiotic, which was first isolated by Élie Metchnikoff over a hundred years ago after he studied what was in the Bulgarians' fermented dairy.

Bifidobacterium bifidum

This bacterium promotes a healthy balance of intestinal flora, enhances immune system response, and keeps the pH at its optimum level. Bifidobacteria are the major component of the intestines, but as the body ages, or because of illness, bifidobacteria levels drop precipitously.

Bifidobacterium infantis

This important probiotic is found in mothers' milk, which is yet another illustration of why breastfeeding is so important to babies' health.

You can receive these examples of the probiotics through: eating lacto-fermented foods such as yogurt, cheese, and kefir; consuming fermented foods such as sauerkraut and Korean *kimchi*; and through consuming probiotic nutritional supplements available in natural food stores.

I first became aware of cultured dairy products and probiotics when I was battling my digestive troubles in the mid-1990s. Sure, I ate cultured dairy products like yogurt growing up. Didn't everyone? But my parents didn't ply me with probiotic supplements because they simply weren't on people's radar or generally available in health food stores during the 1980s and early 1990s. The only supplements that I remember taking as a boy were barley grass juice, bee pollen, and several vitamins and minerals.

I'll bet you that I was probably the one kid on the block who took nutritional supplements, though. That's because my parents were quite health conscious since Dad was a naturopathic physician and Mom was vitally interested in healthy living. My Baby Boomer parents were part of the back-to-nature generation that came of age in the 1960s, and you could say they raised me as a "granola kid." If my neighborhood friends were looking for something to drink, Mom was apt to give them each a glass of fresh-squeezed carrot juice when we invaded the kitchen. I don't remember many takers, though.

When I became very ill in the summer of 1994 at Camp Swan, my parents left no stone unturned as we sought a treatment that could save my life. Since I had horrible digestive and bowel problems, Dad did some checking around and heard that this "new thing" called probiotics could increase the beneficial flora in my gut and drive harmful bacteria out of my digestive tract. Since I was suffering from around-the-clock diarrhea and stabbing gut pains, probiotics sounded like just the ticket to improve my digestive health.

Dad had me try over 30 different brands of probiotics, including one brand that had three probiotic products containing *lactobacillus acidophilus, lactobacillus bulgaricus,* and *bifidobacterium,* all in a powder form. For a period of over one month, I took an entire bottle of each per day. In addition, I consumed the three organisms combined in special oil matrix capsules that cost $2 each capsule. Since I was taking between 30 to 60 probiotic pills each day, you can imagine what this was costing my parents.

After 29 more brands of probiotics proved unsuccessful, I stopped taking probiotics altogether. We still thought the theory about probiotics made perfect sense, but we figured that we hadn't found the right probiotics just yet.

A year later, we did find correct probiotics that sealed my recovery, but I'm getting ahead of my story. (I'll tell you more about those probiotics in the next chapter.) In the meantime, I moved to San Diego in the spring of 1995 to be near a San Diego nutrition expert named William "Bud" Keith. A mutual acquaintance had told him about my sad fight against a variety of gastrointestinal diseases, so he called my father and suggested I come out to the West Coast and stay with his family.

Intrigued, and figuring I had nothing to lose, I flew out to San Diego and met with Bud, who recommended that I consume healthy "live" foods that were rich in vitamins, minerals, and enzymes, as well as those friendly microorganisms called probiotics. Sounded good to me.

After staying with the Keith family a few weeks to get settled, they recommended that I buy—well, it was my parents' money—a well-used RV so I could get around and prepare my own meals from purchases of wild-caught fish, grass-fed beef, raw goat's or cow's milk in the form of fermented kefir, raw cheeses, organic fruits and vegetables, and carrot and other vegetable juices.

Gradually, I regained my strength—and began putting on weight. Over a 40-day period, I added 29 much-needed pounds and topped 150 pounds for the first time in nearly two years. When I left San Diego, I returned to South Florida with a renewed sense of purpose and the confidence that I had conquered the digestive illnesses that nearly killed me.

Loving Cultured Dairy

That life-changing experience in San Diego made me a lover of cultured dairy products to this day, and stories like Élie Metchnikoff and his interest in the long-living villagers in the Bulgarian backwoods have intrigued me ever since. One of my dreams is

THE HISTORY OF CULTURED DAIRY

Although the term "probiotics" is just a century old, the probiotics in cultured dairy have been consumed in nations since time immemorial. Abraham, the father of many nations, brought some "cheese curds and milk" in Genesis 18:8 (NLT) and fed it to others. Assyrians ate cultured dairy for their health, and according to Pliny, the ancient Roman nobleman, Persian women believed fermented dairy worked wonders for their skin. Cleopatra, the Queen of Egypt, bathed in "asses' milk," which, I would presume, would be donkey or burro milk.[8]

Cultured dairy has been around for thousands of years, from Iran to Greece to Finland, but we get our word *yogurt* from the Turkish word *yoğurt*. Up until Metchnikoff's time, about the only people

to someday travel to the Caucasus Mountains and be introduced to the Bulgarian farmers and peasants who still consume cultured dairy like their ancestors—and live just as long as they did. I would love to bring an interpreter along and ask questions about what they eat and sample the famous "sour milk" that Metchnikoff drank. I almost made the long journey to the Ukrainian steppes in 2007, but pressing commitments elsewhere forced me to cancel the trip.

I still love traveling to Europe, though, and one of the reasons why is their cultural love for cultured dairy. Nicki and I have been fortunate to visit the Continent three or four times since we got married, and one of the first things we do after we arrive in a new city is search for the closest *laiterie*—a store that sells fresh dairy products.

You know how most couples go to France and fall in love? Well, I went to France and fell in love all right—with *brebis* yogurt, which is yogurt made from raw sheep's milk. Talk about a creamy, delicious cultured dairy product that is nearly impossible to find in the States (unless you order online). While in France, Germany, Switzerland, and

Italy, I love stocking up on a dozen brebis yogurts and taking them back to the refrigerator in our hotel room.

One of the amazing things about France is walking into a huge super-marché—one is called Carrefour and they're as oversized as our Wal-marts—and finding the refrigerated yogurt section that's as big as a supermarket aisle here in the States. You can browse for cow's milk yogurt, sheep's milk yogurt, goat's milk yogurt, a hundred varieties of cheeses, various flavors of kefir and "bifidophilus" drinks—pasteurized and not pasteurized, *comme vous voulez*—like you want.

Shop at a Publix or a Kroger's back in the States and you'll be lucky to find a couple of rows of yogurts in the dairy section, and they're probably fat-free or "light," which means the milk has been nutrition-ally neutered. What's worse is that our U.S.-made yogurt doesn't taste good. I'll grant you that it tastes sweet—*Would you like to sample our light, fat-free blueberry cheese-cake yogurt loaded with artificial sweeteners, preservatives, thicken-ers, and artificial colors?*—but it's not very palatable. No thanks.

eating cultured yogurt in abundance were farmers and their families in Eastern Europe and Central Asia. Then Metchnikoff single-handedly started a yogurt craze in Western Europe. The first industrial production of yogurt was recorded in 1919 in Barcelona, Spain, when an enterprising Spaniard named Isaac Carasso began using bacterial cultures obtained from the Pasteur Institute. In 1929, Carasso opened a plant in Paris and named his company Danone, a Catalan diminutive of the name of his son, Daniel. His sales pitch: eat the "Dessert of Happy Digestion."

But commercial yogurt, which came in only two flavors in those early days—plain and plainer—wasn't an overnight success. The tart taste that puckered lips wasn't an immediate hit with city dwellers, who were discovering another form of dairy, thanks to the rising availability of refrigeration.

I'm talking about ice cream and its sweet flavors: vanilla, chocolate, strawberry, and pistachio.

In the mid-1950s, yogurt caught the fancy of the French—nobody is sure why—and Carasso gained a beachhead in the United States when he opened a factory in New York. He changed the brand name to Dannon to make it sound more American.

Plain yogurt was a tough sell in the United States until the late 1960s, when yogurt manufacturers like Dannon tore a page from the ice cream playbook: *Let's make it sweeter!* They added fruit, often pre-sweetened, and *voilà*, instead of a pasteurized tangy product languishing in a specialty market, yogurt was a sweet sensation with a pleasing tart aftertaste. Suddenly, you had yogurt manufacturers falling over themselves to create new flavors using natural and artificial sweeteners, and consumers could buy yogurt in flavors

So imagine my excitement a few years ago when Nicki and I pulled off the autostrada and drove into Lugano, a lovely lakeside Swiss town surrounded by hills and mountains right on Switzerland's southern border with Italy. As is often the case when we travel in Europe, I prefer to picnic at lunchtime instead of frequenting a restaurant so that we can eat healthier and eat what we want. Nicki and I were directed to a Manor store in downtown Lugano, which is a lot like a Macy's but with a gourmet market in the basement that sells beautiful foods.

There in the dairy section were choices galore for sheep's yogurt, marked in the three official languages in Switzerland: *Schaf* in German, *pecore* in Italian, and *brebis* in French. (I always look for the French name since I first discovered brebis yogurt in Paris.) At any rate, I must have excitedly scooped up a dozen single-serving *brebis* yogurts into my arms because Nicki's basket was full of cheeses and breads for the picnic. Before we reached the checkout lanes, however, four containers of sheep's yogurt tumbled out of my arms and splattered across the linoleum floor. What a scene! A young Swiss woman in a Manor smock glared at me, and moments later, I heard the Swiss equivalent of "Clean Up on Aisle 4" broadcast on the PA system. Very embarrassing.

The reason I got excited about brebis yogurt is because it's so much better—and healthier—than the commercial yogurt back in the States because it has different lactic acid bacteria, or probiotics. You see, American yogurt must have two strains of lactic acid bacteria: otherwise, it can't be sold as yogurt, and that bothers me.

The two strains are *Lactobacillus bulgaricus* and *Streptococcus thermophilus*, the latter being an organism that I don't like very much because *thermophil* means "heat-seeking" or "heat-friendly." The reason why *Streptococcus thermophilus* is used in this country is because *thermophil* can function better in milk that's been pasteurized—or heated—than other lactic acid bacteria. *Streptococcus thermophilus* also speeds up fermentation, and as everyone knows in today's economic climate, time saved is money earned. Another downside is that these forms of lactic acid bacteria are very fragile.

like maple syrup, coconut cream, cinnamon, and piña colada.

The latest *trend du jour* is the commercial yogurt makers intentionally adding "probiotics" to their yogurt and selling them at a premium to cash in on the increasing interest in adding probiotics to your diet. Dannon has three lines—DanActive, Activia, and Activia Light—with labels touting the addition of "Bifidus Regularis" for its "beneficial role in your intestinal ecosystem."

I like how Dannon used the *au courant* word "ecosystem," but while adding probiotics to commercial yogurt is nice, the truth is that the *real* beneficial probiotics were lost during the pasteurization process. Furthermore, the wrong probiotics are in those yogurts. That's why I consider Élie Metchnikoff the father of *commercial* probiotics.

Look what Metchnikoff has wrought, though. More than 150 different probiotic products—drinks, snacks, and supplements—have hit the stores in recent years, and by 2010, probiotic food is projected to be a $1 billion a year business.[9] I know that the sale of probiotics is the fastest-growing segment in the Natural Products industry, and in a down economy, grew at an explosive 18 percent rate in 2008. Granted, the Natural Products industry is a niche market, comprising independent health food stores, natural grocers like Whole Foods and Wild Oats, and vitamin outlets like Vitamin Shoppe, but this industry is usually ten years ahead of the mainstream, which bodes well for the future of probiotics and further cements the need for a book like The Probiotic Diet.

I'm betting that you haven't heard any of this stuff, but I've been studying probiotics extensively for over two decades as well as consuming them for better health, so I've learned a few things. While I believe that cultured foods are beneficial, I've now come to the conclusion that Metchnikoff's Lactobacillus bulgaricus and, in fact, lactic acid bacterium are not the probiotics that we should be focusing on to get our terrain restored and our health back on track.

I'll say it in a different way: even though a huge multibillion-dollar industry that makes cultured dairy products like yogurt and crème fraîche sprang up out of Metchnikoff's impassioned research into lactic acid bacteria, much like Louis Pasteur's "germ theory," the real truth is found elsewhere.

Élie Metchnikoff had the right idea about lactic acid bacteria improving digestive health, but he didn't discover the very best probiotics to affect and improve the terrain. In our next chapter, you'll learn about three probiotic organisms with a long-storied history, and about an English professor—still alive and well today—who's devoted his life to getting the word out about these three microorganisms.

These three probiotic organisms—*Bacillus subtilis*, *Bacillus coagulans*, and *Saccharomyces boulardii* are what I took to regain my health more than ten years ago and what Dr. Brasco uses in his Alabama clinic today. You'll learn about these true probiotic heroes in the pages ahead.

PRONUNCIATION GUIDE

While pronouncing long, imposing terms like *Lactobacillus bulgaricus* should be rather straightforward—once you figure out where to break up the word—the following three probiotics are more difficult to pronounce. Here's a guide for these three probiotic heroes:

- *Bacillus subtilis is bah-sill-us subtle-is. Just think of the way you normally pronounce "subtle" and you're more than halfway home.*

- *Bacillus coagulans has its roots in the verb "coagulate," which means to congeal, clot, or thicken: bah-sill-us coh-adg-u-lans.*

- *Saccharomyces boulardii may be the most difficult: sack-a-row-my-sees boo-lahr-dee.*

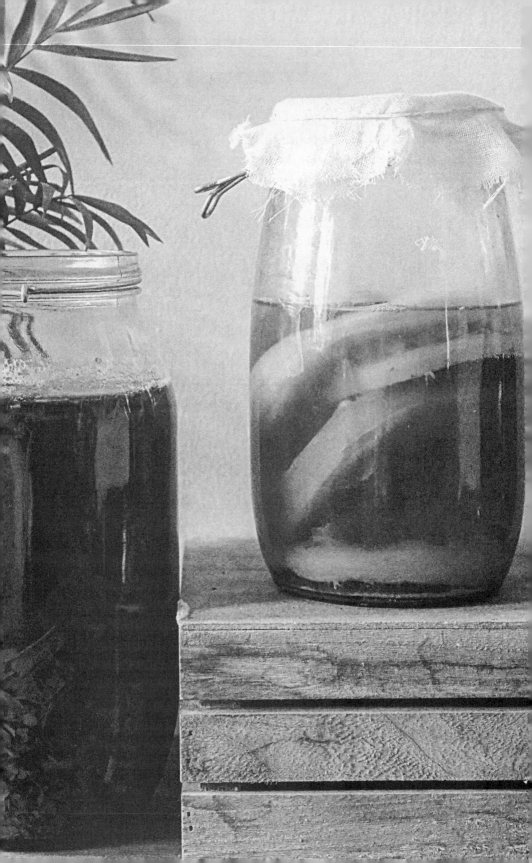

5

THE TRUE PROBIOTIC HEROES

talked about my love affair with brebis yogurt in the last chapter and how when Nicki and I travel to Europe, we enjoy shopping in local markets for breakfast and lunch. Since organic foods are marked "bio" in Europe, we've never had much difficulty finding organic breads, cheese, butter, yogurt (brebis!), and fresh fruits to hold us over till dinner time, when we look forward to a romantic dinner *al fresco*.

On the same trip to Lugano, Nicki and I spent a couple of nights in iconic Venice, where we entered a labyrinth of narrow passageways and alleys only to discover an enchanting city of meandering canals punctuated by picturesque bridges. One afternoon, Nicki explored Venice's Jewish Ghetto, which really isn't a ghetto but used to be hundreds of years ago. When Jews were kicked out of cities all over Europe during the Middle Ages and Renaissance, they were "tolerated" and allowed to live in a *quartiere* of Venice that was not the most desirable part of town. Today, the Jewish Ghetto is home to several synagogues and scintillating shops that are off the beaten—and I'm talking well beaten—tourist path.

While Nicki was window-shopping for a cute sweater or fashionable Italian leather pumps, I did some shopping of my own at the Piazzale Roma, which is the terminus for buses arriving from the Italian mainland. I was searching for a decent market or upscale grocery store, and then I spotted the orange sign for Coop, a large supermarket chain headquartered in Switzerland and much like a Publix or Safeway in the States. I had heard that Coop sold nearly half of all the organic food sold in Switzerland, so that knowledge raised my hopes that I'd find some *bio* foods at the Coop Piazzale Roma. This Venetian outlet, where it looked like the locals shopped, appeared to be medium-sized and well-appointed.

I'm always interested in what I'll find whenever I step into a grocery store in Western Europe, and on this occasion, I wasn't disappointed. I drifted over to the nutritional supplement section—strictly professional curiosity—and checked out some labels. And then I saw it: a dark bottle whose title escapes me, but the only bottle of probiotics in the entire Coop.

As a probiotic researcher and nutritional supplement formulator who stays apprised of the market, I'm rarely surprised by any nutritional products that I find on store shelves—including what's new. But what I held in my hands genuinely stunned me. This dark bottle of probiotics listed three ingredients with tongue-twisting names: *Bacillus subtilis*, *Bacillus coagulans*, and *Saccharomyces boulardii*.

I doubted that these multisyllabic Latin names (see the Pronunciation Guide at the end of the previous chapter) meant anything to the 100,000 tourists who had set foot in Venice that day—or any of the local populace as well. But I had heard that the Italians were on the forefront of probiotics, and this bottle of 90 capsules was proof to me of their forward thinking. I had never seen probiotics with these three ingredients for sale back in the States.

I smiled when I read the first listed ingredient, *Bacillus subtilis,* because this was *the* probiotic organism that sealed my return to good health. It was like greeting an old friend.

What—a probiotic worked for you, Jordan?

I wouldn't blame you for asking that, especially since I mentioned in the last chapter that I took 30 different probiotic supplements in my search for a cure, but all I had to show for it was the world's most expensive urine. Yes, that happened, but later on, I was introduced to an obscure microorganism called *Bacillus subtilis,* and that probiotic, as well as *Bacillus coagulans* and *Saccharomyces boulardii,* became my true "probiotic heroes."

It's a story that I must recount.

After I traveled out to San Diego in the spring of 1995 to live near nutrition expert William "Bud" Keith and his family, I received a package in the mail from my father. I rolled my eyes; Dad was always sending me a health magazine or some interesting clips to read, and occasionally he enclosed a new nutritional supplement for me to try. Ever since I fell deathly ill and had to come home from Florida State University, Dad chased down every lead to get me better. I would say that he had me try 500 different treatments: gadgets, gizmos, pills, and potions that ranged from conventional drugs like prednisone to some pretty edgy stuff.

There was the time I took an extract of the Venus flytrap through an IV. Another occasion I was injected with sheep cells from embryos. The worst experience had to be the cabbage juice diet; I think I lasted two days drinking quarts of that awful-tasting concoction. Then Dad plied me with supplements made from Chinese and Peruvian herbs, Japanese kampo, and olive leaf extract, but that was nothing compared to the horrible-tasting shark cartilage or the painful IVs of adrenal cortical extract, or ACE, that was derived from bovine adrenal glands.

Why all the weird stuff? My battery of conventional medical physicians, including gastrointestinal specialists and immunologists, were stymied to cure what ailed me, and several doctors coldly informed me that I suffered from the worst case of Crohn's disease they had ever seen. Since traditional medicine wasn't working—and my parents believed the horrible side effects of medications like prednisone were hurting more than helping—they were open to alternative medical approaches to my digestive ills. That's why I subjected myself to these unconventional treatments.

When Dad's "care package" arrived in the mail from Florida, I could only imagine what was inside. Sure enough, he had enclosed a recent issue of the *Bio/Tech News,* a monthly newsletter featuring articles about alternatives to conventional medicine. In this particular volume, Dad wanted me to read a lengthy article about using beneficial microorganisms to dramatically improve intestinal health. The title of the article: "Critters!"

I had traveled down this road before, but Dad's letter urged me to study the 12-page article and consider taking something else he had enclosed: a Ziploc baggy filled with a dark-colored powder. He finished his letter with the following sentence: "I know I promised not to send you anything more to try, but I really think you should add this to your diet. Love, Dad."

I held up the baggy of black powder to the light, then tossed it into the air and caught it. Figuring I had nothing to lose, I started reading the *Bio/Tech News* article, which noted that most people were generally aware of the beneficial effects of commonly known intestinal microorganisms like *Lactobacillus acidophilus*, as well as other lacto-bacilli, that were readily found in the human intestinal tract. Every time we consume soured milk products like cultured yogurt, cottage cheese, or whey, we repopulate the gut with these *Lactobacillus* bacteria.

Following that preamble, the *Bio/Tech News* author said "we have been hearing about an amazing new all-natural health product" that was "proving itself to be effective in stimulating the body to heal itself from serious illness and disease." I was invited to read on and learn more about this breakthrough in digestive and immune therapy.

The story then introduced Peter Rothschild, an M.D. and Ph.D., who was described as one of the world's foremost experts on human immune response and its relation to beneficial microorganisms. The first quote from Dr. Rothschild caused me to sit up straighter and pay attention.

"It's a crying shame," Dr. Rothschild thundered, "that most health-minded Americans today have been brainwashed into thinking that their beloved holy St. Acidophilus is the only microorganism that can benefit their health. In truth, there are many bacterial microorganisms in existence that can stimulate phenomenal health and immune system benefits when ingested as dietary supplements—even though they are in no way indigenous to the human system."

Knowing what I know now, I would say that was a shot across the bow of the *SS Metchnikoff.*

Dr. Rothschild was just getting warmed up. He believed that a bacterial microorganism, known as *Bacillus subtilis* but not well known by modern science, could dramatically benefit the human body. Since this bacterium didn't normally take up residence in the human gastrointestinal tract or was found in common foods consumed by Americans, you had to take it in supplement form.

Curious and eager to learn more, I continued reading. Dr. Rothschild next shared an account about the discovery of *Bacillus subtilis* that sounded like one of Paul Harvey's "The Rest of the Story" radio segments.

A Desert Battlefield

Dr. Rothschild said the narrative of *Bacillus subtilis* began on the battlefields of North Africa during World War II. Field Marshal Erwin Rommel, who would become known around the world as the "Desert Fox," arrived in Libya in early 1941 with his vaunted Afrika Korps to support the Italians after their Axis partner had been routed by the British Eighth Army.

Rommel's crack Panzer divisions reclaimed territory in a counteroffensive, and by late summer of 1941, the borders of the Thousand-Year Reich extended from the sands of North Africa to the south, most of continental Europe to the west and north, and east all the way to the outskirts of Moscow.

The German High Command noticed something different about the North Africa campaign, however. The Afrika Korps was losing hundreds of soldiers each week—from dysentery. The casualties from repelling British General Montgomery's bombing attacks and shrapnel explosions were expected; soldiers dying from severe diarrhea caused by a massive infection of the digestive system was another. Dysentery turned their watery feces into a smelly mass of mucus, blood, and pus. The suffering soldiers then experienced sharp abdominal pains before complications set in: delirium, convulsions, and coma.

German doctors were aware that dysentery was caused by disease-causing bacteria found in local water and foods, which was to be expected in remote, barely civilized North Africa. If you're wondering why the Afrika Korps didn't ask for a shipload of penicillin to fight dysentery, antibiotics weren't generally available to the Axis side at that time. The reason why is that after Sir Alexander Fleming discovered penicillin in England in 1928, he and fellow scientists couldn't figure out a way to produce enough penicillin for medical use.

Indeed, penicillin remained nothing more than a laboratory curiosity throughout the 1930s, and it wasn't until the United States joined World War II following Pearl Harbor that American scientists saw the potential in resurrecting Fleming's ground-breaking work to make a germ-killing medicine that would save the lives of Allied soldiers. They received a kick in the pants when the U.S. government challenged the American pharmaceutical industry to come up with a way to manufacture penicillin—in a hurry.

Meanwhile, in North Africa, Rommel was receiving reports about hundreds of his soldiers dying not on the battlefield but in army hospital tents after contracting this ghastly disease. German doctors didn't have any medications in their black bags to fight the dysentery outbreaks. The problem was serious enough for the German High Command back in Berlin to order a battalion of physicians, chemists, bacteriologists, and other experts to North Africa. The first question they asked was this: why are our soldiers dying while millions of Arabs living in the region survive just fine drinking the bacteria-infected water and eating the bacteria-filled meats and dairy products?

The German scientists, always very thorough, closely scrutinized the locals for an answer. What they discovered is that the Arabs caught dysentery, too, just like everyone else. But after the first round of squirts—the number one symptom of dysentery—they would immediately follow a horse or a camel until it pooped in the street or the field. Then the getting-sicker-by-the-minute Arab would grab a handful of dung and eat it! *Yikes!* And the next day, they were back to normal. No more dysentery.

We can only imagine how prim-and-proper Germans reacted after witnessing a local Arab gulping a handful of warm camel dung. Shock? Revulsion? The German scientists recovered enough to ask the locals some questions; after all, *something* had to be in the animal dung that was killing off the dysentery. The

Arab men said they had no idea why eating fresh dung got rid of their diarrhea and dysentery, but it had worked for their fathers, and their fathers before that, so it had to work for them. All they knew was that they had to eat the dung fresh—moments after it plopped on the ground. Dried dung didn't work at all on their stomach problems.

The German scientists put clothespins on their noses and examined the dung under a microscope. What they discovered was a powerful microorganism that would later be named *Bacillus subtilis*. What this microorganism did was feast on harmful microorganisms and pathogenic bacteria like dysentery, which, in effect, was a cure. The German microbiologists began producing active *Bacillus subtilis* cultures for their troops, who had no problem agreeing to take the microorganisms since word got around that it was either swallow the capsules of *Bacillus subtilis* or eat camel dung!

The *Bacillus subtilis* worked like a charm, and Rommel's Afrika Korps returned to full battle strength. They fought valiantly before U.S. General George Patton's Operation Torch crushed the Nazi forces and set the stage for the Italian campaign in 1943. (As a side note, the Afrika Korps were never charged with war crimes following the conclusion of the war with Germany's unconditional surrender.)

Following World War II, Dr. Rothschild continued in the *Bio/Tech News*, cultures of *Bacillus subtilis* were sold worldwide as a medicinal product, mainly for dysentery and other intestinal problems. Here in the U.S., you could purchase *Bacillus subtilis* under the brand name Bacti-Subtil. That all began to change in the 1950s and 1960s as antibiotics heavily touted by giant pharmaceutical companies captured the fancy of American consumers. Physicians were on board, of course: they felt these potent bacterial fighters gave them additional weapons in their arsenal. *Bacillus subtilis* fell into disfavor and was almost forgotten, but Dr. Rothschild contended that a comeback was in order.

I scanned the rest of the *Bio/Tech News* issue until I came to the page that described what *Bacillus subtilis* did once it's ingested. After you swallow *Bacillus subtilis*, the microorganisms travel down the gullet and into the stomach, where potent gastric acids are waiting to burn up these beneficial microorganisms. But *Bacillus subtilis* are impervious to stomach acids.

After successfully marching through the stomach, the *Bacillus subtilis* move into the small and large intestines, where they attach themselves to the intestinal walls. The *Bacillus subtilis* multiply like crazy, and within a short period of time, the beneficial microorganisms populate—or colonize—the entire length of the gastrointestinal tract.

What happens next really caught my attention. These microscopic organisms turn into microscopic Pac-Mans, looking for pathogenic or disease-causing organisms to devour. Any putrefied fecal matter that have accumulated are fair game for the *Bacillus subtilis*, which also chip away at the putrefaction stuck to the walls of the colon like plaster of Paris. The bits and pieces of putrefaction are then flushed out by the intestinal tract through the body's normal elimination process.

Bacillus subtilis also performs these tasks inside the gastrointestinal tract:

- Breaks down the hydrocarbons in foods, which means that the body is now receiving nearly all the nutritive elements in the food, thereby dramatically increasing overall nutrition and rapidly enhancing cellular growth and development

- Stimulates the immune system to produce huge quantities of antibodies over and above the amount the immune system would normally need to ward off disease and illness

- Acts aggressively against pathological molds, yeast, fungi, and viruses that could otherwise infect the body and cause serious illness and even chronic degenerative disease

Reading this great information in San Diego caused me to sit up straighter again. I could only imagine what the creepy crawlers that had taken up residence in my gut and made my life an absolute misery for the last 18 months were like. Then again, I had been around Dad's merry-go-round of "You gotta try this" dozens of times. Would placing my hopes in *Bacillus subtilis* set me up for yet another crushing disappointment?

I talked through my concerns with Dad via a long-distance phone call. After hearing me out, he remained confident that the black powder was just the nature-based elixir I needed. He said the Ziploc baggy was composed of *Bacillus subtilis* in a base of specific micronutrients from single-celled plants and organic substances.

I considered my options. I was already feeling a lot better in America's Finest City—my new diet of raw goat's milk, raw sauerkraut, organic fruits and vegetables, and wild-caught fish was helping immensely—but I still suffered major digestive setbacks. Maybe *Bacillus subtilis* would be the final piece of the puzzle.

That day, I mixed some of the black powder in a glass of water and drank my new sunset cocktail. I can't tell you that I could feel the Pac-Man action happening in my gut, but within hours I did feel it working. The next time I talked to Dad, I told him we were on to something. In fact, I believe *Bacillus subtilis*—and two other probiotics that I started taking later on called *Bacillus coagulans* and *Saccharomyces boulardii,* completed my comeback. They are the reason I have been essentially free of medication for decades and the symptoms of Crohn's disease and a host of other digestive and immune system ailments are a thing of the past.

My Probiotics Mentor

A couple of years after I started taking *Bacillus subtilis*, I met Dr. Peter Rothschild as I was enrolling at the People's University of the Americas in Ponce, Puerto Rico, to study naturopathic medicine. Dr. Rothschild was a teaching professor at the school, and he took such a liking to me that he granted my request to stay in Florida and complete my schoolwork on nutrition, phytotherapy (herbal studies), homeopathy, clinical evaluation and treatment, and additional subjects from home. That was a first for the school.

I asked for a residency waiver because I had launched into a career researching and formulating dietary programs and nutritional supplements—using knowledge I gained from what brought me back from the brink of death. I wanted to study under Dr. Rothschild, even if we were separated by the Florida Straits, because I was hungry to learn all that I could about the incredibly complex human body that God had created.

Dr. Rothschild was a larger-than-life character: the rumor among students was that this noted linguist had been married as many times as the number of languages he spoke. (We're talking around a half-dozen.) We had a spiritual connection as well: even though he was born a Jew and raised in a Jewish home, Dr. Rothschild became a follower of Yeshua Ha Mashiach, Jesus the Messiah, just like me. Small in stature, no more than five feet, five inches tall, he spoke English with a French accent (at least to my unsophisticated ears) even though he was reportedly born in Austria in the 1930s.

Growing up in a Jewish family while living under Hitler's jack-boot had to be exceedingly dangerous, but I never heard how Dr. Rothschild escaped the Holocaust. It was a topic we never discussed but I wish we had. The Holocaust personally resonated with me because Grandma Rose was 13 years old when she and her parents, along with a few other family members, immigrated to the United States in 1935 and escaped almost certain death. They were among the last wave of European Jews to arrive in America prior to World War II.

Two older sisters, Sonya and Dora, who were married with their own families, stayed behind in Poland, which was not a good place to be if you happened to be Jewish in 1939. Following the Nazi *blitzkrieg,* her sisters and their families were rounded up and shipped off to the death camps. No *Schindler's* list could save them. We believe that my great-aunts and families were shot to death by the Nazi SS.

Back to happier thoughts and Dr. Rothschild's story.

As a young man, Peter Rothschild earned a medical degree, a doctorate, a theology doctorate, and a naturopathic medical doctorate, so he was learned as well as someone who could converse—and write medical research articles—in a half-dozen languages. With a well-deserved reputation as one of the early pioneers of integrative medicine, Dr. Rothschild was a highly intelligent Renaissance Man.

Dr. Rothschild was also quite generous with his time, and we spoke often over the phone with questions I had about microorganisms like *Mycobacterium avium subspecies paratuberulosis* (MAP), which caused chronic and fatal intestinal disease in cows and other livestock. His science curriculum at People's University of the Americas was called The Maker's Science, and you better believe that Dr. Rothschild wasn't a proponent of evolution. I took his dietary nutrition course that he called The Maker's Diet, and I liked the name so much that five years later, when I was writing my first book, he allowed me to borrow the name for the book title. *The Maker's Diet*, released in 2004, went on to become a *New York Times* best-selling book with more than two million copies in print.

So now I think you can understand why I have a soft place in my heart for Dr. Rothschild, who is no longer with us, having died in 2005 at the age of 74. I wanted to use Dr. Rothschild as our expert on *Bacillus subtilis*, but since he has passed away, I've made acquaintance with an academic who's generally regarded today to be the world's leading expert on *Bacillus subtilis*. His name is Simon Cutting, and this British researcher agreed to be interviewed for *The Probiotic Diet* book and share his expertise about a probiotic that you need to really think about adding to your diet.

Introducing Dr. Simon Cutting

Whenever the British tabloids need a quote on probiotics and friendly bacteria, Simon Cutting, Ph.D., usually gets the call.

That's because Dr. Cutting, a professor at the School of Biological Sciences at Royal Holloway, University of London, has spent his entire career working with *Bacillus subtilis*, a spore-forming species of rod-shaped bacillus found in soil and decomposing organic matter. The researcher knows how to take a complicated topic like *Bacillus subtilis* and give the media the "sound bites" it needs to flesh out a newspaper article. For the hot medium of television, it doesn't hurt that Dr. Cutting looks a bit like Russell Crowe (from his *Gladiator* days) and even sounds a bit like him.

Dr. Cutting says his life mission is to share the benefits of using bacterial spores like *Bacillus subtilis* as probiotics. "As food supplements and in one case, an over-the-counter medicine, the ingestion of spores appears to confer significant health benefits," he said, adding that he wants to—and must—be very careful about any medical claims attached to *Bacillus subtilis*.

Dr. Cutting has been studying *Bacillus subtilis* ever since he made this bacterium the focus of his doctorate program at Oxford University 30 years ago. After finishing his Ph.D. at Oxford, he spent seven years at Harvard University, where he focused on the genetics of spore formation and spore germination. Now he's back at Royal Holloway, which is part of the University of London. You can tell that he has the academic chops.

I asked him a set of questions regarding *Bacillus subtilis*, and I think you'll be interested in what he had to say about this important component of the Probiotic Diet:

> **Jordan**: Why do you believe bacillus species, particularly *Bacillus subtilis*, are superior as human probiotics to the commonly used lactic acid bacteria such as *Lactobacillus* and *Bifidobacteria*?

> **Dr. Cutting**: The advantage is heat stability. *Bacillus subtilis* is an organism that forms a spore. A spore is a dormant life form. We are alive, obviously, and because we are alive, we are actively metabolizing and aspiring. But a spore is a hibernating-type bacteria, not crystallized but dormant.
>
> So *Lactobacillus* and *Bifidobacteria*, which are common probiotics found in yogurts and fermented foods, are not dormant, which means you have to keep them alive, and the way you do that is to keep them refrigerated. This costs money and can be inconvenient, especially if you are traveling. Since *Bacillus subtilis* is a spore-forming organism, it can be stored at room temperature forever and never lose its potency.

Another important difference between *Bacillus subtilis* and *Lactobacillus* is that the former is gastric stable, and by that, I mean the spores are completely resistant to stomach acids. When you eat a yogurt with *Lactobacillus*, however, anywhere from 10 to 30 percent of the bacteria will be immediately destroyed in the stomach. The manufacturers of commercial dairy products know how strong and powerful stomach acids are.

So imagine what happens when you take a huge swallow of lactobacillus supplements. We know that a portion of those bacteria is instantly destroyed when it reaches the stomach. But with a spore product like *Bacillus subtilis*, we also know that all those spores will survive their encounter with the stomach's gastric acids. When two billion spores of *Bacillus subtilis*, which is a normal dose, are swallowed, you can be confident that the entire amount will pass through your stomach and reach the area of your gut where it's needed. If you consumed fermented milk products or ate yogurt, however, you couldn't say that would happen with any degree of confidence.

Jordan: What role do you feel bacillus species, particular *Bacillus subtilis*, have played in the microflora of humans throughout history?

Dr. Cutting: We know that *Bacillus subtilis* is a spore-forming organism. If you were to go online and type *Bacillus subtilis* into a search engine, one of the first links would tell you that you were dealing with a soil organism. When I started working on bacillus in the mid-1980s, my professors told me it was a soil organism. They were correct. If you stepped outside and turned up a spade of farm soil, it would be full of bacterial spores.

This part has always been very mysterious to me, but we know that when you eat bacterial spores, they pass through the stomach untouched. Inside the small intestine, or ileum, they germinate and grow in part of the body where all the action happens. The small intestine is where we interact with foods, interact with probiotics, and even get disease. Stuff like that happens all the time in the small intestine.

When bacillus spores germinate, that means they hatch like plant seeds, but of course, they are microscopic. They start to grow, and the reason they grow in this area is because the environment is full of nutrients—like a soup. You eat your hamburger or whatever, and when it gets broken down in the stomach, you soon have an enormous soup filling your small intestine.

While your body is absorbing all the nutrients, it's also making decisions and has a clever way of doing this. The body is saying, "You're a food... you're a bad bacteria ...and you're potentially beneficial." When you consume bacillus spores, your body says, "We see that a large number of these spores have entered our body. They are growing like crazy. We are now being stimulated in the immune system." The body then mounts an immune response, which is like turning up a dial on an amplifier. You're activating your body while the bacteria keep moving through your gut.

Everyone knows you have to use the bathroom X number of times a day, and there's a reason for that. Your body has a natural rhythm. *Bacillus subtilis* bacteria now grow in your small intestine, and they will eventually reach the colon, the large intestine. That's an area where not much happens physiologically, but your body still must deal with the end result of what you've eaten in the last 24 hours. In simple parlance, this digestive matter turns into stool.

I know this can be complicated, so let me recap: you've consumed *Bacillus subtilis* spores, which germinate. They pass through your stomach. They grow. They hatch out. They grow some more in the small intestine. Then they are pushed toward the large colon, where they form spores again because that is a survival mechanism.

Of course, these spores will come out in the stool, and for humans, that fecal matter enters the sewage system. But for animals, which are doing the same exact thing, those spores enter the environment when they hit the ground. That's why they eventually become what we call "soil organisms."

Let's say zucchinis or broccolis are planted in that soil, or manure is spread over a farm field. Every time you eat zucchini or broccoli, depending on how well you wash the vegetables when you eat them, there are considerable numbers of spore-forming bacteria present on these foods. Potatoes would be a classic case. Even if you scrub your potatoes, you're still going to have leftover spores present in the food.

Since time began, humans have been eating plants and vegetables that have been extracted from the soil, and by eating those plants, spores enter your body—unless your diet is heavy in processed foods. That's why eating fresh fruits and vegetables is so healthy for you. This was backed up by the good work done at Loyola University in Chicago, where one of my colleagues proved that spore-forming bacteria are essential for developing a robust immune system in baby rabbits.

If you think of Marie Antoinette, the Queen of France who lost her head during the French Revolution, you probably know that she said, "Let them eat cake." We need to modify this statement to, "Let them eat dirt." The logic is that human beings need to eat dirt so that we can expose our bodies to bacteria. Because we don't do that very much these days, America and England are some of the worst places in the world for allergies, unless you are brought up in the countryside or live on a farm.

Since World War II, there's been a steady increase in allergies and asthmatic conditions in children, and it hasn't been an accident. The reason we have so many allergies is because we are bringing up our children in a sheltered, clinical environment. Our food is processed and sterilized, and we are no longer exposing ourselves to bacteria because we've been taught that bacteria are bad.

Jordan: What is the history of *Bacillus subtilis* for human use?

Dr. Cutting: To my knowledge, places like Southeast Asia, including Vietnam, seem to have a link between *Bacillus subtilis* and a history of eating vegetables full of this bacterium. In Japan they have a food called natto, which are fermented soybeans, that is full of *Bacillus subtilis* spores. The same story is true for *kimchi*, a Korean food.

Even though Asian people have a long history of eating bacillus spores, they wouldn't have known what bacillus was a hundred years ago—or even today. You can't go back and say one thousand years ago that people in China, Thailand, and Vietnam were deliberately culturing *Bacillus subtilis* because that was impossible. They were getting their *Bacillus subtilis* from their vegetables because there was a little bit of dirt on them.

Jordan: What is the safety of bacillus-based products for humans?

Dr. Cutting: *Bacillus subtilis* is a safe organism to eat, although one has to be careful and say that not everything is completely safe. I, myself, have done safety tests with some species of bacillus with no adverse affects at all.

Jordan: What applications have you seen bacillus-based probiotics used in? Foods? Supplements? Pharmaceuticals? What conditions have they been used to treat or as an adjunct in treatment?

Dr. Cutting: There are different species and different types of bacilli. There's one spore product that's manufactured in Italy by a company called Sanofi-Aventis, the sixth-largest pharmaceutical company in the world. It's an over-the-counter medicine, which is a drug. It comes with a plastic ampoule containing two billion spores of a *bacillus* species and is GMP produced, meaning Good Manufacturing Practices, which means it was produced as a drug by people wearing facemasks and white suits. Since this *bacillus* specie is used medicinally, they can make a specific health claim, and in this situation, they can say that if you eat two billion spores a day, you will not get childhood diarrhea, which is caused by the rotavirus. They've performed clinical trials to support this.

About 75 percent of childhood diarrhea is caused by the rotavirus. In developed countries, the rotavirus won't kill anyone, although it will give you bad diarrhea. But for people who live in developing countries, rotavirus kills about a million children a year, which is astonishing. The disease is transmitted by fecal-oral routes, so when children go to the toilet and don't have good hygiene, they still have fecal matter on their hands. Then they play with their friends, have close personal contact, and their friends contract diarrhea from them.

Taking *Bacillus* spores can prevent the spread of rotavirus, and medical trials show quite effectively that if you take a thousand parents or a thousand children, give them probiotics every day, they will have less diarrhea against a parallel group that didn't take probiotics. I've seen very clearly that *Bacillus* prevents diarrhea, including "traveler's diarrhea," because the bacillus boosts the immune system.

Jordan: Why do you think the concept of using bacillus species in probiotic applications has been largely ignored by the general scientific community?

Dr. Cutting: I don't know. You have large dairy food companies that have jumped on the lactobacillus bandwagon, companies like Danone and Unilever here in the United Kingdom, that are very hard to compete against. I think a lot of it is marketing, but things are changing, no doubt about it. I predict that we'll see food companies in Europe adding bacillus spores to certain foods because they are heat stable.

That said, I was responsible for preparing the dossier that the United Kingdom Food Standards Agency used to give approval for *Bacillus subtilis* to be sold as a food supplement in the UK And in Italy, it's already being sold as a food supplement, as you discovered in Venice. The Italians take their bacillus spores seriously, and the joke is, they pour it into their cappuccinos in the morning.

Since the Italians have approved the use of *Bacillus subtilis* for humans, it's been automatically approved for use in other European Union countries—as long as that country makes an application. That hasn't happened yet, though, in another EU country.

I see another potential market for *Bacillus subtilis*—with pets. I've had some companies tell me that the way to go, where the money is, is with goldfish. It sounds ridiculous, but tropical fish are a big industry here in England. People will pay any amount of money to prevent their fish from getting secondary infections from fungi and bacteria, which are present in the water. So some people say use bacillus spores for feeding goldfish and tropical fish.

Jordan: I understand that you discovered another bacillus species. Can you tell us about it?

Dr. Cutting: I discovered an organism that I named *Bacillus indicus*, which is yellow or orange in color because it produces carotenoids. We've sequenced its genome and proved that it is gastric stable.

Jordan: How come you didn't name it *Bacillus simoncuttingis*?

Dr. Cutting: After myself? In the old days, scientists used to do that. In the last hundred years, we've become more modest, although that could be changing in this celebrity-obsessed age.

I appreciate Dr. Cutting's modesty, but when it comes to devoting decades to *Bacillus subtilis*, I think he should get his props and be awarded with a bacillus named after him. (After all, we immortalized Louis Pasteur.)

I really liked what Dr. Cutting had to say about billion-dollar food companies having a protective and proprietary interest in dairy-based probiotics. They've invested millions and millions of dollars to convince you that the lactic acid bacteria in their yogurts and supplements can perform wondrous things in your gut. Hollywood actress Jamie Lee Curtis plunked herself down on a green couch with just the right amount of gray hair and just the right amount of commercial spunk to pitch Dannon's Activia yogurt with its special probiotic ingredient, *Bifidus Regularis*.

I'm glad that a celebrity like Jamie Lee Curtis is jump-starting the American conversation on probiotics, but I'm in Dr. Cutting's court: I believe that *spore-forming* bacteria such as *Bacillus subtilis* are the *better* probiotics for your body because they survive your stomach's acid bath and deliver up to *ten times* more probiotics than most yogurts. I like the way these hardy probiotics pass Go and collect $200 on their way to your gut, where they get to work multiplying and chomping on harmful bacterial bad guys lining the small and large intestines.

Bacillus subtilis is not the only probiotic capable of leaving the stomach unscathed and helping re-train your terrain. I've been studying probiotics for nearly three decades, and during that time, I've found two other probiotic species that need to be part of the discussion; they're called *Bacillus coagulans* and *Saccharomyces boulardii*.

Introducing *Bacillus Coagulans* and *Saccharomyces boulardii*

I first heard about *Bacillus coagulans* in 1995 when I read abstracts of human clinical studies conducted in India using this probiotic. Similar to *Bacillus subtilis, bacillus coagulans* is a spore-forming bacterium that survives the hostile environment of the stomach, colonizes the intestines, and produces lactic acid, which are all components to the success of a good probiotic. *Bacillus coagulans* was first isolated in 1932 by German scientists L.M. Horowitz-Wlassowa and N.W. Nowotelnow. Further research confirmed that upon activation of spore formation in the acidic environment of the stomach, *Bacillus coagulans* can germinate and proliferate in the intestines and produce lactic acid, which are critical factors to the success of a probiotic.

Bacillus coagulans isn't entirely unknown in the popular culture. Remember how I quoted Oprah at the very start of the book—"Pro-by-what?" That was during her interview of Dr. Mehmet Oz, a once-regular guest on her iconic show and mega-selling author (along with Dr. Michael F. Roizen) of the *You: The Manual* series. I must give the good doctor some credit for outlining the importance of having beneficial bacteria in your gut for maintaining digestive and immune health. In *You: Staying Young*, Dr. Oz recommended taking "two billion cells of healthy bowel bacteria like bacillus coagulans" as a choice to consider.

Dr. Oz really went to bat for probiotics, echoing what I've been saying all along in *The Probiotic Diet*. Here's an excerpt:

> **Dr. Oz:** In a basic sense, you have a war inside your intestine between your good and your bad bacteria—in fact over 90 percent of the cells in your body are not yours. Probiotics are living bacteria that help you stack the war's outcome in favor of good or bad health-promoting bacteria.
>
> Probiotics can be found either as tablets or as capsules or in certain foods like yogurts. Eating bacteria may seem like a rather strange idea, because when we think of bacteria, we often think about the "bad"

bacteria or "germs" that can make us sick—things like salmonella in under-cooked chicken or bacterial infections. But you have and you rely on trillions and trillions of "good" bacteria to keep your digestive and immune systems functioning properly. However, the levels of these "good" bacteria can decline due to factors such as age, diet, stress, and even with the use of antibiotics. When this happens, you can run into digestive problems and your immune system can be weakened.

This is where probiotics really come in. Probiotics are reinforcements to restore the level of "good" bacteria in your body. That's one of the reasons why a pharmacist or your physician may suggest taking probiotics or eating specific yogurts after taking a course of antibiotics.

By this point, you might be ready to go out and look for probiotics to add to your daily routine. Interestingly, this simple act may be the most difficult aspect of probiotics to grasp—isn't yogurt all around us? Not so fast. The important thing to remember is to provide benefits to you, probiotics must survive not only sitting on the shelf in your home and in the store, but they must also make their way past the harsh stomach acids to reach your intestinal tract where they then must grow and thrive. Thus it isn't the number contained in the pill or in the container, it's the number that survive into your intestine (notice I said *your*).

Different strains of probiotics differ greatly in their abilities to do this. Most conventional forms of lactobacilli, found in many probiotic yogurt mixes, are inactivated by stomach acids, while Bifidobacteria, another popular strain found in some yogurts and supplements, is often inactivated by high heat.

Bacillus coagulans, a probiotic that protects itself by developing its own protective shell, is one of the most exciting strains of "good" bacteria to come around. Why? Because it can withstand extreme temperatures and the harsh acid in the stomach. Because of its unique ability to survive these conditions, bacillus coagulans is even being added into foods that were not otherwise possibilities, like baked goods and dry soup mixes. Those are in addition to the normal supplements that *bacillus coagulans* can be found in.[1]

The other probiotic I recommend, *Saccharomyces boulardii*, is *not* a spore-forming bacteria but a friendly yeast that supports healthy digestion. *Saccharomyces boulardii* is often used to counter antibiotic therapy or fight diarrhea since this live microorganism has been shown to destroy pathogenic bacteria in the bowels.

The story of how *Saccharomyces boulardii* was discovered sounds like the one told by Dr. Rothschild about the Afrika Korps. A French microbiologist named Henri Boulard traveled to Indochina in the 1920s, a long, arduous journey to be sure, but one driven by Dr. Boulard's drive to find a heat-resistant yeast that could be used to ferment beverages above 70° Fahrenheit. Like the German Army scientists who studied what the locals were doing to keep from dying from dysentery, Dr. Boulard observed what the local population ate and drank when they got diarrhea. He happened to observe the Vietnamese drinking a tea from litchi fruit skins to combat a cholera epidemic, which is marked by severe diarrhea.

Intrigued, Dr. Boulard studied the litchi fruit tea and conducted painstaking research before managing to isolate the yeast responsible for curing the locals' diarrhea. Since he performed the original microbiological detective work—and had a bigger ego than Dr. Cutting—Dr. Boulard named the yeast after himself: *Saccharomyces boulardii*.

Mais bien sur! But of course.

Saccharomyces boulardii became commercialized after World War II in Europe before reaching American shores around 50 years ago. Medical studies over the intervening decades have confirmed what Vietnamese folklore has known for centuries: if you have bad diarrhea, then *Saccharomyces boulardii* can help. This friendly yeast can also relieve the bloating and gas that often go with unbalanced terrain. Further research also highlighted *Saccharomyces boulardii*'s ability to repair the mucous membranes lining the intestinal walls and strengthen immune function in the digestive tract.

I first heard of *Saccharomyces boulardii* when I was introduced to a third-generation baker and fermentation expert from Australia in 1999. I immediately began researching and consuming this organism and noticed excellent benefits. I highly recommend and strongly urge that you make these spore-formed probiotics and friendly yeast part of your daily nutritional regimen.

It's a Question of Potency

I love traveling to the West Coast, and whenever I arrive in Southern California, the first thing I do is ask the locals where to find a raw food or health food restaurant. It seems like I always get directed to one of those quintessential New Age restaurants—the ones filled with chakras, Buddhas, wind chimes, and more crystals than you could shake a talisman at. The tattooed staff—and clientele—may have a lot of piercings and dreadlocks, but the yummy-for-the-tummy organic entrees are to die for.

I also ask directions to the nearest health food store, where I stock up on raw snacks—nuts, dairy, salads, and drinks—and take them back to my hotel room for dessert and breakfast the following morning. It was on a trip to Orange County when I first heard about a probiotic beverage called Yakult. If the Golden State's reputation as a bellwether state pans out, you could be seeing Yakult's five-pack of 2.7-ounce bottles in your supermarket dairy case soon.

I can see you scratching your head. *What's Yakult?*

Yakult consists of skimmed milk powder, sugar, water, and a bacteria called *Lactobacillus casei shirota*, a probiotic named after its creator, Japanese microbiologist Dr. Minoru Shirota. In 1935, Dr. Shirota was attempting to create a probiotic that would help people during a time when infectious disease mortality rates were high. Yakult has been around ever since, mainly in Asia. Yakult is sold in more than 30 countries, but it didn't reach American shores until late 2008 when a beachhead was established in California, Nevada, and Arizona.

The mixture of skimmed milk powder, sugar, and water is ultra-pasteurized, then fermented using *Lactobacillus casei shirota*. A 65-milliliter plastic bottle (2.7 fluid ounces) contains 6.5 billion—that's not a typo—*Lactobacillus casei shirota* that support maintenance of gut flora and regulate bowel habits and constipation.

We'll see if Yakult generates the necessary buzz to expand its sales territories nationwide, but I can assure you that you won't find Yakult in the Rubin family refrigerator. The skimmed milk powder is missing what I call the "Original Probiotics" following pasteurization. I don't drink beverages with sugar, and I don't think lactobacillus-based probiotics are the best probiotics you can consume.

But that's not what you hear from the marketing campaigns behind the big food companies producing dairy-based probiotics. I hope I've given the impression that I'm not totally down on dairy products and their lactic acid bacteria; you can certainly derive some wonderful nutrients from cultured dairy, preferably unpasteurized and unhomogenized.

It is my belief, however, that the wonderful benefits associated with consuming raw, fermented dairy lies in the predigested proteins, carbohydrates, and fats as well as the organic acids produced by the organisms and not the lactobacillus probiotics that produce the health-giving qualities. So in a sense, Élie Metchnikoff was right about cultured dairy benefiting those healthy Bulgarians, but I believe it was due to the fermented dairy itself and not the lactobacilli. That's why for me, the issue comes down to *potency*. By the time the stomach has had its fun with lactic acid bacteria, these dairy-based probiotics are weakened and compromised—perhaps decimated—as they travel on to the small intestine.

The reason why consuming lactic acid bacteria doesn't work in the long run can be told through a parable about sea turtles. I used to live in South Florida, where sea turtles fall under the state's Marine Turtle Protection Program. Florida loves their sea turtles, and you can even select an attractive sea turtle license plate for your car that features a loggerhead hatchling crawling on the beige sand toward the blue water.

That image is apropos because very few—very, very few—baby sea turtles ever make it back to the water and grow to maturity. Marine biologists say that mama sea turtles may lay a thousand eggs during mating season, but only *one* survives to adulthood. You wouldn't want to take those odds to Las Vegas.

The period between nesting and the first year of life is the most treacherous for sea turtles. It all begins when Mama Sea Turtle leaves the sea and digs a nest in the sand. She lays hundreds and hundreds of eggs in a pile, then covers the nest and returns to the sea. She will never see her babies. Meanwhile, the sun keeps the sand and therefore the eggs warm and dry.

The turtle eggs are defenseless. A dog's keen sense of smell can steer it to any sea turtle eggs buried in the sand, and if Rover discovers the nest, the entire clutch of turtle eggs can be quickly destroyed. In some areas of the world, humans comb the beaches for nests because sea turtle eggs are a culinary delicacy.

If the turtle eggs remain unmolested, they eventually hatch, and here's where things get tricky. The tiny turtles must get to the sea, but they're exposed to predators. Sea gulls circle high in the sky and swoop down. Raccoons are looking to poach a quick meal. Crabs are waiting at the water's edge for a morning snack. If the baby turtles manage to avoid these predators and reach the ocean, all sorts of sea creatures are waiting to pounce on their next meal.

As I said, only one of those thousand turtles will survive to reproduce and start the whole process over again, but that's how the species propagates itself.

And that's what the world's largest food companies are doing when they create probiotic products. They are producing Activia yogurts, Yakult drinks, and encapsulated probiotic supplements with billions of lactic acid probiotics, but untold millions of bacteria fail to survive the rough-water ride through the churning rapids inside the stomach.

Bacillus subtilis, Bacillus coagulans, and *Saccharomyces boulardii* don't have that problem because they are not destroyed by heat (don't forget that the body's core temperature is 98.6 degrees), gastric acids in the stomach, and unfriendly bacteria residing in the gut. Lactic acid bacteria, on the other hand, have too many natural enemies in your body.

Most lactic acid bacteria are not strong enough or resilient enough to produce the right chemicals to combat the horrific conditions in your gut. I've already mentioned that researchers believe that a healthy person needs at least 85 percent beneficial microbes and 15 percent pathogenic or negative microbes. Eating today's modern diet usually results in a colon that's alkaline and not acidic, which reverses that ratio. If you send wimpy lactic acid bacteria into the gut to that ratio around, that's like fighting a forest fire with a garden hose—naked.

The reason I like this analogy is because it relates to *Lactobacillus acidophilus*, which is acid-friendly dairy-based bacteria. People think *acidophilus*, which is the most popular probiotic species in the world, produces lactic acid that will lower your pH levels in your colon, but in reality, *Lactobacillus acidophilus* doesn't lower your colon's pH because it *needs* an acidic environment to thrive. So if your colon is alkaline, and you're sending acidophilus down the hatch, it's not going to survive the journey.

Acidophilus needs an acidic medium to survive and thrive. Furthermore, it doesn't automatically produce B vitamins; it *uses* B vitamins in its metabolism. So without B vitamins and an alkaline colon, which is what most unhealthy people have, eating or drinking a lot of *Lactobacillus acidophilus* is like trying to fight a raging forest fire wearing nothing more than a smile and a garden hose in your hand.

Probiotics are the right answer to many of your health issues, and they *have* to be intentionally included in your diet. But taking probiotics willy nilly—much like I did when I gulped down 30 brands and multiple bottles of expensive probiotics each day—won't do you any good if they are not getting where they need to go. So why play a game with probiotics when you can consume something that was created to go into the body and make it to the gastrointestinal tract, where it can set up shop and begin to do a number of wonderful things for the body?

Bacillus subtilis and *Bacillus coagulans* can be looked at as bio-remediation agents. They're like those guys in white hazmat suits working an oil spill during the clean-up stages. Actually, if there is an oil spill in your garage and you go over to Home Depot to buy a cleaning agent—one of those commercial industrial products—you'll find that the manufacturer uses bacillus microbes to break down that carbon-based oil dirtying your garage floor.

In the same manner, your colon could be plugged with undigested carbohydrates. Carbohydrates, as you would expect for a word with a Latin prefix *carbo*, have lots of carbon, and when these undigested carbohydrates float around your intestines, they feed and multiply bad bacteria. *Bacillus subtilis* and *Bacillus coagulans* can go in there and secrete compounds that eat away at the encrusted fecal matter and toxins.

In a sense, consuming the right probiotics is another way to "cleanse" the body. In natural health circles, those who know about cleansing say that most people carry about five to ten pounds of impacted fecal matter in their colon. That's because they've seen what comes out after colon hydrotherapy—think of an enema on steroids—that infuses the colon with pressurized water. This is the old autointoxication theory at work: you can't eat three meals a day and go to the bathroom three times a week. Something is not right with this picture because the equation doesn't compute. So where does all that stuff go? It sits around in your colon and clogs your pipes.

There's an urban legend that's swirled around natural health circles for four decades, and it's that when Hollywood star John Wayne died in 1979, he had 25 pounds of impacted fecal matter in his colon.

I've heard the John Wayne story told and retold, but it's an urban legend that's been deemed false by fact checkers. No autopsy was performed after The Duke succumbed to cancer

CHECK IT OUT

Italy isn't the only place you can find a probiotic supplement containing *Bacillus subtilis*, *Bacillus coagulans,* and *Saccharomyces boulardii.* You should be able to walk into your local health food store and find a nutritional supplement containing these three remarkable ingredients, or you can shop online.

in 1979, which meant no one could "run his gut" and weigh the amount of fecal matter trapped inside his intestinal tract.

Though we'll never know what John Wayne's colon was like when he died, to my manner of thinking he was a quintessential American, and America's love affair with the "goo and glue" diet—cheeseburgers, French fries, bacon-topped sandwiches, blueberry muffins, sugar-frosted cereals, and 31 flavors of ice cream—all contribute to a carbohydrate overload that gets everything backed up in the gastrointestinal tract.

With regards to the Probiotic Diet, it's great to have organisms like *Bacillus subtilis, Bacillus coagulans,* and *Saccharomyces boulardii* break down this industrial-strength sludge, but what about dealing with unhealthy carbohydrates in the first place? What if you can cut off the problem at its source?

One of my greatest health lessons came from a noted author named Elaine Gottschall, who took an interest in my digestive health and me at a pivotal moment during my comeback. She made several recommendations about eating carbohydrates that, when combined with a probiotic supplement containing *Bacillus subtilis, Bacillus coagulans* and *Saccharomyces boulardii*, made a major difference in how I felt *when* I ate and *after* I ate. You'll learn more about this amazing woman and her theories in our next chapter.

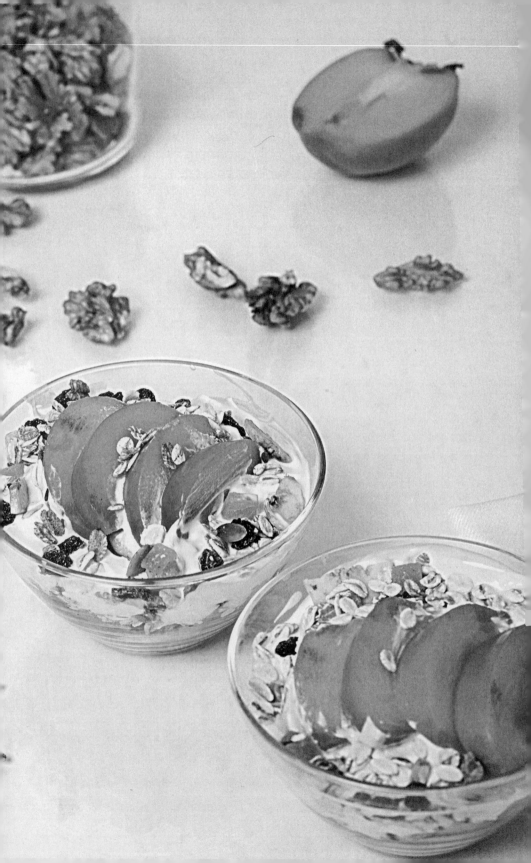

6

THEY ARE WHAT YOU EAT

After my body broke down at Camp Swan when I was a 19-year-old church camp counselor, my worried parents escorted me to a local family doctor who basically patted me on the head and wrote me a prescription for antibiotics. I felt sicker than a dog, but life had to go on, right? I was already enrolled for the fall semester at Florida State University.

"I know of no reason preventing you from returning to school," my doctor replied when I asked him what I should do. "Just continue taking your medicine, and we'll monitor your situation and see what happens."

I returned to Tallahassee and moved into a six-bedroom house with seven other roommates. One of them, Todd Oden, had the dream job. He worked part time at the Kappa Delta sorority as a food runner. The Kappa Delts—known as a sorority with some of the prettiest girls on campus—had a sit-down dinner every evening at six o'clock at their sorority house on West Jefferson. We teased Todd unmercifully about subjecting himself to the rigors of serving 100 beautiful women each night. It's amazing he survived.

Meanwhile, I was in a survival test of my own. Just a couple of weeks into the fall semester, a package arrived in the mail—from Dad. This was the first of many mailings that I would receive from him over the next two years. (Remember the black powder that arrived in San Diego?)

Inside the package was a dog-eared book called *Food and the Gut Reaction* by Elaine Gottschall and a letter in Dad's handwriting saying I needed to read this book because of the diet she recommended for people with digestive issues like me. Dad said he had been exposed to *Food and the Gut Reaction* several years earlier when studying up on natural treatments for digestive disorders, and he had kept the book in his personal library.

"Study what she says," Dad directed. "I think her Specific Carbohydrate Diet makes a lot of sense for you."

The book began with a recounting of how Mrs. Gottschall, in 1958, had an eight-year-old daughter, Judy, whose digestive system could not tolerate any food. Whatever she ate would pass rapidly right through her, almost completely unabsorbed. Since kindergarten, the poor girl had endured nosebleeds, night sweats, and persistent diarrhea. She screamed when she filled the toilet with blood.

A parade of doctors shook their heads and regretfully told Herb and Elaine Gottschall that their daughter suffered from incurable ulcerative colitis. After years of treatment with cortisone and sulfonamides, plus innumerable other medical approaches, their medical team said surgery was imminent.

You have to know that major abdominal surgeries like a colostomy—the surgical removal the colon and sometimes the rectum—were just being developed in the 1950s. Compared to today's high-tech approaches, with sophisticated laparoscopic instruments and refined techniques, colostomy surgeries 50 years ago were in their infancy.

This is what happens during a basic colostomy surgery: after the entire colon is removed, the surgeon creates an opening in the abdominal wall, though which the ileum (or small intestine) is rerouted to the outside of the body, creating a stoma. To collect stool as it exits the ileum, a disposable pouch is attached to the skin around the stoma with a medical adhesive. Back in the 1950s, patients had to fashion their own pouches to collect their fecal waste, using pasted-on water bottles or jerry-built devices. They would leak and smell, and the corrosion on their skin was absolutely horrendous.

This was the type of surgery I was confronting if my digestive problems, later diagnosed as Crohn's disease, didn't get better. My gastroenterologist said I wasn't there yet, but the severity—and the quickness!—of my symptoms were taking me down that dark road.

I can only imagine what Mrs. Gottschall, a stay-at-home mother of two small daughters living in a leafy New Jersey suburb, was going through at that time. She wrote that she desperately wanted to save her precious daughter from a lifetime of changing messy pouches of fecal waste, as well as the constant embarrassment that comes with it. Her quest took her to the medical offices of Sidney and Merrill Haas, medical doctors and brothers who shared a practice at 91st and Park Avenue in Manhattan. They had published a book titled *Management of Celiac Disease*, which documented their experiences in treating and curing hundreds of patients though a well-balanced diet that was highly specific as to the types of sugars and starches allowed. When patients followed their "Specific Carbohydrate Diet," they were put on a path toward freedom from the digestive diseases that ailed them.

In *Food and the Gut Reaction*, Mrs. Gottschall described how the Specific Carbohydrate Diet saved her daughter from the surgeon's scalpel and allowed the young girl to live a normal life—and ultimately experience a total cure. Mrs. Gottschall had bonded with Dr. Sidney Haas, Judy's principal physician, but when the kindly doctor died a few years later at the age of 94, Mrs. Gottschall feared that unless someone acted to carry on his legacy, his simple but effective remedy for digestive maladies would follow him to the grave, depriving others of the chance to recover from debilitating digestive diseases.

That thought, plus the investment of so much emotional energy in seeing her daughter through, prompted Mrs. Gottschall, with her husband's blessing, to enroll at Montclair State College in Montclair, New Jersey, and later, Rutgers in New Brunswick, New Jersey, where she earned degrees in biology, nutritional biochemistry, and cellular biology at the age of 47.

Because Dad was so passionate about me reading *Food and the Gut Reaction*—that's all he talked about whenever he and Mom called to see how I was doing—I carved out some time to read the book. Actually, I should say that I *tried* to read *Food and the Gut Reaction*. I couldn't grasp any of the concepts, and the vocabulary—words like amylopectin, ismolatose, and microvilli—seemed to have come from another planet. At 19, I didn't know much about health or the physiology of the human body. The only things I knew about nutrition were from an Intro to Nutrition class I took in high school and what I had picked up from my dad over the years.

In many ways, Elaine Gottschall was my first teacher on the subject of digestive health, and for that, I owe a debt of gratitude.

Carbohydrates that Compromise Health

This is what the Specific Carbohydrate Diet, as explained by Mrs. Gottschall, was all about:

You begin with the foods used to fuel your body—protein, fats, and carbohydrates—and the premise that undigested carbohydrates can compromise the body's health and immunity. When carbohydrates are not properly digested, they do not pass harmlessly through the small intestine and colon, where they are eventually eliminated. Instead, the undigested carbohydrates remain in the gut, where they have the potential to feed harmful microbes.

The overgrowth of unfriendly bacteria, yeasts, and parasites in the digestive tract can really clog up the works. As unhealthy intestinal flora multiplies, the walls of the intestines are "coated" with destructive bacteria that further impair and compromise the digestive tract. Even worse, these injurious bacteria have even more undigested carbohydrates to feed on, and the tailspin continues.

Mrs. Gottschall called this a "vicious cycle" in which the bacteria keep getting stronger as they have more and more undigested carbohydrates to feed on. (In fact, she would change the title *Food and the Gut Reaction* to *Breaking the Vicious Cycle* when the book became a wild success from word-of-mouth support.) The Specific Carbohydrate Diet, she said, was designed to put an end to this vicious cycle, and you did that by *changing* the type of carbohydrates you eat each day.

Wait—aren't all carbohydrates "carbohydrates"?

The answer is no because all carbohydrates are not created equal, which is an important concept that relates to understanding the Probiotic Diet. Carbohydrates are one of the three macronutrients, or basic food groups; the other two are protein and fats. Everything you eat—good or bad—is a protein, a fat, or a carbohydrate.

Protein builds body organs, muscles, and nerves and provides for the transport of nutrients, oxygen, and waste throughout your body. Your main sources of protein are from animals:

chicken, beef, lamb, dairy, eggs, and so on. Fish from lakes, rivers, and oceans are another notable source of healthy protein.

The next macronutrient is fats, which are a concentrated source of energy and source material for cell membranes and various hormones. Fats play a vital role in the health of your bones, enhance the immune system, and guard against harmful microorganisms in the digestive tract, so you can see why fats are important to the Probiotic Diet.

Last, carbohydrates are the sugars and starches produced by plant foods, and when they are consumed, the digestive tract breaks them down and converts the starches into mainly glucose, which is a source of immediate energy. Sugars and starches aren't necessarily bad for you, but the problem is that most Americans eat sugar-laden foods with every meal: break-fast with its sweet cereals and Danish, break time with soda or "mocha coffees" mixed with sugary additives, lunch with its chocolate chip cookies, and dinner with its sugar-crusted pies, candied cakes, and syrupy ice cream for dessert.

There are three types of carbohydrates that we consume, and they are all 50 cent words: monosaccharides, disaccharides, and polysaccharides. To help you understand these three long-lettered words, remember your Latin prefixes: "mono" means single or one, which in this context means that monosaccha-rides are comprised of a single sugar. Most fruits, vegetables, natural cheeses, cultured yogurts, nuts, and raw honey contain carbohydrates that are mainly in the form of monosaccharides. The gastrointestinal tract finds monosaccharide foods easier to digest because this single-molecule carbohydrate can be absorbed through the lining of the small intestine without hav-ing to be broken down first.

Disaccharides, with the Latin prefix of *di*, meaning two, refers to any substance that is composed of *two* molecules of simple sugars that are linked together. Examples of disaccharides are sugar, sugar, and sugar. Okay, I'm exaggerating, but any sort of food with refined white or brown sugar—ranging from cookies, cupcakes, and Double Stuf Oreos to ketchup, peanut butter, and teriyaki sauce—are examples of disaccharide carbohydrates. Processed grains like boxed cereal, bread, bagels, dinner rolls, muffins, and Cinnabons also have disaccharides. Milk sugars, or lactose, are the disaccharides found in certain dairy products such as ice cream.

Polysaccharides, as you would expect with a prefix of *poly*, which means many, have many sugar molecules. Rice, potatoes, corn, wheat, and soy products can be put in the polysaccharide camp, as well as some grains, beans, and legumes. To simplify things for the rest of this chapter, though, I will refer to carbohydrates with multiple sugars such as disaccharides and polysaccharides as simply disaccharides since they basically have the same effect on the body.

Disaccharides are *much* more difficult to digest and stack up in the gut like an army of toy soldiers marching into a blind alley. When unabsorbed carbohydrates remain in the large intestine undigested, they feed harmful bacteria and upset the balance of the intestinal flora—prompting digestive problems to strike. Eating disaccharide foods can also lead to malabsorption in the gastrointestinal tract, which means that food travels too rapidly through the digestive tract, which is what happened to Judy Gottschall. The "end" result: bouts of diarrhea and painful cramps, as well as malabsorption that can lead to stunted growth and development. Since the gastrointestinal tract has less time to break down the starch and sugars into various enzymes, their absorption into the bloodstream is severely impaired. Since the digestive system can't keep up, it just lets them go.

Mrs. Gottschall explained in her book that people who have digestive problems are often in a fix because of what happens to the hair-like protrusions that line the small intestine. Known as microvilli, these hair-like sensors extend from goblet cells in the intestinal wall. The microvilli are designed to make contact with digestive enzymes that attack disaccharides and split them into monosaccharides, or simple sugars. When this happens as it should, the disaccharides become monosaccharides and are much easier for the small intestine to absorb through the intestinal walls.

Her theory stated that people with digestive problems usually have flattened or blunted microvilli, which prevents their digestive system from making contact with the enzymes leaving the disaccharide carbohydrates passing through the small intestine. Since no contact is made, the undigested carbohydrates sail down the intestinal tract in full disaccharide mode—since they weren't broken down into monosaccharides.

When these disaccharides reach the large intestine and colon, they haven't been "chopped down" to size by the microvilli. What happens next is that these undigested carbohydrates set up camp in the colon and are feasted on by any bacteria, parasites, yeast, and viruses floating around in the large intestine. The heavily bloated disaccharides putrefy in the gut, and if you were Élie Metchnikoff, you'd chalk it up to another case of autointoxication.

Mrs. Gottschall was sure that if you specifically consumed only monosaccharide-rich carbohydrates, along with liberal amounts of proteins and fat and restricted disaccharides and polysaccharides, then you'd be starving the bad guys and allowing the good guys to grow. That was the way you would restore the balance of bacteria in the gut.

The diet plan made all the sense in the world to my father, who boiled it down to two sentences:

Single sugars: good.

Double sugars: bad.

The Specific Carbohydrate Diet was just what it was advertised to be: a restrictive diet where you were allowed to eat only certain specific carbohydrates—the ones that were single sugars. In real world terms, this meant proteins like meat, fish, eggs, natural cheeses, and a homemade yogurt made according to her recipe. Fresh or frozen fruits and vegetables (there were a few exceptions) along with some nuts and juices were also okay since they were monosaccharide carbohydrates.

The list of what I *could not* eat was a lot longer. No processed meats like hot dogs or bologna, no milk or other fluid dairy products, and no grain foods like breakfast cereal, store-bought breads, and baked goods. The long list of banned disaccharide carbohydrates caused my throat to gulp. For one month, I had to say goodbye to:

- grains such as wheat, barley, corn, rye, oats, rice, buckwheat, millet, bulgur, and spelt. Cross off cereals, breads, and flour made from these grains as well.

- potatoes (white and sweet), rice, yams, okra, chickpeas, bean sprouts, soybeans, fava beans, and turnips

This would be a significant change in what I was used to eating. Even though I wasn't the typical college student who survived on the three B's—burgers, burritos, and beer—I didn't have the greatest nutritional habits either. I ate pretty much what everyone else in my rental house did, except I didn't go overboard on sweets and sugar. I had learned a few things growing up in a home where white sugar was banned from the cupboard.

One nice thing about having a roommate who worked at a sorority house during dinnertime was that he could bring back any leftovers. The Kappa Delts, picky about how much they ate to maintain their petite figures, apparently didn't eat much, so the kitchen always had leftovers. Todd could pack it up and bring home the leftovers. Half an hour later, we were feasting on barbecue chicken, broiled fish, beef strips, mashed potatoes, fluffy rice, and sautéed veggies. Not a bad diet for a college kid when Todd brought home a couple sacks of doggie bags.

But Elaine Gottschalk's Specific Carbohydrate Diet sounded like a fate worse than death. Not only was the list of approved foods not too exciting, the soft-serve frozen yogurt sundaes for lunch and late-night delivery pizza were over. Following the Specific Carbohydrate Diet meant doing my own shopping, my own cooking, and my own cleanup.

I resisted Dad's entreaties to give it a whirl, but then he raised the ante by calling Elaine Gottschall on the phone and becoming her New Best Friend in these pre-Facebook days. From what Dad told me, Elaine was a very nice Jewish lady, a grandmotherly type in her mid-seventies who wanted to help as many hurting people as she could. Dad, like hundreds of other parents I later learned, had tracked her down in Canada, where she had become a member of the Department of Cell Science at the University of Western Ontario in London, Ontario.

That sealed the decision for Dad, who was running the show. I *had* to try the Specific Carbohydrate Diet, and he brooked no discussion. Since I had no choice, I was a dutiful son and gave it a shot. Remember, my digestive problems were getting worse each day, and I was game to try anything.

Fanatical Adherence

While at Florida State in the fall of 1994, I adopted every aspect of Elaine Gottschall's diet plan, crossed every T, and dotted every i. I had to, especially after she wrote that the "strictness of the diet cannot be overemphasized nor should the difficulty of adhering to it be minimized." Mrs. Gottschall also said that wandering off the reservation "will seriously delay recovery, and it is unwise to undertake this regimen unless you are willing to follow it with **fanatical adherence**."[1]

Yes, those last two words were in boldface italics in her book, so I think she meant it. Sobered, I gave it everything I had when I followed the Specific Carbohydrate Plan on four separate occasions over the next 18 months—once in Tallahassee and three times at my parents' home in West Palm Beach. The results were always the same: my digestive problems didn't get better, and my health continued to deteriorate despite my "fanatical adherence" to her strict regimen.

It wasn't for a lack of effort, though. In fact, after Dad made contact with Mrs. Gottschall, she took a vital interest in my health and was also always available when Dad called. We developed a friendship over the phone, too. There were weeks when I called Canada nearly every day and talked to her about what was happening. Mrs. Gottschall couldn't have been more concerned or more loving whenever I interrupted her busy schedule. She took the time to ask me what I had for breakfast that morning or what happened after dinner the previous night.

I didn't want to hurt Mrs. Gottschall's feelings, so I never told her how boring her diet was, having to eat the same things over and over. A typical breakfast was a cheese omelet and a baked apple. I couldn't have any toast since grains weren't permitted. I *could* have eaten a slice of bread or a muffin made from either pecan or almond flour, but that involved a lot of kitchen work for Mom. I remember one time when Mom went to the trouble of making me some almond flour muffins. I tried those heavy-in-the-gut pastries twice—the first and the last time.

Lunch would be a beef patty or a skinless chicken breast with some kind of soft veggies, or I could mix things up with home-made chicken soup. When I was really, really sick and watching the pounds melt off, Mrs. Gottschall told my parents to prepare pureed peas or butternut squash so I could put some meat on my bones, but the squishy baby food was awful to eat and didn't help me put on weight.

Dinner might be homemade spaghetti sauce made with ground beef, onions, and garlic but served on a bed of boiled beans. Any form of pasta was strictly forbidden. My plate was usually garnished with peas and carrots—preferably not pureed. A green salad with tomatoes was okay to eat, but the dressing had to be oil and vinegar. Dessert was fresh fruit.

The only "dairy" products I could have were dry-curd cottage cheese and her homemade "24-hour yogurt." Mrs. Gottschall said wet cottage cheese had lactose, so if I wanted the taste of dairy, my parents had to purchase dry curds and moisten them with her homemade yogurt, which was a complicated two-page recipe in her book.

On the occasions when I stayed at Grandma Rose's house to give my parents a break, my beloved grandmother tried to lift my spirits by following Mrs. Gottschall's recipe for "pizza." To make the crust, Grandma Rose grated three cups of zucchini, added three eggs, almond flour, and grated cheese, mixed everything together, and then spread the crust on an oiled pizza pan. Then she topped the crust with a thick tomato sauce.

Whipping up a zucchini pizza was a lot of work, but Grandma Rose never complained, even when she made her famous chicken soup, which involved cooking a chicken carcass all day long and chopping a lot of vegetables. Both meals broke the monotony. Even though most of the foods permitted on the Specific Carbohydrate Diet tasted okay, even good, I still found the limited carbohydrate plan tedious.

And unproductive as well. I'm afraid the Specific Carbohydrate Diet, which was said to have helped thousands and thousands of hurting, desperate, and mostly young people, never brought me to the Promised Land of good health no matter how slavishly

I followed the four-week program. Each time Mrs. Gottschall heard the bad news, she couldn't have been more gracious. She always said that if her diet wasn't working after one month, then it wasn't going to work at all. So while Mrs. Gottschall's diet didn't help me in and of itself, it did give me a foundation that I could build on during my health comeback.

After studying probiotic health for nearly 15 years, I now know why the Specific Carbohydrate Diet didn't work for me, and, presumably, thousands of others who gave the disciplined diet a go. You see, Mrs. Gottschall certainly had the right idea—getting rid of the bad guys by eating monosaccharides to help build a healthy terrain—but if you're not infusing your body with healing foods, particularly organically raised meats and cultured dairy that's unpasteurized and unhomogenized, then there's a strong possibility that you won't regain any ground that you lost.

The flaw in the Specific Carbohydrate Diet is that it focuses on foods that you *can't* have instead of emphasizing healing foods you *should* have. I'm talking about grass-fed beef, wild-caught fatty fish, eggs high in omega-3 fatty acids, grass-fed butter, cultured dairy such as yogurt and kefir, and organic fruits and vegetables—foods that are part of the Probiotic Diet Eating Plan.

Mrs. Gottschall did so much good for a lot of people, but her blind spot was not recognizing the value of organic foods, high omega-3 foods, raw foods, cultured or fermented foods, *and* the introduction of the spore-forming organisms like *Bacillus subtilis*. Later on, after I had published my first books and was starting to make a name for myself in health circles, Mrs. Gottschall and I talked about probiotic supplements, including one that I formulated with *Saccharomyces boulardii* and *Bacillus subtilis*. She was adamantly opposed to those probiotic supplements, however, saying, "Look, I know the exact program that helped my daughter, and I'm not going to switch one iota."

I appreciate the way she stood for her principles until her death in 2005 at the age of 84, but in my experience, if you're not consuming the right nutritional supplements, the right live foods, and the right healthy fats—all integral parts of the Probiotic Diet—then your health will never be where you want it be, whether you're suffering from a serious digestive disease or looking to improve your already good health.

Having laid down that marker, I still want to carry the torch for Mrs. Gottschall, just as this remarkable woman carried on the legacy of Dr. Sidney Haas. We both agree that what you eat determines the balance of organisms in your terrain. It's just that I believe the Probiotic Diet takes the Specific Carbohydrate Diet to the next level. Your diet should simply not be about consuming monosaccharide-based carbohydrates and excluding disaccharides; it should be about consuming quality probiotic-rich foods and adding the right probiotic supplements to the program.

Introducing the Probiotic Diet Eating Plan

I believe throughout *The Probiotic Diet* that I've made the case that excellent health in the gastrointestinal tract is imperative for overall wellness. Unfortunately, the typical American diet infuses all sorts of junk into the digestive system. Eating the wrong foods—like greasy fries and sticky sweets—is like filling your car's fuel tank with crude oil instead of 93-octane fuel. This is the time to change your focus to naturally raised organic meats, cultured dairy, and organically grown fruits and vegetables. The Probiotic Diet Eating Plan means waving goodbye to processed foods, which strain the gut by causing the digestive system to work harder to extract nutrients that were raided during the growing and manufacturing process.

I agree that disaccharide starches such as bread, pasta, rice, corn, and potatoes are "double sugars" that are the most difficult carbs for the digestive system to break down. When left undigested, these unabsorbed carbohydrates linger in the intestinal tract, where they give sustenance to harmful bacteria, yeast, viruses, and parasites, and upset the delicate balance of the intestinal flora, causing gas, bloating, and abdominal pains.

Following the Probiotic Diet Eating Plan will promote the growth of beneficial bacteria and other microbes in your intestines while starving the bad guys, leaving you feeling energized. You'll notice that many of the healing foods I recommend have gone through a fermentation process, which means they were cultured through the intentional growth of bacteria, yeast, or mold, a process as old as biblical times. Since refrigeration hadn't been invented back then—and foods weren't known to have a "shelf life"—people in ancient times didn't have the option of freezing food or storing any foodstuffs inside a cool box. Instead, they learned how to preserve foods for a short time through the process of fermentation.

Our ancestors knew the value of fermented food, if for no other reason than fermented foods kept them from starving between harvests. They fermented milk and vegetables not only to preserve these foods—don't forget that you couldn't run down to your local Walmart in 300 BC if you needed a gallon of milk—but to take advantage of the health benefits of fermentation. I would imagine that the Bulgarians of Metchnikoff's day who consumed "sour milk" did so because they instinctively knew that cultured milk promoted intestinal health. Although they knew nothing about helpful flora, they listened to their gut and knew they felt better—and lived longer—when they consumed gourds of cultured dairy.

Other cultures employed fermentation techniques long before the Bulgarians inhabited the Caucasus Mountains. The

WHEN YOU NEED TO SNACK

It's okay to snack when you're on the Probiotic Diet. In fact, snacking is a wise strategy because eating between meals can keep things moving in the digestive tract and help you satisfy hunger pangs before they become overwhelming.

What you don't want to do is reach for one of the bad old snacks—honey-roasted peanuts, mesquite-flavored potato chips, crème-filled cookies, vanilla ice cream bars dipped in chocolate, and store-bought snack cakes. These commercially produced snack foods are loaded with refined sugars, chemical preservatives, artificial sweeteners, and processed ingredients that can give you a stomachache and set you back two steps after making a stride forward.

The better snacking alternative is to consume probiotic snacks, which

Chinese have fermented cabbage for centuries. The Romans also learned to ferment cabbage, which is known today as sauerkraut. Eastern Europeans discovered ways to pickle green tomatoes, peppers, and lettuce. The lactobacilli in these fermented vegetables contain digestive enzymes that break down food in the gut. Lactobacilli makes the vitamins more potent and increases the digestibility of food.

The three-phase, 12-week Probiotic Diet Eating Plan, which you will find on page 237, lists in great detail the foods you can enjoy and foods you should avoid. You will be asked to limit your carbohydrate sources during Phase I of the Probiotic Diet, which is the most restrictive phase. Actually, Phase I cuts off all sources of disaccharides, but we gradually reintroduce them in Phases II and III.

We still want you to consume the monosaccharide carbohydrates found in salads and vegetables like squash, asparagus, broccoli, and cauliflower, but Phase I will have you cut back on your starches considerably by having you avoid sugar and its sweet relatives—high fructose corn syrup, sucrose, molasses, and maple syrup. By choosing to eat high-fiber fruits, vegetables, nuts, seeds, and some legumes, plus a small amount of whole grain products (sprouted, soaked, or sour-leavened), which are always better for you than refined carbohydrates that have been stripped of their vital fiber, vitamin, and mineral components, you shouldn't go hungry.

When it comes to making the most of the Probiotic Diet, carbohydrate control will be key, and restricting carbohydrates may reduce bloating and other gastrointestinal problems. While "counting carbs" is not necessary on this program, you do have to be mindful about picking the right foods and sticking to the approved items found on the Probiotic Diet Eating Plan.

provide a healthy environment for your gut to thrive. These include yogurt, cottage cheese, almonds, and even coconut macaroons—made with organic ingredients, of course.

Healing Foods to Focus On

In general terms, here's an outline of foods that you need to be focusing on when you're on the Probiotic Diet:

1. Healthy meats

I strongly urge that you purchase and prepare meat from organically raised cattle, sheep, goats, buffalo, and venison that graze on nature's bountiful grasses and fish caught in the wild like salmon, tuna, or sea bass. Grass-fed meat is leaner and is lower in calories than grain-fed beef. Organic and grass-fed beef is higher in gut-friendly omega-3 fatty acids and important vitamins like B_{12} and vitamin E, and way better for you than assembly-line cuts of flank steak from hormone-injected cattle eating pesticide-sprayed feed laced with antibiotics.

Fish with fins and scales caught from oceans and rivers are lean sources of protein and provide essential amino acids in abundance. Wild-caught fish are a great source of omega-3 fatty acids DHA and EPA, which can reduce inflammation in diseases of the gut such as Crohn's disease and ulcerative colitis. Wild-caught fish can be purchased in natural food stores and fish markets, but supermarkets are stocking these types of foods in greater quantities these days. Some of the best fish to eat are wild-caught salmon, high omega-3 tuna, sardines, mackerel, and herring.

2. Raw milk and cultured dairy products from cows, goats, and sheep

The consumption of cultured dairy is absolutely critical to the success of the Probiotic Diet. Raw milk provides important enzymes and good bacteria that are crucial to probiotic support for the gut. These enzymes and bacteria aren't found in pasteurized milk since they're inconveniently destroyed during the pasteurization process. Raw milk contains lactic acid bacteria that can kill certain pathogens and thereby prevent disease, and provide more calcium, magnesium, phosphorus, and sulfur than pasteurized, homogenized dairy.

The best dairy products are the lacto-fermented kind—yogurt, kefir, hard cheeses (preferably aged), cream cheese, cottage cheese, and cultured cream. You can shop for them at natural food supermarkets in certain states, but the best sources of raw cultured dairy are found at local farms. (Visit www.RealMilk.com for a farm near you.)

Another advantage to eating cultured dairy is that those who are lactose-intolerant—and many with digestive issues such as irritable bowel syndrome are sensitive to lactose—can often stomach fermented dairy products because they contain little or no residual lactose, which is the type of sugar in milk that many find hard to digest.

Certified organic whole milk kefir, sold in ready-to-drink quart bottles, is a tart-tasting, thick beverage containing naturally occurring bacteria and yeasts that work synergistically to provide superior health benefits. Kefir is also a great base ingredient to build smoothies around: just add eight ounces of kefir into a blender, an assortment of frozen berries or fruits, a spoonful of raw honey, maybe some multi collagen or bone broth protein powder, and you're well on the way to churning up a delicious, satisfying smoothie.

As for yogurt, if you shop at a health food store, I prefer you consume yogurts not made from cow's milk. You'll be better off purchasing yogurts derived from goat's milk and sheep's milk, which are easier on stomachs as well as less allergenic because they do not contain the same complex proteins found in pasteurized cow's milk. Goat's milk and sheep's milk yogurts are readily available at natural grocers, although my personal favorite—the yogurt made from sheep's milk—is more difficult to find in stock but can often be ordered if you ask the store dairy manager. If you are able to find raw cow's milk yogurt, it can be wonderful for your health.

One thing I don't like in *Breaking the Vicious Cycle* is that Elaine Gottschall never discussed the differences between pasteurized dairy and raw dairy from grass-fed organic sources and which was better for you. In fact, she stressed that you *should* consume pasteurized dairy, presumably because of the conventional wisdom that pasteurization kills unwanted or deadly microbes when, in reality, heating milk to 161 degrees also destroys the beneficial bacteria and probiotics in the milk or yogurt product.

Mrs. Gottschall's mindset—and I know this from having many over-the-phone conversations with her (we never met in person)—was that she wanted the Specific Carbohydrate Diet to be user-friendly for the masses. That's why she recommended foods that you could pick up at any corner supermarket: conventional eggs, pasteurized and homogenized dairy, conventionally raised chicken and beef, and fruits and vegetables from "agribusiness"—the huge conglomerations that boost yields (and therefore profits) by using persistent pesticides and fertilizers that leave toxic residues in the fruits and vegetables you consume.

Mrs. Gottschall was also not overly concerned with artificial colors and artificial sweeteners, and she even said it was okay to "add a crushed saccharin tablet" to sweeten a glass of wine.[2] I hold the opposite view: low-calorie artificial sweeteners like aspartame, saccharine, and sucralose (found in those blue, pink, and yellow packets on restaurant tables) are practically poison in my eyes because of their alleged link to many health problems, including cancer. From all the studies I've seen, I think you'd be crazy to get within ten feet of them.

3. High omega-3 eggs

Free-range eggs from hens that roam around a pasture instead of being caged throughout their short lives have the highest-quality protein of any food, except for mothers' breast milk. But the main reason I'm a huge fan of eggs in the Probiotic Diet is because of their high concentration of omega-3 fats.

So what are omega-3 fatty acids? Omega-3s are a type of fat that the body needs to run the gastrointestinal system. They manufacture and repair cell membranes and hormones, balance the nervous system, and expel harmful waste products. They are essential to health because the body cannot naturally manufacture its own omega-3 fatty acids.

The Probiotic Diet is designed to increase your consumption of omega-3 fats and *decrease* your consumption of another fatty acid known as omega-6s. Omega-3s and omega-6s are the only two essential fatty acids (EFAs) that our bodies must have because they regulate body functions such as heart rate, blood pressure, fertility, and conception. The problem is that ever since Élie Metchnikoff was alive, our diets have flip-flopped. We receive very little omega-3s (because we don't eat foods like wild-caught fish and pasture-raised eggs) and *too many* omega-6 fatty acids because omega-6s are found in sunflower, safflower, corn, cottonseed, and soybean oils, which, in turn, are found in processed foods and refined grains. If your favorite meal is chicken nuggets and French fries, then you're eating a ton of omega-6 fatty acids, and that's not good for you or your digestive tract.

Since the typical American diet is weighted heavily toward omega-6 fatty acids instead of omega-3s, we typically have a ratio of 20 omega-6s to one omega-3, or 20:1. That's way too high and increases the likelihood of inflammatory and autoimmune disease, which strains your terrain. Following the Probiotic Diet should greatly improve your omega-6 to omega-3 ratio to something like 4:1, which is the bull's eye you want to shoot for.

4. Extra-virgin coconut oil and grass-fed butter

These two important foods have anti-microbial saturated fats that can work wonders for people with digestive disorders. Coconut oil is so beneficial to digestive health that years ago a person suffering from Crohn's disease wrote "Dear Abby" and insisted that eating macaroons eliminated symptoms of the disease. She was talking about your standard-recipe macaroons, the ones with white sugar, white flour, bad oils containing omega-6 fatty acids... but she included six to eight grams of coconut oil! Just the addition of extra-virgin coconut oil to a recipe that would normally be anathema to the Probiotic Diet helped out someone with Crohn's disease, and the reason why was because of the anti-microbial fatty acids in coconut oil.

Coconut oil, a miracle food that few people have heard of, has healthy fats that slow the absorption of sugar into the bloodstream, thereby keeping blood sugar levels on an even keel. It's easy to add to your diet; all you have to do is think intentionally about adding extra-virgin coconut oil whenever you pull out a saucepan to cook scrambled eggs, glaze diced onions, or heat up leftovers. I even add a tablespoon of coconut oil to my Vitamix blender when I whip up a delicious smoothie for breakfast.

Extra-virgin coconut oil contains medium-chain fatty acids such as lauric, caprylic, and capric acids, which are anti-viral and anti-fungal. Since most people suffering from digestive problems have an overgrowth of yeast and potentially high levels of virus in their systems, this obscure food can work wonders. I recommend those with digestive problems consume two to four tablespoons of extra-virgin coconut oil per day. A side benefit of extra-virgin coconut oil is that it helps you balance your weight whether you are under- or overweight. Consuming extra-virgin coconut oil to the tune of four tablespoons per day is a great way for those who are underweight to pack on the pounds.

Grass-fed butter, or raw butter, is good for your digestion because it has compounds that help repair the gut lining. Organic butter also contains anti-microbial fatty acids, including butyric acid, which has strong anti-fungal effects in the digestive tract. The superb fatty acids in butter help heal the mucosal lining and provide an environment for beneficial microflora to colonize. Butter also contains *glycosphingolipids*, which protect you against infection.

5. Cultured and fermented vegetables and other "living" foods

Raw cultured or fermented vegetables such as sauerkraut, pickled carrots, beets, or cucumbers supply the body with lots of probiotics. Although these fermented vegetables are often greeted with upturned noses at the dinner table, these foods help reestablish natural balance to your digestive system. Cultured vegetables like sauerkraut are brimming with vitamins, such as vitamin C, and contain almost four times the nutrients as unfermented cabbage. The lactobacilli in fermented vegetables contain digestive enzymes that help break down food and increase its digestibility.

I'll have a lot more to say about fermented vegetables in the next chapter, "Probiotic Foods from Around the World," but let me put a plug in for three raw foods that are essential to the Probiotic Diet. They are avocados and chia and flaxseeds.

I'll grant you that a lot of raw veggies can give you a problem if you have an acute inflammatory condition or an ulceration in the gut, but avocados and chia and flaxseeds are foods high in healthy fats such as monounsaturated fats (in the case of avocados) and omega-3 fatty acids from chia and flax. Indeed, chia's fiber-rich seeds have the highest percentage of omega-3s of any plant, including flaxseeds. These three foods are high in protein, too, so if you're a vegetarian, make sure you're eating plenty of avocados and chia and flaxseeds. Natural food stores carry wonderful chia seed and flaxseed products.

6. Bone broth

Your entire gut lining is made up of collagen, which means you need to consume foods that support collagen production. Bone broth can help repair the gut lining, and it's also easy to digest, because it's in an amino acid form. Bone broth is high in proline, glycine, and hydroxyproline, as well as glucosamine, chondroitin, and hyaluronic acid—all of which help heal and reseal your gut lining.

7. Herbs and spices

Some cultures consume a lot more spices per capita than we do in a lot of westernized countries. Nutrient density-wise, herbs are powerful. Ginger is the ultimate healing herb for your gut. It's slightly warming and anti-inflammatory. Peppermint is also excellent. You can consume peppermint as an essential oil, adding a drop or two to a smoothie or other recipe, to help cool and soothe the digestive lining. You can also add a little cardamon to your coffee or a smoothie, as well as consider taking licorice root and fennel.

8. Sprouted, soaked, or sour-leavened grains

I totally agree with Mrs. Gottschall that grains are problematic to those with gut issues. But there are ways to neutralize these disaccharides and that's through consuming grains that have sprouted, been soaked overnight in water, or leavened with a sourdough culture. A whole grain sourdough bread, for instance, would have *less* disaccharides and be in a form that most people can tolerate. The issue with grains doesn't have to be an all-or-nothing approach.

CHICKEN SOUP IS GOOD FOR THE SOUL... AH, GUT

I've referred a couple of times to the homemade chicken soup that my Grandma Rose used to make for me with her loving hands. There's something about slurping a zesty soup made from scratch with fiber-rich vegetables such as celery, carrots, onion, and zucchini, which can help digestion by attracting stomach acids. By acidifying the gut, these vegetable fibers make proteins and minerals more bioavailable and put the brakes on bloating, indigestion, and constipation.

The gelatin in the chicken soup stock is what prevents the buildup of too much acid in the digestive tract. That's why I recommend you listen to my Grandma Rose and make a great stock by cooking the chicken or chicken pieces in a large stainless-steel pot and letting it simmer for eight to 12 hours before proceeding with the rest of the recipe. That soup stock is a great addition to the Probiotic Diet.

Rose's Healing Chicken Soup

Ingredients

- 1 whole chicken
  (free-range, pastured, or organic chicken)
- 3–4 quarts filtered water

1 tablespoon raw apple cider vinegar

4 medium-sized onions, coarsely chopped

8 carrots, peeled and coarsely chopped

6 celery stalks, coarsely chopped

2–4 zucchinis chopped

1 pound green beans

4 tablespoons of extra-virgin coconut oil

1 bunch parsley

1 cup fresh or frozen green peas

5 garlic cloves

4 inches grated ginger

2–4 tablespoons of Celtic sea salt

1/4 teaspoon cayenne pepper (optional)

Directions

If you are using a whole chicken, remove giblets, neck, and any loose fat from the cavity. Place chicken or chicken pieces in a large stainless-steel pot with the water, vinegar, and all vegetables except parsley. Let stand for 10 minutes before heating. Bring to a boil and remove scum that rises to the top. Cover and simmer for 8-12 hours. The longer you cook the stock, the more cleansing it will be and the better for your digestive health. About 15 minutes before finishing the stock, add parsley. This will impart additional mineral ions to the broth.

Remove from heat and take out the chicken. Let it cool and remove chicken meat from the carcass, discarding the bones. Drop the meat back into the soup. You may purée for even easier digestion.

9. Drink water and probiotic beverages

When an overloaded gastrointestinal system gets backed up, fecal matter can ferment in the colon and cause painful bowel problems. The colon wall absorbs the remaining water in the feces, turning the stool hard as stone pebbles. The harder the feces, the more difficult it is to eliminate. This same scenario can cause explosive diarrhea in those who are prone to it.

A crucial cog of the Probiotic Diet is drinking abundant amounts of water because many digestive diseases can be attributed to dehydration. The digestive tract needs essential hydration to perform as it should, just as the body needs water to maintain the cardiovascular system.

You should be drinking half an ounce of water for every pound of body weight. In other words, divide your weight in two and that's the number of ounces of water you should drink throughout the course of the day. For example, if you weigh 160 pounds, that means you should drink 80 ounces of water per day, or around ten eight-ounce glasses.

CHEAT IF YOU MUST, BUT UNDERSTAND THE COST

Lifetime habits are hard to change. Many cannot quit eating junk food cold turkey; some feel like they "deserve" a nutritional indulgence for even trying. Others chafe at restrictions or being told what to do, so they cheat.

You will be tempted to cheat on the Probiotic Diet as well. That's human nature. My advice is to exercise discipline and not cheat when you have serious digestive issues because cheating exacts a heavy price. If you absolutely, positively must cheat, however, then cheat wisely and limit your "cheat treats" to weekends, a time when most families and couples socialize anyway.

Cheating wisely means limiting your damage by not eating any of the foods marked "Avoid" in Phase I of the Probiotic Diet Eating

Plan. This may be a problem for some. Perhaps you're thinking, *Wait a minute. Are you telling me that cocktail wienies, Boston Crème Rolls, chocolate-covered pretzels, and Lucky Charms cereal are off limits?*

Yes, that's what I've been saying all along. You begin by taking steps to remove temptation from your path. You'll find the route to wellness easier if your pantry isn't stocked with snack cakes, chocolate-covered candy bars, or all your old favorite breakfast cereals. Toss that junk food into the trash. Clean out your cupboards. Scour through the deep recesses of your freezer. Rummage through your refrigerator.

Then replenish your pantry with organic treats purchased at the health food store: dates rolled in coconut, flaxseed crackers, and raw cashews, to name a few items. Organic "sprouted" cereals are readily available these days. Dried fruits (unsulfured

Fruit juice, sports drinks like Gatorade, or coffee and tea should not be substituted to meet the daily hydration requirements. Instead, you should be adventurous and sample a probiotic drink called kombucha, or mushroom tea. Kombucha (pronounced *kom-BOO-cha*) is a fermented beverage made from black or green tea and a fungus culture.

I'll have a lot more to say about kombucha in my next chapter, which describes some other probiotic foods and beverages that aren't familiar to American taste buds, but they should be. Examples are cultured or fermented soy products such as *kimchi*, natto, miso, and unpasteurized soy sauce, as well as cultured vegetables such as sauerkraut. Throughout history, people around the world have consumed probiotic-rich foods, not knowing *why* these types of foods were good for them but certain they derived great health benefits from consuming them.

Even if you aren't the adventurous type when it comes to trying new foods, you should know about them, and you'll get your chance in the next chapter.

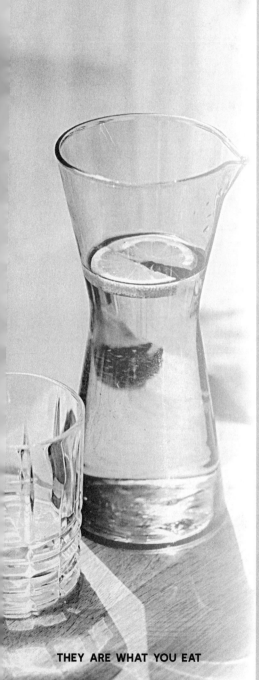

are best) such as apricots, peaches, prunes, and raisins are known as "nature's candy" and are ready to eat at any time. These convenient, healthy snacks pack almost as much a nutritious punch as their fresh counterparts.

What about those occasions when you're invited over to a friend's Fourth of July barbecue or Super Bowl party, and all the old pleasure foods are beckoning from the buffet table? Your resistance melts like a Hershey bar in the warm sun. Within minutes, you're filling a paper plate with hogs in a sleeping blanket, gooey nachos dripping in melted American cheese, and Swedish meatballs drowning in a pool of sweet molasses sauce. You know you're cheating, but you can't stop yourself.

Well, there's good news to report. If you're going to cheat in the scenario just described, just make sure you do all your cheating in a one-hour time frame. Why 60 minutes? Because if you can keep your cheating within a 60-minute time window, your digestive tract will not have to work overtime to digest foods that keep coming down the hatch. This 60-minute time frame is not a license to binge, however. Don't eat past fullness.

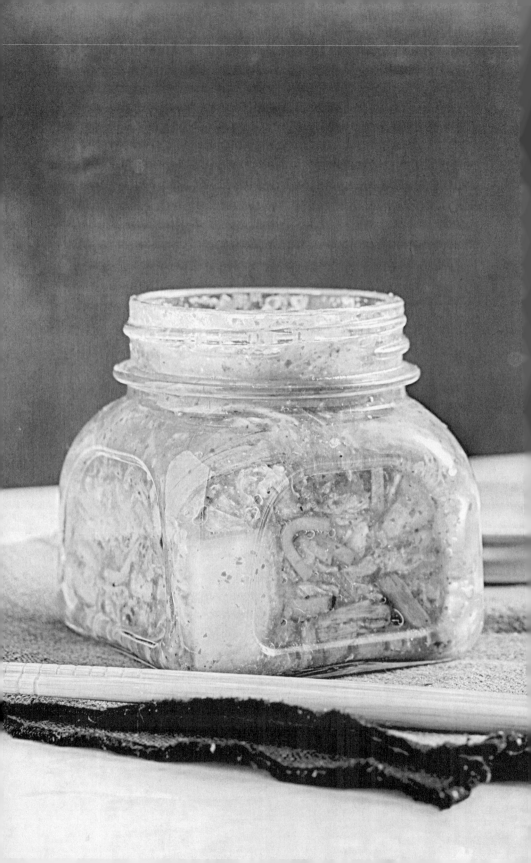

7

PROBIOTIC FOODS AROUND THE WORLD

When I traveled out to San Diego to be near William "Bud" Keith in the spring of 1995, the first thing the nutritionist did was give me some homework.

"Here, read these," he said, dropping three books in my arms. I glanced at the titles, which were:

- *God's Key to Health and Happiness* by Elmer A. Josephson
- *None of These Diseases* by S.I. McMillen, M.D., and David E. Stern, M.D.
- *The Milk Book: The Milk of Human Kindness Is Not Pasteurized* by William Campbell Douglass II, M.D.

I was unfamiliar with all three, but each book would profoundly impact me, none more so than *The Milk Book* by Dr. Douglass.

The first recommendation, *God's Key to Health and Happiness*, convinced me that too many people coast through life without realizing that at least 80 percent of diseases are lifestyle related. When discussing the question of why we are not as healthy as we should be, Mr. Josephson shared a Bible verse that has stuck in my brain for nearly 15 years: "My people are destroyed for lack of knowledge." This verse from Hosea 4:6 (NKJV) means that we're not thinking about the significance of what we eat, the quantities we consume, or the necessity of getting off our duffs and exercising our limbs.

Two medical physicians, Dr. S.I. McMillen and Dr. David Stern, pointed out in *None of These Diseases* that medical science is coming to the same conclusions about healthy living that God revealed to us in the Bible. An example: the American Academy of Pediatrics was forced to retract their declaration that circumcision had no medical benefit.

While the first two books were important *and* excellent reads, it was a book about milk—of all things—that blew me away. If you ever get a chance to read *The Milk Book*, take the time to peruse this entertaining and clever volume. Dr. Douglass has a keen storytelling ability and wit, which made this page-turner about dairy products uniquely interesting and fun to read.

"Don't skim over this book about milk" was the pun that opened the book, and for the next 271 pages, the author added little asides—like stage whispers—in footnotes at the bottom of the pages. For instance, in one section Dr. Douglass wrote: "Many restaurants keep their cooking oil and reheat it, adding additional oil as needed. That's a lot cheaper than starting over every day. But prolonged heating and reheating of unsaturated oil causes 'polymerization,' which turns the oil into shellac and varnish. Pinckney reported that animals fed these oils often develop intestinal blockage.*"

When your eyes followed the asterisk to the bottom of the page, Dr. Douglass had a footnote waiting for the obedient reader. "No wonder everyone is constipated," he quipped.

After deconstructing the "udder menace" of pasteurization, Dr. Douglass declared that cultured dairy—yogurt, kefir, and koumiss (a drink made from fermented mare's milk)—were the finest sources of protein in the world because they are predigested. This means that the fat, sugar, and protein have been partially broken down, making them much easier to digest.

Even though I talked about yogurt and kefir in the previous chapter, I want to add a few more thoughts about these cultured dairy foods as well as introduce you to some probiotic-rich foods from beyond our borders. When you adopt the Probiotic Diet, you need to intentionally look for ways to include a wide variety of fermented foods in your diet, including fermented beverages, fermented snacks, and fermented condiments. In fact, as you will see in the Probiotic Diet Eating Plan, I recommend that you consume a fermented dairy product sometime during the day, drink a probiotic beverage with a meal, consume a probiotic snack, and intentionally add a probiotic condiment to your dinner plate.

Krazy About Kefir

When I was just starting elementary school, my only sibling, Jenna, joined our family. Like any young mother of a newborn, Mom liked to get out of the house every now and then, so she would take Jenna and me to the Palm Beach Mall in West Palm Beach to stroll around in air-conditioned comfort.

Even at the age of six or seven, I knew that a mall outing was a great time to hit up Mom for a treat. My mother wasn't about to get me a vanilla soft-serve ice cream cone or a gooey chocolate sundae, though. My health-conscious parents were teaching me that anything with white sugar was bad for me and should be avoided at all costs.

There weren't many health food stores in those days, especially in malls, but Mom knew that the General Nutrition Center store at the Palm Beach Mall carried a small selection of health foods and snacks. That wouldn't be the case today. GNCs have reinvented themselves as mainly sports nutrition stores with a ton of weight loss and bodybuilding supplements—and become a convenient whipping boy whenever a professional athlete fails a drug test. (Alex Rodriguez, the former Yankee third baseman, once implied that he could have tested positive from something he bought at GNC. Yeah, right, A-Rod.)

Back when I was a Little Leaguer, though, our local GNC offered some great health foods and healthy snacks. At any rate, since Mom didn't want to buy me a chocolate-and-vanilla swirl cone, she steered the baby carriage into the mall's GNC because she knew they sold pints of blueberry goat's milk kefir. That "treat" became my earliest memory of kefir. I didn't mind the effervescent, tangy taste of those blueberry goat's milk kefirs at all.

The next time I sampled kefir was when I was a 20-year-old on the comeback trail in San Diego, where I had purchased a well-used RV so I could live near the beach, soaking up sunshine and breathing in ocean air while overcoming my digestive illness. After Bud Keith directed me to read *The Milk Book* by Dr. Douglass, I was "all in" regarding the virtues of raw cultured dairy. Following Dr. Douglass's advice, I started drinking not one but *two* quarts a day of raw milk kefir. I had no problem with the slightly sour taste because my taste buds remembered the pints of GNC blueberry kefirs I drank back in my elementary school years.

Since I didn't have a refrigerator in my RV, I purchased a cooler and kept it filled with ice—and my cartons of raw kefir. There was only one brand of raw kefir in those days—Steuve's natural raw-certified kefir, and the joke was that I could purchase their raw kefir in any flavor I wanted as long as it was plain. My goal, as I said, was two quarts a day, so I pounded those cardboard containers all day long.

Finding enough Steuve's raw kefir was a greater challenge than drinking it. Boney's Market in Pacific Beach (now a Henry's Farmers Market) usually had a shipment arrive every Thursday, but that was hit or miss since there was a statewide battle to shut down the sale of raw dairy in the Golden State. If Boney's didn't have my raw kefir, I could sometimes find it at Grossmont Nutrition Center in El Cajon, but using a pay phone to place an order or check on inventory in those pre-cell phone days was a hassle.

It was worth the effort, though. I think all the great enzymes and billions of live, friendly bacteria in the raw kefir did their part to "crowd out" the lethal bacteria that had been colonizing my gut. Kefir contains vitamins A, B, and C, lactic acid, antibiotics, antiviral agents, anti-cancer agents and even the tiniest hint of alcohol—0.1 percent. But it was the healthy omega-pre-digested proteins, carbohydrates, and fats in kefir that helped me add 29 pounds to my emaciated frame during a 40-day period that spring.

You'd think the opposite would be true, but I'm afraid that it's become even *more* difficult to find raw kefir these days. Your best bet

YOU CAN MAKE YOUR OWN KEFIR

Because raw kefir is difficult to find, consider making your own, but the process is not for the faint of heart.

My father used to make homemade kefir when I was a boy. You start with something called "kefir grains." You pour a pint or quart of raw milk into a glass container, add the kefir starter (powder or grains), cover with a lid, and allow the mixture to stand at room temperature for a day or two. Tiny soft, cauliflower-like grains begin to grow in the cultured milk, which can be gathered when you pour the milk through a cheesecloth strainer. These kefir grains are a combination of proteins and carbohydrates filled with friendly bacteria and yeasts.

When you have enough kefir grains, you use them to start another batch of kefir. (Refrigerate any leftover grains in a small amount of milk for later use or to share with friends.) The best kefir is made when you tightly cover a glass jar and set it out for 12 to 24 hours but not in direct sunlight. Careful: in hot weather, the milk ferments faster. Shake the jar a couple of times a day, then release any carbon dioxide (CO_2) gas buildup by opening the lid and then tightening it again.

Dad always knew the kefir was ready when the milk began to thicken. To separate the newly made kefir and retrieve the kefir grains, he would pour the liquid through a cheesecloth strainer or colander. We could drink the kefir as it was, or we could refrigerate it for up to a couple of weeks.

It takes some practice to get a feel for making kefir, and a lot depends upon the temperature inside the house and the type of milk you use. Keep this thought in mind: you can increase the thickness of your kefir by using more kefir grains,

is to ask around and find local dairy farms to seek out a source near you, but the fact of the matter is that today's commercial kefir is usually made from pasteurized low-fat milk, flavored with various sugars and sweeteners, and thickened with fibers that may have deleterious effects on the gut. Even in natural grocers, you'll have a hard time finding super-healthy kefirs, although Greek-style, whole milk plain kefir with no added thickeners would be an acceptable alternative.

If you can't find any raw kefir, and you don't want to deal with the aggravation or the expense of mail order, then I would take this intermediate step: shop for and consume sheep's milk yogurt, even if it's pasteurized (which it usually is). This recommendation demonstrates how highly I think of this probiotic-rich cultured dairy product. I would even go for pasteurized sheep's milk yogurt over pasteurized cow's milk kefir from whole milk, but make sure it's unflavored. Sheep's milk yogurt has been a hit around our house for years; my kids loved it when they were little and still eat it today.

I like to drink a quart of raw kefir each day when I'm around the house, and it's because I believe kefir trumps yogurt when it comes to the Probiotic Diet. When people ask me the difference between the two fermented dairy products, my reply is that yogurt must use two lactic acid bacteria, *Lactobacillus bulgaricus* (from our old friend Élie Metchnikoff) and *Streptococcus thermophilus*. Otherwise, the product cannot legally be labeled "yogurt." Dairy producers like to use *Streptococcus thermophilus* because it speeds up the fermentation process, but I'm not so sure it's a good thing to speed up something entrenched in nature.

Kefir differs from yogurt in that it has healthy yeasts in addition to healthy bacteria. The yeast component is why kefir cultures differently than yogurt and why, according to Dr. Douglass, it can be called the "champagne of milk." Besides the beneficial bacteria and yeast, kefir contains calcium, phosphorus, magnesium, and vitamins A, B2, B12, D, and K. Tryptophan, one of the essential amino acids abundant in kefir, is well known for its relaxing effect on the nervous system.

Whatever you add to your diet—yogurt or kefir or both—you'll be consuming a healthy product that's

and you can increase its tartness by increasing the fermenting time.

The amount of time for fermentation should be between 24 and 48 hours. If you tend to have loose bowels, ferment the milk for 48 hours. If you have a tendency toward constipation, then consume or refrigerate the kefir after 24 hours.

more nutritious than milk. Cultured dairy is much higher in vitamin B content and vitamin C, and the protein is the very highest quality available in human consumption. Dr. Douglass wrote that yogurt and kefir protect against infection because of the built-in antibodies, and "they are protective against hardening of the arteries, and there is a potent anti-cancer effect."[1]

History of Fermentation

We refrigerate our yogurt and kefir, and think nothing of it, but in developing countries, as well as in significant pockets of Europe, Asia, Central America, South America, and Africa, refrigeration is reserved for the well-to-do. Because practically every American family has a refrigerator, I doubt many of your neighbors can explain what fermentation is all about. Very few of us are aware that it's even possible to intentionally grow certain bacteria, yeasts, or molds to preserve unrefrigerated foods and beverages so that they can be safely consumed at a later date.

The culturing or natural processing of foods has a history as long as mankind itself. You could start a heated debate by asking which was fermented first—grape juice into wine, grains and water into beer, goat's milk into kefir, or vegetables into relish—but it doesn't matter. "Fermented foods were very likely the first foods consumed by human beings," wrote Robert W. Hutkins, author of *Microbiology and Technology of Fermented Food.* "This was not because early humans had actually planned on or had intended to make a particular fermented food, but rather because fermentation was simply the inevitable outcome that resulted when raw food materials were left in an otherwise unpreserved state."[2]

Although the first fermentations were certainly trial and error, you can be sure that our forebears eventually learned how to intentionally produce fermented foods. "When, where, and how this discovery occurred have been elusive questions since written records do not exist," said Hutkins.[3]

Nonetheless, we know that fermented foods and beverages date back to at least Noah's time. In Genesis, Noah is described as a "man of the soil" who planted a vineyard following the Flood. "When he drank some of its wine, he became drunk and lay uncovered inside his tent," says Genesis 9:21 (NIV), which was an inauspicious first mention of wine in the Bible.

Somewhere along the way, Noah and his contemporaries learned that grape juice, a sugary fruit beverage, could be fermented through the action of yeasts found naturally on the grape skin. As time passed, wine became something to drink when fresh water was unsafe or unavailable, as an ailment for stomachaches, and as a libation for religious and celebratory occasions, such as weddings and feasts.

We can only speculate when another fermented beverage—beer—reared its foamy head. The ancient Mesopotamians are said to have discovered beer when water leaked into a vessel containing grain harvested from some wild crop; the result was a fermented drink with a pleasant and intoxicating taste. For the Egyptians, beer became a divine drink with medicinal value. "There is a whole series of Egyptian pharmacopoeias [medicine books] that talk about things beer can help with," said George Armelagos, an anthropologist at Emory University in Atlanta, Georgia.[4]

The ancient Chinese must have done a lot of experimenting with fermentation because their culture came up with three alcoholic beverages thousands of years ago: *chang*, an herbal wine; *li*, a sweet, low-alcoholic rice beverage; and *jui*, a fully fermented rice or millet beverage with 10 percent to 15 percent alcohol by weight.[5]

When the Greeks heated wine—what they called "the nectar of the gods"—they discovered that the alcohol could be separated from the other substances in the liquid. The Greek philosopher Aristotle coined the term "spirits" for the cooled distillate, probably because he felt his "spirits" were lifted after downing a tall glass of Grecian hooch.

I hope all this talk about fermented beverages like wine and beer isn't making you thirsty because I recommend staying away from any form of alcoholic beverages—wine, beer, and mixed drinks—during the first two phases of the 12-week Probiotic Diet. If you do drink alcohol, which I don't and certainly don't recommend on a regular basis, make sure you consume raw, unpasteurized organic wine or beer with no sulfites. As for the healthy benefits of wine, your health needs will be better served by consuming any non-alcoholic cultures/fermented beverages.

That said, I understand that many people enjoy a glass of wine or a cold beer after a round of golf. I'm well aware that moderate consumption of wine has been shown to offer health benefits such as reducing the risk for heart disease and cancer. Beer is brewed with beneficial bacteria and yeast, although commercial beer is pasteurized to keep the beer "fresh" on cross-country shipments in refrigerated railcars, which means the beneficial probiotics are as flat as day-old beer.

If I were a beer drinker (and I'm not), I would be checking out microbrews and craft beers, which are unpasteurized. Modern wine techniques do not use pasteurization, but some vintners add a small amount of sulfur to prevent the wild yeast from starting up.

When it comes to imbibing, my drink of choice is kombucha, which I mentioned in the last chapter. Russian in origin and tart as a Granny Smith apple, kombucha is a lacto-fermented beverage with probiotics and enzymes that delivers a cidery flavor and a kick of fizziness. Kombucha is made from black or green tea and a fungus culture—a kombucha "mushroom," which is a pancake-shaped mass of bacteria and yeast. The mixture ferments for a week, resulting in a slightly sweet and slightly sour beverage containing a long list of amino acids, B vitamins, and living things like *Acetobacter* bacteria and *Brettanomyces bruxellensis*, *Candida stellata*, *Schizosaccharomyces pombe*, *Torulaspora delbrueckii* and other yeasts, including my favorite discovered by Henry Boulard himself, *Saccharomyces boulardii*.

Kombucha became popular in the mid-1990s when I was going through my health struggles. Dad— who loved checking out the latest new thing in health—made some homemade kombucha in the family kitchen, but I politely refused to give it a try. I didn't think my tender stomach could handle the fizziness, and besides, this would have been the 501st "treatment" I received for my digestive ills.

But I certainly knew what kombucha was when this murky drink began getting a word-of-mouth buzz around 2002. I was introduced to kombucha a year later and came to enjoy its sweet and sour effervescent taste. I soon figured out that

WHAT ABOUT SPARKLING APPLE CIDER?

You might think I've forgotten another fermented drink—apple cider. Sure, old-fashioned "hard cider" has probiotic benefits, but you can hardly find fresh fermented cider that has not undergone pasteurization or a filtration process that removes coarse particles of pulp or sediment, which is where all the good stuff lies. About the only places you can find unpasteurized cider, which is traditionally made each fall from late-harvest and windfall apples, are farmers' markets or roadside stands near apple orchards.

As for the popular "sparkling cider" that's often served at weddings and festive occasions instead of wine, it's nothing but regular old apple juice concentrate mixed with carbonated water to give it a cider-like fizz.

One great fermented food/beverage that you can make at home with ingredients purchased at any health food store is an apple cider vinegar tonic. Using two tablespoons of raw apple cider vinegar mixed into eight to 12 ounces of water, along with one to two tablespoons of raw honey, this beverage has a long history of use by natural foods enthusiasts, thanks in large part to the writings of natural health pioneer Paul Bragg, who wrote the quintessential book on the subject.

kombucha is not a drink you guzzle down on a hot summer's day. You sip slowly, not sucking down more than four ounces at a time.

Since then, I've become a kombucha fan who gulps—slowly—a couple of bottles a week or day, if I'm in the mood. Kombucha has developed a cult following in the last decade as health food stores stock this "sparkling Himalayan tonic" in the refrigerated case. My favorite brand of kombucha comes from Katalyst Kombucha, a "living elixir" brewed in Maine and distributed only in the Northeast currently. My favorite flavor is Bliss-Berry, which is raw kombucha with added juice of fresh-pressed wild organic blueberries from Maine and fresh ginger. The other flavor I like is Schizandra-berry, which is a "five-flavor" prized herb from China known for its complex flavors.

Besides being an acquired taste, kombucha isn't cheap at more than four bucks a bottle. You also don't want to give kombucha a firm shake and then screw off the lid. "The resulting spew made my car smell like a marinated artichoke for days," wrote Jim Ridley with the *Nashville Scene* newspaper, who said kombucha tasted like a "smelly sock steeped in salad dressing and Fresca."[6]

Believe me, if kombucha tasted that bad, no one would drink it.

Moving on to Cultured Vegetables

Scientists call the process of preserving vegetables for a long period of time a form of "lacto-fermentation," even though you might think that dairy products are involved. What is that?

Here's what author Sally Fallon had to say in her book *Nourishing Traditions: The Cookbook that Challenges Politically Correct Nutrition and the Diet Dictocrats*:

> Lactic acid is a natural preservative that inhibits putrefying bacteria. Starches and sugars in vegetables and fruits are converted into lactic acid by the many species of lactic acid-producing bacteria. These lactobacilli are ubiquitous, present on the surface of

Another early example of preservation is the practice of salting meat to preserve it from microbial deterioration. Ancient cultures had no way of knowing *why* meat spoiled so rapidly, but anthropologists believe that the ancient Egyptians began salting meat back in 1500 BC, followed by the Greeks and Romans. Then it was discovered that pounding or stripping meat into thinner slices and then leaving them out in the sun to dry turned the meat into "jerky" that could be eaten later.

Salt enhances the flavor of meat by suppressing undesirable or unpalatable savors and extending shelf life. Centuries ago, the Italians started wrapping ground meats, or sausage, into casings made from intestines to make salami, whose prefix comes from the Italian word *sal* for salt.

living things and especially numerous on leaves and roots of plants growing in or near the ground... The proliferation of lactobacilli in fermented vegetables enhances their digestibility and increases vitamin levels. These beneficial organisms produce numerous helpful enzymes as well as antibiotic and anti-carcinogenic substances. Their main byproduct, lactic acid, not only keeps vegetables and fruits in a state of perfect preservation but also promotes the growth of healthy flora throughout the intestine.[7]

When I read Sally Fallon's book *Nourishing Traditions* a couple of years after I got well, she convinced me that cultured vegetables could help my gut, which piqued my interest for more information. My search led me to *The Complete Guide to Raw Cultured Vegetables* by Evan Richards, who made the case that raw cultured vegetables were a rejuvenating source of non-dairy lactobacilli, including *acidophilus* and *Lactobacillus plantarum*, which were important for the maintenance of healthy intestinal flora and the alleviation of digestive disorders.

Talk about a fermented food right up my alley.

Shortly after I read *The Complete Guide to Raw Cultured Vegetables*, I met Evan Richards, who was the CEO and founder of Rejuvenative Foods, a Santa Cruz, California-based company that produces a wide range of live foods. Evan—who's since become a friend—suggested that I try a combination of red cabbage, beets, carrots, and garlic called Vegi-Delight Live Zing Salad. The fresh, raw vegetables were ground up, put into a stainless-steel container, and left to culture for five to seven days. Because the Vegi-Delight Live Zing Salad was not pasteurized, the healthy lactobacilli and enzymes contained exciting health benefits.

Since Evan and I met, I've had boxes of Vegi-Delight shipped to me, but sometimes the long journey takes its toll on my fermented foods. I can remember opening boxes and getting smacked with a sulfur-like smell that filled the entire house. What happened is that a bottle or two of Vegi-Delight broke during shipment, but the raw veggies continued to ferment. Phew!

I soon found out that I had better open my bottles of Vegi-Delight in the kitchen sink because sometimes the cultured veggies would rise up like a volcano and drip over the side like lava on the loose. Whenever that happened, it reminded me of my junior high volcano experiment in science class.

I quickly developed a taste for Vegi-Delight, and today I regularly eat it as a condiment—a side dish to the fish or meat on my plate. Now that I'm a Rejuvenative Foods fan, I stock my pantry with Vegi-Delight, Organic Sauerkraut, and Organic Salsa. Their sauerkraut is a mixture of cabbage, lemon juice, and dill that's cultured for five to seven days, and it's delicious.

But the real taste treat is their probiotic Organic Salsa, which is nothing like the spicy tomato-based salsa served at Mexican restaurants with a bowl of chips. The Rejuvenative Foods salsa has cabbage,

JUST PEACHY IN ATLANTA

I travel to Atlanta a great deal, and when I do go there on business, it's always a good excuse to visit my sister, Jenna, and her husband, Christian. One of my very favorite restaurants in the world is R. Thomas Deluxe Grill, the Peachtree eatery that started as an offbeat burger joint when it opened nearly 35 years ago under the direction of Richard Thomas.

Two decades ago, Richard saw the light and ditched the junk food menu for all-organic fare. We're talking Thai Express Bowls (a sauté of broccoli, red cabbage, carrots, scallions, red onions, and cilantro in a spicy peanut sauce), Cajun Sauté (blue corn pestle with a sauté of free-range chicken, rosemary potatoes, onions, and red peppers in a spicy marinara sauce), and Organic Salmon Piccata (salmon sautéed in lemon and clarified butter sauce and topped with a dollop of lemon dill coconut kefir).

In fact, all the entrees are served with raw cultured vegetables because Richard—who's become a good friend of mine—wanted a fermentation-rich menu. No one is more surprised than he at the turnaround. "I used to be president of the Kentucky Fried Chicken operation company," he said, "and now I drink kefir and eat cultured red cabbage every day!"[8]

Their cultured cabbage, seasoned with dill, garlic, and lemon, is so popular in the Atlanta area that local supermarkets and health food stores buy it for resale. "We put it on almost anything," Richard said.

I can't wait for my next trip to Atlanta.

tomatillos, carrots, hot peppers, and the obligatory cilantro. I must confess that the look, smell, and taste is completely different from commercial salsa, and that's a good thing. (You can usually find Rejuvenative Foods fermented products in some natural foods stores, or you can do what I do—order online through the Rejuvenative.com website.)

Raw cultured or fermented vegetables such as Rejuvenative's Vegi-Delight or Organic Salsa can supply your gut with plenty of probiotics. Although fermented vegetables such as pickled carrots, beets, cucumbers, or sauerkraut are often greeted with upturned noses at the dinner table, these foods help reestablish natural balance to your digestive system. Cultured vegetables such as sauerkraut are brimming with vitamins like vitamin C, and they contain almost four times the anti-cancer properties as unfermented cabbage. The lactobacilli in fermented vegetables contain digestive enzymes that help break down food and increase its digestibility.

When you embark on the Probiotic Diet, I would like you to work up the courage to try raw cultured vegetables, preferably as a condiment during dinner. The following examples of fermented vegetables from foreign lands are prime examples of cultured foods that rarely find their way onto American plates. They are:

- *kimchi* from South Korea
- natto, miso, and soy sauce from Japan
- sauerkraut from Germany

It's a shame that these foods—except for sauerkraut—are nearly invisible in the United States. In fact, I could joke that just about the only non-dairy fermented foods that Americans eat these days are pickles in their Big Mac hamburgers. (And guess what—American pickles are not true fermented foods.)

At any rate, each of these cultured foods has a long history in a traditional culture far beyond our borders. Let's take a closer look at each of them.

South Korea's Kimchi

It could be the final question to win a million bucks on *Who Wants to Be a Millionaire*, but you better have a South Korean friend as a lifeline. Here's the query:

Who was the first Korean astronaut in space?

The final answer: Yi So-yeon, a 30-year-old computer science engineer who beat out 36,000 contestants to become the first South Korean space traveler. She blasted into space in April 2008 aboard a Russian Soyuz spaceship bound for the International Space Station, together with two Russian cosmonauts. Onboard the Soyuz spaceship was a ten-day supply of Korea's national dish, *kimchi*, which is a spicy blend of fermented cabbage and other veggies.

Kimchi? Most Westerners have never heard of this type of fermented vegetables, but Koreans say they must eat *kimchi* wherever they are—even if it's 220 miles above Earth. So it was only natural for Korean space officials to think that their first astronaut must have their beloved national dish while in orbit, even if that meant creating a special "space *kimchi*."

"If a Korean goes into space, *kimchi* must go there, too," said Kim Sung Soo, a Korean Food Research Institute scientist. "Without *kimchi*, Koreans feel flabby. *Kimchi* first came to our mind when we began discussing what Korean food should go into space."[9] The Korean Food Research Institute was one of three research facilities that devoted three years and millions of dollars to create a special version of the fermented vegetables dish that was suitable for space travel.

You may think that the Koreans were going overboard with this *kimchi* thing, but we're talking about something a lot more than an ordinary *banchan* (side dish) next to the steamed seasoned fish or shredded beef marinated in soy sauce. "*Kimchi* is a national icon, a cultural treasure, a palpable expression of the country's feisty spirit and determination throughout history to grow and protect its own unique soul—to resist wholesale assimilation into the more megalithic cultures of Asia, through culinary defense. *Kimchi* is a cure-all, a protective shield, a magic balm, and a goddess of plenty," explained a long-winded Joel McConvey, a Canadian teaching English to kindergartners on Jeju-do, an island in South Korea.[10]

Kimchi has been a staple of the Korean diet for centuries. The development of *kimchi*, a peppery fermented cabbage, is reportedly rooted in the agrarian culture that began before the era of the Three Kingdoms on the Korean peninsula. Due to the cold Korean winter, they had to come up with a way to store vegetables so they could eat them in the middle of January.

Koreans serve *kimchi* at almost every meal, and few Koreans can last more than a few days before cravings get the better of them. The South Koreans, who eat 1.6 tons of this side dish each year, like to spice up their Korean version of sauerkraut with other vegetables like onions, garlic, and red-hot chili peppers.

It's the pungent peppers that did a number on my terrain when I tried *kimchi* a few years ago. I'm not a spicy-food kind of guy, so I'm not a big *kimchi* fan. One thing I know is that *kimchi* will clear your sinuses in a hurry. The gut, too, if you can stomach the taste going down.

I've tried the Rejuvenative Foods *kimchi* (they make five different versions), however, and so should you. Low in calories, high in dietary fiber, *kimchi* is rich in vitamin A, thiamine (B1), riboflavin (B2), calcium, and iron and is an excellent resource for lactic acid bacteria that aids in digestion.

While we're on the topic of Korean foods, another Korean dish I didn't particularly care for was fish eyeballs. I attended a conference on probiotics one time, and the person putting on the conference—a Korean—planned the banquet menu for the conferees. We were served a traditional Korean meal, including a dish with a large fish cooked whole on the plate. Once the fish was served family style, the three Koreans sitting at the table argued over who would get to eat the eyeballs. All I can remember is that all I could see was white globes—and you couldn't see any sort of pupil.

I prefer food without eyeballs, but if you're feeling adventurous the next time you're in an Asian restaurant, skip the fish eyeballs but ask your wait person if they serve *kimchi* as a side dish. You may have a greater affinity for the spicy food than I do, and if so, you've discovered an incredibly healthy food to eat.

Japan's Natto, Miso, and Soy Sauce

If this is your first time hearing about natto, relax because not too many people outside of Japan have heard of this traditional food made from soaked and fermented soybeans.

The origins of natto date back a thousand years to Japan's Edo period. According to an old story, one day in 1083 while on a war campaign, a group of Japanese soldiers were boiling soybeans for their horses. An ambush attack forced them to wrap up the beans in a hurry in straw bags and throw them on their horses. After hightailing it out of camp, they forgot the sacks of soybeans were still tethered to their horses for a few days. When someone noticed the pungent smell coming from one of the horses, he opened a sack of fermented beans. Despite the ghastly smell, some of the soldiers ate the gooey mess anyway, no doubt because they were hungry and there wasn't anything else to eat. Some liked the taste and continued eating. The rest is history.

Since then, natto has gained a reputation in Japan as an extremely healthy food that has medicinal uses backed by years of research and studies. If you've ever wondered why the Japanese population has one of the highest life expectancy rates in the world, then natto must take partial credit for the way it prevents heart attack, strokes, cancer, osteoporosis, obesity, and digestive system ailments. Natto is considered Japan's "miracle food."

The sticking point, so to speak, is taste and aroma. There's no doubt that natto's stinky smell can be a stumbling block for those not used to the unpleasant aroma—even in Japan. For example, natto is universally disliked in the Osaka area but remains popular in Tokyo and the northern part of the main island. If you're going to give it a try, then natto is best eaten when served over rice, and many claim it's better tasting than its Limburger cheese-like smell indicates.

I wouldn't know because I think I've tried natto just one time. My recollection is that it wasn't the tastiest thing I've ever tried, and the slimy part got to me. But if you get past the gag reflex, then you'll be rewarded with wonderful probiotic nutrients. Natto contains *Bacillus subtilis*—yes, the same *Bacillus subtilis* that Drs. Rothschild and Cutting talked about in Chapter 5—as well as a subspecies called *Bacillus natto*. Natto is also packed with phytoestrogens that have anti-cancer attributes.

Natto is hard to find in the United States, mainly because it's just about impossible to import from Japan because this stinky fermented paste doesn't travel well. But if you shop at Asian markets or well-stocked natural foods stores, you should be able to find the fermented soybean mass, which is sometimes sold frozen and must be thawed before consumption.

Miso is another form of fermented soybeans from Japan that is often mixed with rice or used as a seasoning in this country. When combined with sea salt and another grain like barley, miso develops a complex and distinct flavor, and its level of saltiness and sweetness can also vary. When purchased as a thick paste, miso can be used for sauces and spreads or as a condiment to pickle vegetables and meats.

Most Japanese restaurants in this country serve miso soup in which diluted miso is added to a vegetable broth along with tofu. Rich in fiber, protein, vitamins, and minerals, miso soup is a good way to introduce fermented foods to your diet, especially if you're not used to eating cultured foods.

I'm much more comfortable around miso than natto. Mom and Dad served miso over my rice when I was a kid because they knew how healthy it was. When I go to Japanese restaurants these days, I almost always have the wonderful miso broth as my appetizer.

I hope I have not scared you from trying natto or miso. I'm sure you've tried fermented soybeans before... in soy sauce.

Several microbes, including yeast and *Lactobacillus acidophilus*, are used in the fermentation process of soy sauce, which produces a probiotic-rich food. The problem is that commercial soy sauce—the handful of brands that dominate our supermarket shelves—is manufactured from inorganic acids and not living microbes, presumably to lower the manufacturing costs. We all know what pasteurization does to the good as well as the bad bacteria.

That's why I make sure I use a non-pasteurized brand called Nama Shoyu, a soy sauce made from organic soybeans, mountain spring water, organic whole wheat, and sea salt. Nama Shoyu—"nama" means raw or unpasteurized in Japanese—is the only soy sauce that's aged for years in cedar kegs by a unique double-brew process, which gives this soy sauce a full-bodied flavor and delicate bouquet. Nama Shoyu is the only raw soy sauce that I'm aware of that is available in North America.

Say Jawohl to Sauerkraut

If I asked you what comes to mind when I say the word "sauerkraut," you might think of heavyset waitresses slinging plates heaped high with bratwurst, boiled potatoes, and sauerkraut in an ethnic German restaurant. Yet sauerkraut is not a German invention. The first sauerkraut was made in China at the time when Christ was born. During the building of the Great Wall, that 1,500-mile structure across Asia, coolies subsisted on rice and a type of cabbage pickled in wine.

One thousand years later, Genghis Kahn plundered China and discovered the recipe for pickled cabbage. In time, his Mongolian hordes transported the fermented food to Europe. The Germans took to the cabbage-pickling idea, and by the 16th century, had learned to omit the wine. The process of fermenting cabbage with just salt was born. Salt inhibits putrefying bacteria for several days until enough lactic acid is produced to preserve the vegetables for many months. In the case of fermenting cabbage, salt, and a few spices, the result is known today as sauerkraut, which, in German, means "sour cabbage."

Outside of an ethnic German restaurant, you won't find sauerkraut on Americans' plates very often, unless you're a fan of Reuben sandwiches or love going to your local Oktoberfest celebration. If you've never eaten sauerkraut, though, that's a pity because sauerkraut is one of the few foods that contain the bacterium *Lactobacilli plantarum*, which is a digestive All-Star that should be penciled into your food lineup whenever possible.

Don't run down to your local supermarket and pull a bottle of commercially prepared sauerkraut off the shelf, however. The Food and Drug Administration recommends that commercial sauerkraut be pasteurized, which effectively destroys all the beneficial bacteria. You should look for raw, unpasteurized sauerkraut in health foods stores, or, if you're industrious, make your own.

PICKLED GINGER

Pickled ginger, the world's most widely cultivated spice, contains chemicals that inhibit toxic bacteria in the digestive tract while it promotes friendly bacteria, which is why this spice is effective in treating conditions ranging from constipation to diarrhea. Ginger reduces the total volume of gastric juices, stimulates fat-digesting bile, and restores balance to proper digestive function.

You've probably seen a dab of pink pickled ginger whenever your sushi order arrives at a Japanese restaurant. Careful: pickled ginger should be tan or beige, so the eye-pleasing pink means that it was artificially colored. The same holds true for wasabi, which is not a traditional fermented food since it's horseradish. That's dyed a green color, again for "presentation" purposes.

PASS THE KETCHUP

The Chinese are generally credited with inventing ketchup, which started out as a fermented fish brine sauce known as *ke-tsiap*. When sailors brought stone jars of *ke-tsiap* home to England, they added pickled cucumbers (another fermented food) with kidney beans and oysters. Then English settlers in New England added tomatoes in the late 1700s, and before you knew it, McDonald's was handing out ten-gram packets of ketchup by the millions.

Ketchup is a wonderful condiment, but today's commercial ketchup is no longer a fermented food. Manufacturers add vinegar to the production process, which short-circuits the fermentation process. Vinegar preserves more quickly but produces condiments that have no probiotic benefit.

Less Is More

Keep in mind that fermented vegetables such as *kimchi*, natto, and sauerkraut are not meant to be eaten in large quantities but as condiments. This really is a situation where less is more.

Every condiment has its beginnings as a fermented food, and throughout history has always been healthy. When beginning to eat cultured or fermented vegetables, remember that a little bit goes a long way. Start with small amounts to allow your digestive system time to adjust to these cleansing foods. Depending on the strength of your stomach, a forkful or two accompanying your meal is all you need early on. You can work your way up to three or four forkfuls a day after a week or two. These condiments work beautifully with meats and fish as well as bland starches like rice.

If you've purchased probiotic condiments from Rejuvenative Foods, all you have to do is open the jar. Just make sure you hold your nose and set that jar in a sink before you pop the lid.

Coming Next

In our next chapter, we turn away from what probiotic foods and beverages you should consume to taking a closer look at the special needs of women vis-à-vis probiotics.

After all, women have *two* terrains, not just one.

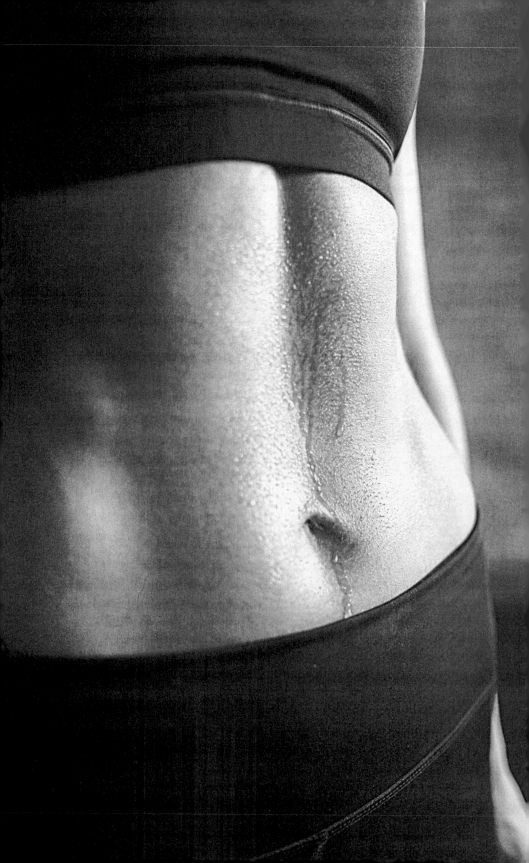

8

LADIES AND GERMS

I was into acting as a kid—remember, I played the lead role of Oliver Twist in a community stage production—so whenever my grandparents and relatives came over, I cajoled and wheedled them into watching a "performance."

Grandma Rose was my most enthusiastic fan, and her face always lit up when I earnestly pleaded with her to watch me act and sing on my "stage"—the living room.

"Ladies and Germs," she would announce to my parents and other relatives in the house. "Now performing, Jordan Rubin!"

My parents and relatives would quietly chuckle at Grandma Rose's humorous introduction—and in my mind, I can still hear her saying "Ladies and Germs" almost four decades later. Thanks to Google, I know where she got the catchphrase. After Grandma Rose married in the late 1940s, an invention called television invaded homes. An acerbic, cigar-smoking vaudevillian who eagerly embraced the new medium was none other than comedian Milton Berle, who staged a live variety show on Tuesday nights. In the days when you could count the number of channels on two hands, "Uncle Miltie" ruled the roost.

"Good evening, ladies and germs," he would announce at the start of every show. "I mean ladies and gentlemen. I call you ladies and gentlemen, but you know who you really are."[1]

Cue the laugh track.

When it comes to probiotic health, "ladies and germs" is no laughing matter. If you're a guy reading this chapter, then count your blessings because the only terrain you must worry about is between the mouth and the bowels. Women, on the other hand, have *two* major areas of the body to be concerned about: their digestive tracts *and* their reproductive areas.

The reason why women are more vulnerable to having an unbalanced terrain in their nether regions is because of the physiological fact that their vaginal orifices are (1) exposed to the outside world and (2) are warm incubators of good and bad bacteria. These days, bad bacteria inside their vaginas seem to be gaining the upper hand, causing urinary tract infections (UTIs), overgrowth of a yeast called *Candida albicans*, and smelly, itchy conditions such as bacterial vaginosis. Add to that the fact that women experience constipation and irritable bowel syndrome in greater numbers than men, and I'm confident that I can make the case that women need the Probiotic Diet more than men.

There's no doubt that the female reproductive anatomy is one of God's most awesome creations. I have no idea why some women grow up hearing that their vaginas are dirty or full of germs. From everything I've read, vaginas should be full of *good* germs that keep the bad bacteria at bay inside their reproductive systems.

The bacteria charged with protecting the vagina are *Lactobacilli*, and if you're doing a double take, it's because you've remembered that *Lactobacilli* are the same bacteria found in cultured dairy products like yogurt. *Lactobacilli* provide a natural disinfectant while helping women maintain a healthy balance of microorganisms that prevent the overgrowth of yeast. The main competition inside the vagina is a yeast cell called *Candida albicans*, although there are other microorganisms intent on wreaking havoc.

Here's an example of another microorganism: Do you remember the toxic shock syndrome (TSS) that killed dozens of women in the 1980s? The syndrome was linked to overabsorbent tampons that created a breeding ground for the bacteria called *Staphylococcus aureas*.

Normally, the vagina naturally takes care of anything that comes its way and cleanses itself daily with a non-odorous clear or milky discharge, no doubt related to the *Lactobacilli* swirling in the vagina. But when the "terrain" of the vagina experiences a shift in the delicate balance between competing organisms, yeast cells such as *Candida albicans* grow like thickets and rapidly overwhelm the friendly bacteria. When there is an overgrowth of yeast and fungus in the vagina, the medical condition is known as vaginitis.

Bacteria, yeast, viruses, chemicals in creams or sprays, or even tight or wet clothing can cause bacterial vaginitis. According to the Mayo Clinic, the most common types of vaginitis are:

- **Bacterial vaginosis.** This type of vaginitis results from overgrowth of one of several organisms normally present in your vagina, upsetting the natural balance of vaginal bacteria.

- **Yeast infections.** You now know that the naturally occurring fungus called *Candida albicans* causes yeast infections. The U.S. National Women's Health estimates that 75 percent of women will suffer an irritation of the vagina and vulva due to yeast overgrowth during their lives.

- **Trichomoniasis.** This type of vaginitis, also nicknamed "trich," is caused by a one-celled parasite and is commonly transmitted by sexual intercourse.

- **Chlamydia.** Known as one of the most common sexually transmitted diseases in the United States, chlamydia often leads to pelvic inflammatory disease (PID), which increases a woman's risk of infertility, pelvic adhesions, and chronic pelvic pain. This form of vaginitis often goes undiagnosed.

- **Atrophic vaginitis.** This type results from reduced estrogen levels after menopause. The vaginal tissues become thinner and drier, which may lead to itching, burning, or pain.[2]

Why are far too many women experiencing unhealthy terrains in the vaginal areas, leading to an overgrowth of yeast and other microorganisms? I pin the blame on several factors:

- The synthetic estrogens found in birth control pills or hormone replacement therapy destroy good bacteria and decrease microflora populations.

- Feminine hygiene products, such as panty liners, scented tampons, and vaginal washes, wipe out the natural and healthy organisms normally present in the vagina.

- The consumption of caffeine, which lowers the immune system and allows candida yeasts to thrive.

- Eating conventionally raised beef, chicken, and dairy products from livestock and poultry fattened up with antibiotic-laced feed.

- The proximity of the vagina and anus, where harmful bacteria left over from a bowel movement can infect the vagina when women wipe from back to front and spread intestinal bacteria from the rectum to the urinary tract and vagina.

We know that one of the principle causes of bacterial vaginosis is the presence of *E. coli*, which is normally found in the rectum. The failure to "reverse wipe" following a bowel elimination is the leading reason why bacterial vaginosis is the most frequently occurring vaginal infection, affecting up to 64 percent of the female population at any given time. If left untreated, bacterial vaginosis may increase a woman's risk of pelvic inflammatory disease, cervicitis, endometriosis, and pregnancy complications.[3]

So what can be done to prevent vaginitis or eliminate its occurrence? Here are other steps you can take:

- Shower daily to keep the vulval area clean.
- Wipe from front to back after a bowel movement.
- Keep the vaginal area dry. If you work out, don't linger long before taking a shower, especially if you're wearing Spandex. If you're swimming, don't stay out in a wet suit too long.
- Wear cotton underwear and avoid nylon pantyhose. Skintight jeans and leotards also foster a warm, moist environment that candida loves.
- Avoid using perfumed, chemical-laden feminine hygiene products—tampons and sanitary napkins— that can leave a chemical residue in the vaginal area. Most conventional feminine care products are made with absorbent fibers that have been bleached with chlorine, which is a toxin you want to avoid. Tampons, as well as toilet paper, made from 100-percent organic cotton and whitened without chlorine are safer for those sensitive areas and free of irritating dyes or fragrances.

- If you're using oral contraceptives, consider having your husband use protection instead.

If you think you have a form of vaginitis and schedule an appointment with your gynecologist, he or she will commonly recommend over-the-counter medications such as miconazole (Monistat) and clotrimazole (Gyne-Lotrimin), but these medications aren't necessarily equipped for re-establishing the right levels of microorganisms in your terrain. In fact, these over-the-counter antifungal agents as well as potent prescriptions like fluconazole (Diflucan) can be harmful to the liver and the immune system.

"Treating the vagina alone is often a waste of time and money," said William Crook, M.D., author of *The Yeast Connection and Women's Health*. In his excellent book, which I recommend if you're fighting a stubborn candidal infection, Dr. Crook argues that your terrain needs a yeast-fighting diet that calls for organic meats and fish, fresh vegetables, nuts, seeds, and pure water.

I'm glad that Dr. Crook and I are on the same page, but I further stipulate that adding probiotic-rich foods such as cultured dairy—yogurt and kefir—to your diet, as well as raw sauerkraut, can mitigate candida overgrowth. These foods are part of the Probiotic Diet Eating Plan on page 237.

Nicki and Her Starbucks

When I learned in researching this chapter that bacterial vaginosis may increase a woman's risk of endometriosis—and that the consumption of caffeine could wreak havoc in a woman's terrain—I nodded my head in agreement. Allow me to explain.

After Nicki and I had been married several years, we were ready to bring a child into the world. Nothing unusual about that. We were like hundreds of millions of young couples around the world who cherished the idea of starting a family and believed in the inestimable worth of children. We thought the timing was right, especially because Nicki was in her early thirties. Nicki was in superb health after making a major diet switcheroo during our first year of marriage. After being around me, I suppose, Nicki totally bought into the importance of eating grass-fed beef and bison, free-range chicken, organically grown fruits and vegetables, and cultured dairy. She began taking probiotic supplements with *Bacillus subtilis* and *Saccharomyces boulardii* after I told her about their probiotic value.

Each month we tried to conceive, however, resulted in disappointment. After a year without Nicki getting pregnant, we were concerned. After two years, anxiety set in. After two-and-a-half years, it was time to see a doctor.

Our family physician referred us to a fertility specialist, who walked us through a series of embarrassing and personal questions, then poked and prodded before having us submit to several invasive medical tests. When the results came back, I checked out fine. But with Nicki... our doctor flatly declared that she wasn't ovulating—and hadn't been for many months or even years.

The news stunned us. "Why isn't Nicki ovulating?" I asked, knowing that conception was impossible unless Nicki's body could produce an egg during the menstrual cycle.

The fertility specialist turned toward Nicki. "My suspicion is that you have endometriosis, which is one of the major causes of female infertility," he said.

I knew something about endometriosis, but I wanted to hear the doctor's explanation of this condition. He replied that the endometrial tissue—the lining inside the uterus—was growing outside the uterus and attaching itself to other organs, such as the ovaries and fallopian tubes. The presence of these tissues was messing with Nicki's menstrual cycle, which explained why she was not ovulating.

The medical condition sounded serious. Poor Nicki looked petrified, and I wrapped an arm around her in the doctor's office. "What are our options?" I asked, breaking the silence.

"Most likely surgery," the physician replied matter-of-factly. "A laparoscopic procedure would remove any ovarian cysts that we find inside the pelvic cavity. Thoroughly routine these days."

Routine if you're not the one getting cut on.

"You'll have to give us some time to think about this," I replied for the both of us.

When we got home, I had had enough time to think about the fork in the road we were facing. I told Nicki that I thought surgery should be a last-resort measure. Until we decided to go that route, I wanted to explore what could be done through diet. Since Nicki wasn't thrilled with the prospect of going under the knife either, she was willing to try anything if that was what it took to become pregnant.

You could say my wife was motivated.

I asked Nicki if she would consider going on the Maker's Diet 40-day health plan with me—and make an all-out effort to eat as healthy as possible. I had read that the consumption of too many carbohydrates, particularly disaccharide sugars and starches, could raise insulin levels and produce a hormonal imbalance. Perhaps that was throwing her ovulation cycle off-kilter.

Nicki told me later she gulped before saying yes since that meant saying goodbye to her beloved Starbucks Caramel Macchiato drinks. Unbeknownst to me, Nicki drove to a nearby Starbucks nearly every morning, where the friendly baristas could recite her drink order by heart: tall Caramel Macchiato, two shots of espresso, extra caramel sauce, and whipped cream.

That was a pretty good shot of caffeine and sugar to Nicki's terrain.

Caffeine has always been known as a diuretic that stimulates the digestive system because it inhibits an enzyme thought to regulate mucosal secretions in the small intestine. When the secretions go up, the fluid in your bowel rises, and if the amount of fluid in your colon is greater than the amount of fluid you can reabsorb, you better scout out a restroom because diarrhea is on the way.

Nicki came clean about her daily fixes of Caramel Macchiatos, and while her Starbucks trysts weren't the end of the world, they couldn't have been helping my wife's *other* terrain—her reproductive system. Now that I knew all the facts, I had a hunch that her caffeine consumption had been a contributing factor to her endometriosis issues, and hence, her infertility. I found research showing that some caffeine-drinking women could have problems getting pregnant, although I added that modern science had yet to formally establish a link between caffeine and endometriosis.

Nicki determinedly followed the Maker's Diet with me, even though she felt lightheaded during the first few days of "detox." I appreciated her attitude: she put on her accountant's mindset—the one that said there could be no deviation if she expected the correct results. Gone were the forays to Starbucks and occasional "cheat" with strawberry-flavored Twizzlers. Instead, she focused on eating the healthy foods on the Maker's Diet, many of which are part of the Probiotic Diet. Then, just six weeks after she started, a glorious miracle happened. A home pregnancy test revealed that Nicki was pregnant! We thought back to the date when that blessed event could have happened, and we determined that Nicki had conceived on the fortieth day of the Maker's Diet!

The news flabbergasted us. After struggling with infertility, we thought we were doomed to be among the one in eight couples who couldn't conceive. Instead, God showed mercy after a 30-month wait, and we would become parents for the very first time.

The Probiotic Saboteurs

Caffeine and sugar, along with antibiotics, birth control pills, feminine hygiene, and skin and body care products are examples of what I call "probiotic saboteurs" that take dead aim at women. The resulting hormonal imbalance can lead to serious digestive issues and an overgrowth of yeast and other fungi in the reproductive area.

Yeast infections seem to go together with pregnancy since the high estrogen level inside pregnant women's bodies enhances the glycogen level, which makes the vagina a breeding ground for a yeast infection. Thankfully, Nicki avoided any yeast infections during her pregnancy.

Yeasts may sound like creepy crawlers, but they aren't. Yeasts are single-cell organisms that are neither animal nor vegetable—they are a kind of fungus. Mildew, mold, mushrooms, and candida are names of different types of yeast. The yeast particularly associated with women is *Candida albicans*, which thrives in the warm inner creases and crevices of the vagina. The primary symptoms of candidal vaginitis are vulvar itching, which can be quite severe, and a thick, curdy discharge that looks like cottage cheese. A painful, burning sensation often accompanies urination or sexual intercourse. Candida overgrowth can have systemic and local effects, such as hormonal, skin, and immune system disorders. Diabetes and other conditions that suppress the immune system are also associated with frequent yeast and bacterial infections.

Men are very fortunate that we don't have to deal with these type of yeast infections—duh!—but women need to be wary of the balance between good bacteria and disease-causing organisms taking up residence in their vaginas. When this balance is disturbed for any reason—and I've just listed a few of the "saboteurs"—it sets the stage for an overgrowth of *Candida albicans*. Once the "vicious cycle" gets going, as Elaine Gottschall used to say, it's hard to pull yourself out of the tailspin unless you make major changes in your diet, just as Nicki did before getting pregnant. This is where the Probiotic Diet Eating Plan can help.

In the past 20 years, yeast infections caused by candida have increased two-and-a-half times due to several factors, chief among them the increased use of antibiotics, which kill the bacteria that normally protects and balances the yeast in the vagina.[4] Antibiotics may kill everything else, but they do not kill candida yeasts. Since yeast levels are normally present and well balanced in the vagina, you're susceptible to

CANDIDA AND CHRONIC FATIGUE

Candida albicans absolutely *loves* sugar and is thought to contribute heavily to chronic fatigue syndrome and fibromyalgia, a pair of diseases that present themselves through persistent, overwhelming symptoms of fatigue and feelings of exhaustion. Chronic fatigue syndrome and fibromyalgia are much more common in females than in males; some say the ratio is as high as 90 percent female and 10 percent male.

Chronic fatigue syndrome and fibromyalgia are among the most mysterious and controversial maladies of the last few decades. Back in the 1980s, chronic fatigue syndrome was waved off as "yuppie flu" by medical practitioners because the condition seemed to be concentrated among young urban white professionals. Some male doctors dismissed it as a "head case" disease since predominantly women came to their offices complaining about feeling tired all the time. Others call it "a disease with a thousand names."

Doctors find it difficult to diagnose chronic fatigue syndrome or fibromyalgia because there are no lab tests for them. If you enter a doctor's office complaining about feeling tired all the time, he or she will ask about your physical and mental health, perform a physical exam, and order urine and blood tests to see if something else could be causing your symptoms. They often come back empty.

Many theories are floating out there about what causes chronic fatigue and fibromyalgia, but yeast infections zoom to the top of any list of suspected culprits. There's no doubt that *Candida albicans* challenges the immune system and releases toxins into the body, resulting in fatigue and muscle pain.

an infection when antibiotics in a woman's system upset this normal balance.

Also called vaginal thrush when the condition becomes pervasive, candida may trigger premenstrual syndrome (PMS) by activating an autoimmune response to sex hormones, according to Dr. Crook. He believes there is a connection between the systemic overgrowth of *Candida albicans* and PMS and the cyclic rise and fall of estrogen levels that result in fatigue, headaches, irritability, bloating, and depression during the week before the period starts.

Dr. Crook studied the role of sugar—in its various forms—and how it plays in the multiplication of *Candida albicans*. As mentioned in Chapter 6, sugar is a disaccharide carbohydrate that provides a short-term energy burst, but refined white sugar has a way of feeding the candida yeasts in the body. Eat too many sweets, which is easy to do if you follow the Standard American Diet, and you're setting yourself up for some problems south of your navel.

A recurring itch in and around your vagina or unusual discharges are good reasons to suspect an excess of *Candida albicans*, and when those symptoms occur, you should always seek the help of a physician, even though many doctors will reflexively write you a prescription. I guess Louis Pasteur's "germ theory" lives on!

But after you learn what you're dealing with, do your homework by going online and educating yourself on the importance of changing your diet to improve the terrain inside your vagina. If you're not sure whether you have a yeast problem, you can go to Dr. Crook's website at www.yeastconnection.com and appraise the role yeast plays in your chronic health problems by clicking on "Dr. Crook's Famous Yeast Evaluation Questionnaire."

If you are feeling tired, even after sleeping, or muscle pain and aches dog you all day long, you could have chronic fatigue syndrome or fibromyalgia. I believe that Phase I of the Probiotic Diet Eating Plan—which cuts back on starches such as bread, pasta, and rice and *any* foods with sugar and its sweet relatives— high fructose corn syrup, sucrose, molasses, and maple syrup—will go a long way toward bringing some bounce back to your step.

The Gift of Germs

Finally, I would like to end this chapter directed toward women by issuing a challenge to all females of childbearing age: *Please, if possible, try to deliver your baby through the birth canal.* If you can do so, you'll be giving your baby his or her first gift: a dose of probiotics.

How so?

As labor begins and the baby is pushed through the birth canal, the baby is exposed to beneficial bacteria as he or she slips through. Bifidobacteria from the mother's birth canal colonize the infant's terrain and give the baby's immune system its first infusion of beneficial microorganisms, such as *Bifidobacterium lactis ssp infantis*, *Bifidobacteria bifidum*, and *Bifidobacteria breve*.

Look at it as nature's first probiotic bath.

That's what we wanted to do for our child after we learned that Nicki was pregnant following her incredible 40-day health experience with the Maker's Diet. Right from the get-go, we were both committed to Nicki delivering vaginally instead of submitting to a Cesarean section birth, which reminds me of an old joke:

What's the difference between involved and committed?

Answer: In a bacon-and-egg breakfast, the chicken was involved, but the pig was committed.

Okay, so I was involved, and Nicki was committed.

At any rate, Nicki had a difficult pregnancy, marked by several months of morning sickness and a lack of energy that often hits first-time mothers. We took the requisite childbirth classes, and the instructor joked that the best time to get an epidural was right after you find out you're pregnant. We chuckled along with the rest of the class, but later that night, we both agreed that we didn't want her to get an epidural shot, which is an injection of anesthetic relief directly into the spine to numb the legs and lower torso. We didn't like the downside, which is that an epidural makes pushing tricky because you're numb from the waist down, and any medications given during labor can affect the health of the child.

I know: Easy for me say. I was involved and my pregnant wife was committed.

But we wanted the best for Nicki and for our son, since an ultrasound earlier in the pregnancy revealed that we had a Jordan Jr. on the way. As we talked about what kind of delivery we wanted, we discussed the pros and cons of a home birth. My mother had delivered me at home in the presence of four students and a midwife from the National College of Naturopathic Medicine in Portland, Oregon, where my father was a student, so having a home birth wasn't a crazy idea in our household. Even though the idea of a home birth sounded intriguing, Nicki and I both agreed that this was something we weren't willing to do.

So that meant a hospital setting. We were fine with that, but neither of us was sold on the idea of Nicki meekly allowing an obstetrician to run the show—a show that had a one-third chance of ending up with birth via a Cesarean section. We were aware that obstetricians often steered moms to Cesarean sections because they were practicing defensive medicine: they didn't want to be sued in case something tragic happened in the birthing room. Fear of lawsuits is probably the number-one reason why nearly one-third of all pregnancies end up with a Cesarean delivery. According to the Centers for Disease Control and Prevention, 31 percent of American women who gave birth in 2006 had a Cesarean delivery, up from 6 percent in 1970, 17 percent in 1980, and 23 percent in 1990.

What's driving those rising numbers is that the practice of obstetrics has changed a great deal in the last 20 or 30 years as the induction of labor and Cesarean section become the norm. Whether it's fear of litigation, a response to a maternal request, or just plain convenience, more and more mothers are *scheduling* their deliveries rather than allowing labor to begin naturally.

THE PREGNANCY DIET

If you're pregnant and reading this book, then you should know that *The Probiotic Diet* could really be called *The Pregnancy Diet*. I'm sure you had well-meaning friends remind you that you're "eating for two," and you are (or have been). Babies drink the amniotic fluid inside the placenta, and if you're eating plenty of fermented foods, then your body is sending those probiotics right into the umbilical cord.

The same advice goes for nursing mothers. Eat a wide variety of probiotic-rich foods, especially cultured dairy, so that your body can make the healthiest milk possible for the son or daughter suckling at your breast.

We weren't going to schedule Nicki's delivery or have a Cesarean section. While C-sections were promoted as a safe and painless birth option, we knew that a Cesarean section was major abdominal surgery with high complication rates ranging between 20 percent to 50 percent. The complications included hemorrhaging, infection, damage to other organs, and four to seven times increased risk of maternal death.[5] Last, we didn't want Nicki to undergo a Cesarean birth because she would have to have a C-section if she ever gave birth in the future. Our stance on a Cesarean section was that we would only agree to one if it was *absolutely* necessary.

We also knew that slicing Nicki's abdomen to retrieve our first child would deny our son a trip down Probiotic Lane. So we found a compromise that worked for everybody: we would have a nurse/midwife deliver our child in a hospital so if there were complications, trained medical staff were just steps away. We also preferred that Nicki's labor would not be induced, if at all possible, which also went against the grain for us. We wanted to go the natural route for as long as possible because we believed that was best for our child.

We checked around to find a hospital that would be a good fit for our philosophies, and we found one: the Jupiter Medical Center in nearby Jupiter, Florida. We also liked the hospital's billboards posted around town boasting that "Men are from Mars, but babies are from Jupiter."

We met with a prenatal nurse to go over the program and fill out a "birth plan" that stipulated what direction and what medical measures we wanted when Nicki started going into labor. No epidural. No Pitocin to induce labor. No episiotomy. And no Cesarean section.

In the predawn hours of May 29, 2004, Nicki went into labor. We rushed to the hospital as first-time-about-to-be parents, giddy about the Big Day. Because Nicki wanted to go as far as possible without medication, she didn't opt for an infusion of Pitocin to move labor along. But as the contractions lumbered into the early afternoon hours, the labor turned brutal. She pushed for four hard hours without any significant progress. That's when we decided that enough was enough, and we okayed the use of Pitocin. But I have

WOMEN AND THEIR HEALTH

Talk about getting the short straw.

Not only do women have to contend with vaginal yeast infections, but twice as many women suffer from symptoms of irritable bowel syndrome (IBS)—recurring constipation, abdominal pain, digestive discomfort, and bloating—than men. Chronic constipation in women contributes to the development of hemorrhoids, diverticulosis, and polyp formation.

From a strictly personal experience, I can assure you that I'm amazed at the number of women who approach me after I speak, seeking a chance to have a few words with me about their digestive troubles or physical maladies. Women are much more open than men, who grow up hearing that they should "tough it out" when they experience digestive problems.

Guys would rather read a newspaper for two hours on the toilet than admit they're backed up like the Santa Monica Freeway at rush hour.

It's a shame that women are more proactive about their health than men. Women are more likely to visit a doctor, read a health-related book, take nutritional supplements such as vitamins and minerals—and perhaps try out the Probiotic Diet.

to hand it to Nicki: she was determined to push our son into this world without an epidural.

I hate to say this, but poor Nicki pushed so hard that blood vessels in her face almost burst. Her screams could be heard in the hallway by our worried parents. All I could do was stroke her matted hair and offer encouragement. Her face was puffy from exertion, and it was distressing to see my wife suffering such intense pain.

Finally, at 6 p.m., after 20 hours of agony, Nicki managed to push Joshua Michael Rubin into the world. Just before he took his first breath of life, Joshua received his first ingestion of friendly bacteria that his tiny terrain needed when he suckled for the first time at Nicki's breast and received specific oligosaccharides that promoted the growth of bifidobacteria in his squeaky-clean colon.

Even as I'm typing these words, I'm tremendously grateful for what Nicki did in enduring a very difficult delivery—one that resulted in our son's birth and his first dose of probiotics.

9

SAY AH TO ORAL PROBIOTICS

receive my share of natural health newsletters and press releases in my inbox, but many deserve only a cursory glance before I hit the delete button. An e-mail link to an article at the Natural Products Insider website, however, proved to be a worthwhile read from start to finish.

The story outlined how probiotics can promote good *oral* health by inhibiting the growth of bacteria that cause gum disease and tooth decay. In this article, I learned that a Harvard-educated researcher named Jeffrey Hillman, D.M.D, Ph.D., had discovered a way to replenish the "good bacteria" in the mouth through sucking on a probiotic mint that he had developed after years of research and development. Touted as the first complete oral care probiotic, this new product was said to support tooth and gum health, freshen breath, and whiten teeth.

Whoa—talk about something in my probiotic wheelhouse. Learning that an oral probiotic even *existed* was exciting news to me, especially because I was in the throes of writing *The Probiotic Diet*. When I started this book, I knew I wanted to talk about probiotics for the gut and for the female reproductive system, but probiotics for the mouth?

Why not? Oral probiotics make all the sense in the world if you look at the mouth and teeth as the starting point of the alimentary canal, which is a physiological fact. The mouth, teeth, and gums jump-start the digestive process by breaking the food apart, softening each morsel with saliva, and pushing the food into the throat, where the swallowing mechanism sends the partially digested food on to the stomach. All those juices in the mouth contain legions of microorganisms, some good for the body and some not so good. When everything goes as nature intended, the probiotic-type "action" happening inside the oral cavity contributes to our overall health.

I clicked onto Dr. Hillman's online webinar, which was an hour-long presentation regarding the new oral probiotic, called ProBiora3, that he had discovered. While some of the information was dry and technical, I came to the realization that just as there is a gut terrain and a female reproductive terrain, there is also an oral terrain that our bodies must contend with on a 24/7 basis.

Learning about Dr. Hillman's trailblazing development of oral probiotics reminded me of research conducted by Dr. Weston A. Price, who, ironically, had a periodontal background similar to Dr. Hillman. When I was a non-resident naturopathic medical student at the People's University of the Americas under Dr. Rothschild, I studied one of the most significant books ever written on health: *Nutrition and Physical Degeneration* by Dr. Price, a Cleveland dentist who lived from 1870 to 1948. During the Great Depression years, Dr. Price took a sabbatical from his practice and traveled around the world studying indigenous people whose teeth and gums were untouched by processed foods.

After living among these primitive cultures and examining row after row of healthy teeth, Dr. Price wrote that he was convinced that the American "diet of commerce"—defined by the refined flours and refined sugars in foods sold on market shelves—was sending us down the road to perdition. Cavities and gum disease,

Dr. Price said, portended ailments in the digestive tract, which, in his view, were often the underlying reasons behind cardiovascular disease and bone deterioration. In other words, people with serious plaque in their teeth usually had plaque in their arteries. People with enamel deterioration usually had some type of bone deterioration, such as osteoporosis.

It sounded like Dr. Price and Dr. Hillman were on the same page. As I continued reading the Natural Products Insider that day, I learned that Dr. Hillman had devoted most of his professional life to researching the effects of oral microflora on good periodontal health preceding the development of the technology behind his probiotic formula called ProBiora3. I believed—in my gut, which is ironic—that Dr. Hillman was on to something.

Up Close and Personal

Jeffrey Hillman jokes that he was born small and grew up tall and pale. When he turned 18 in 1966, he enrolled at the University of Chicago—a good idea if you didn't want to end up in a Vietnamese rice paddy with an M-16 draped across your shoulders. Jeffrey was an excellent student, and following graduation, he applied to several dental schools. The Harvard School of Dental Medicine accepted him, and Jeffrey was off to Cambridge, Massachusetts.

Upon graduating with a D.M.D. degree, Jeffrey could have gone into private practice. "Early on in dental school, though, I became fairly convinced that I did not want to spend the rest of my life with my fingers in somebody else's mouth," he said.

The research side of periodontal disease and treatment appealed to him, however. He and just one other member of his Harvard graduating class went on to earn Ph.D. degrees from Harvard University Medical School; Dr. Hillman's doctorate was in Microbiology and Molecular Genetics. After eight years of post-graduate schooling, he planted himself in the world of periodontal research at the Harvard-affiliated Forsyth Institute in Boston. Dr. Hillman's main interest was preventing bacterial infections through the use of "replacement therapy" for tooth decay. An example would be working on a mouth rinse that could be administered by a dentist to provide solid protection against cavities. "I decided to take my periodontal and molecular genetics training and use it for researching bacteria in the oral cavity," said Dr. Hillman.

One day, he attended a lecture given by a renowned and revered microbiologist, Sigmund Socransky, Ph.D., who had been associated with the Forsyth Institute for years and acted as the principal investigator on studies that looked into controlling periodontal infections and gingival epithelial cells inside the oral cavity.

"Dr. Socransky talked about a particular bacterium—pathogenic in scope—that was believed to cause periodontal disease," said Dr. Hillman. "He mentioned during the course of his lecture that patients have this organism in their mouths most of the time, if not all of the time. I started to wonder why more of us don't have diseases caused by this pathogenic bacterium. I wondered, too, if there were other bacteria present in the oral cavity that could inhibit the growth of the organism causing this disease."

Back in his laboratory, Dr. Hillman performed several simple experiments to determine which good bacteria inside the mouth inhibited the bad bacteria from initiating the disease process. This was his introduction into oral probiotics research 25 years ago.

"As part of my research into replacement therapy, we would introduce a stream of bacteria into a person's mouth—a living, breathing stream," said Dr. Hillman. "This bacterium had the ability to persistently colonize, which meant a single treatment of this bacteria could provide lifelong protection against tooth decay. My thought was, maybe we could do the same sort of thing with gum organisms, but it turned out that any good bacteria would disappear rather quickly in the mouth. After a while, I felt like I was hitting a brick wall, so I put my probiotic research aside for a while. Besides, no one had ever heard of probiotics at that time anyway."

Several years passed, and Dr. Hillman was in Amsterdam, The Netherlands, attending another medical conference. While on a lunch break, he noticed that his European colleagues were digging into a large, refrigerated barrel and taking out small plastic containers containing several ounces of a dairy-colored liquid. Then they would open and drink the contents of the tiny container.

"I'm a curious sort," Dr. Hillman said. "So I went over and pulled one of the plastic bottles out of the barrel and noticed that the label said the drink was for probiotic health. It struck me that there really were people willing to do something on a day-to-day basis to promote healthy organisms inside their bodies."

Was the probiotic drink in Amsterdam a bottle of Yakult, the Japanese probiotic drink that established a beachhead in Europe a couple of decades ago?

"It could have been," replied Dr. Hillman. "But I do know the drink contained *Lactobacillus* and *Bifidobacteria* and the usual panoply of bacteria for gastrointestinal health. At any rate, when I got home, I decided to resurrect the idea of using beneficial bacteria in the mouth as a probiotic way to promote good health."

In addition to his research work, Dr. Hillman was on the faculty at the Forsyth Institute and at the Harvard Dental School for 15 years, so these were incredibly busy years. He never lost his thirst for learning more about the good *and* bad microorganisms that swim in the nooks and crannies of the oral cavity. Personal health concerns, however, forced him to move from damp and cold Boston to sunny Florida in the early 1990s, where Dr. Hillman became a teaching faculty member at the University of Florida in Gainesville.

Teeming with Bacteria

Even though Dr. Hillman's academic environment changed locales, the flame still burned for finding the right beneficial bacteria in the oral cavity—bacteria that could improve the health of teeth and gums. The concept sounded simple but was incredibly complex, even though every first-year periodontal researcher knew that the human mouth teemed with bacteria. Good bacteria, he knew, lurked around the teeth and gums; otherwise, our mouths would be periodontal cesspools. On the other hand, bad bacteria caused disease when they overpopulated and took over the oral cavity. When gum disease struck, bad bacteria could enter the bloodstream, where they would travel to other parts of the body with mischief on their minds.

Dr. Hillman was aware of research from the Mayo Clinic showing that tooth decay and gum disease could be linked to heart disease, diabetes, osteoporosis, certain cancers, eating disorders, and sexually transmitted diseases. In some cases, like that of HIV/AIDS and osteoporosis, symptoms could show up in the mouth first. In other cases, bad bacteria thriving in the mouth contributed to systemic inflammation, which increased the risk of several life-threatening conditions.

Inspired to continue his scientific quest, Dr. Hillman asked for academic leave from the University of Florida College of Dentistry, where he was a professor of oral microbiology, so that he could devote himself full-time to researching microorganisms and how they worked in the mouth. He wanted to get back to laboratory work isolating the more than 500 species of bacteria, good and bad, swirling around the oral cavity.

And then an "ah-ha" moment—appropriate for someone in his line of work—happened.

Dr. Hillman, after more than a 20-year quest, came across three natural strains of bacteria that—when successfully combined into a single mixture—helped patients maintain healthy gums and teeth. A pair of these beneficial bacteria, known as *Streptococcus oralis* and *Streptococcus uberis,* are normally present in dental plaque. The third strain of beneficial bacteria is called *Streptococcus rattus.* When put together in a single stream, Dr. Hillman determined that they prevented the growth of bacteria responsible for periodontal diseases such as tooth decay and gum disease in clinical testing. The trio of beneficial bacteria exerted its largest influence against a ruinous bacteria known as *Streptococcus mutans*, which produces lactic acid from sugar in the diet. Higher levels of lactic acid bacteria in the mouth are harmful because lactic acid can erode enamel and cause cavities.

Dr. Hillman, who called the three strains of beneficial bacteria ProBiora3, set in motion the wheels to patent the technology and form a company called Oragenics, Inc., taking on the role of chief scientific officer. When I happened to read the Natural Products Insider article that day, Dr. Hillman and his fledgling corporation were announcing the promising results of a clinical trial that established the effects of ProBriora3 on specific disease-causing bacteria in the mouths of a test group of young, healthy adults. The news release declared that ProBiora3 could also "produce a whitening effect and decrease levels of volatile sulfur-containing compounds (SCCs), which contribute to halitosis."

Translation: ProBiora3 could whiten teeth and help bad breath, too.

My excitement extends to what oral probiotics can add to the Probiotic Diet. In my mind, this was a missing piece since the way people have tried to make their teeth, gums, and mouth healthy in the past was strikingly similar to use of antibiotics for the gut or the use of feminine hygiene products for women by simply destroying the bad germs without restoring the good guys.

Probiotic Killers

The "oral care" market, an eight-billion-dollar annual business in the United States, is huge because every single man, woman, and child brushes his or her teeth while just about everyone gargles with mouthwash, uses teeth whiteners, sucks on breath mints, chews gum to overcome bad breath, or plops drops of breath freshener on their tongues.

But as Henny Youngman, another '50s comedian that Grandma Rose loved, would say, "Take your mouthwashes and mints—please!"

The leading, green-colored mouth rinse, which puckers the mouth and makes the tongue tingle, may "kill germs on contact," but it kills bad *and* good germs—just like antibiotics. Dr. Hillman said popular mouthwashes lack "substantivity," which means they act inside the mouth until the moment you spit out the stinging solution into the bathroom sink. "This is different than our probiotic approach, where the bacteria in ProBiora3 stays on the teeth and works continually through-out the day."

The reason why popular mouthwashes burn in your mouth is because they contain a significant amount of alcohol, up to 27 percent of volume to provide that tingly sensation. But a spoonful of sugar helps the medicine go down: mouthwashes are sweetened with sorbitol, sucralose, and sodium saccharine, and there's nothing natural about these artificial sweeteners.

Researchers have been suggesting for years that the high alcohol content in mouthwash acts on the cells lining the mouth in such a way that they clear a path for cancer-causing substances in foods or nicotine to get through. Clinical studies looking at the possible link between mouthwash and cancer have been undertaken for 30 years, and while scientists say nothing conclusive can be gathered from the data, a recent study publishing in the *American Journal of Epidemiology* found that twice-a-day mouthwash use could have a significant risk for head and neck cancer. The Centers for Disease Control and Prevention, however, replied that there is no strong link between alcohol-containing mouthwash and oral cancer, although excessive use "should be discouraged."[1]

I don't think *any* mouthwash with alcohol should be encouraged, and besides, there are alternatives. There are many healthy oral care companies whose products are available at health food stores and progressive groceries nationwide that offer mouthwashes that don't contain dyes, saccharin, artificial flavors or nasty chemicals like phthalates found in other oral care products,

FOOD FOR THOUGHT

When you think about it, it's astonishing that more bad things *don't* happen in the mouth, considering all the downright unhealthy—and probiotic-unfriendly—foods and beverages we send down the gullet.

Dr. Hillman agrees. "You know, it's pretty amazing what we do to the microflora in our mouths on a day-to-day basis, and what we get away with. It's also pretty remarkable how we can disrupt the normal ecology inside the mouth and not wind up with more disease," he said.

such as toothpaste. Phthalates harm the developing testes of young boys and can damage children's lungs, liver, and kidneys.

That's why only natural toothpastes are acceptable for the Rubin family. (Sorry, we don't believe in mouth rinses, so there is no Official Mouthwash either.) Another reason that we're not fans of commercially available toothpastes is because they contain artificial sweeteners, potassium nitrate, sodium mono-fluorophosphate, and trace amounts of fluoride ion. I figured out a long time ago that those red, white, and blue stripes weren't made from fresh strawberries, coconuts, and blueberries.

Our goal is to help our kids get through life cavity-free, which is not a pipe dream. I can still see the grainy black-and-white pictures of the happy Eskimos in the Far North and the isolated Polynesians in the South Pacific pictured in Dr. Price's book, their smiles revealing two rows of pearly-white teeth. If these indige-nous people from the 1930s could get through life with teeth free of decay and cavities, then my kids can do it, too.

I don't think my children will need teeth-whitening products when they grow older either. I put teeth whiteners in a far worse category than mouthwashes. In the blossoming world of cos-metic dentistry, teeth whitening reigns supreme since whiter teeth are associated with beauty and a healthier lifestyle. When people have a thousand-watt smile, they are perceived as being more attractive, friendlier, and trustworthy.

Celebrities' whiter-than-white smiles on *People* magazine covers have spurred sales of teeth-whitening products and cus-tom-made bleaching trays through the roof. Because there's an emphasis on fast results, these teeth-whitening products bleach your smile with high concentrations of a chemically produced hydrogen peroxide or carbamide peroxide gel, which can dam-age gums and cause pitting and etching of teeth enamel.

If you're ever noticed teeth or gum sensitivity after using a teeth-whitening trays or strips, that's because the harshness of the peroxide solution can erode the gum tissues and create inflammation. In addition, most teeth-whitening products pit and roughen the surface of all teeth and can stain veneers and dental crowns. Since teeth that have been pitted and edged are more susceptible to staining in the future, this leads to a whitening-and-re-whitening cycle that can further disrupt the balance of oral health.

The rule of thumb for conventional teeth whiteners is that the shorter the contact time, the harsher and stronger the concentration of hydrogen peroxide must be to whiten the teeth. ProBiora3's *Streptococcus oralis*, on the other hand, produces a very low dose of natural hydrogen peroxide as its natural byproduct. Since the three natural strains of beneficial bacteria in ProBiora3 work around the clock, this long contact time enables a gradual whitening effect of three to four shades in 30 days that is safe and effective while sustaining the natural healthy balance in the mouth. Over-the-counter whitening products and those professionally applied in dental offices, however, are extremely harsh and disrupt the fragile ecosystem in the oral cavity and create an even greater imbalance in the mouth's microflora.

As this good bacteria are replenished daily, they create a gradual tooth whitening that lasts 24 hours a day when the bacteria are replenished twice a day when chewing on the ProBiora3 mints. The long contact time and very low doses of natural hydrogen peroxide create a healthy white smile. This is a much better route than bleaching fragile teeth enamel with high levels of harsh chemicals that create a roughness on the tooth's surface. *Streptococcus oralis* binds to the surface of the teeth, crowding out harmful bacteria by competing for the same nutrients and surfaced spaces. With daily use, the colonization of *Streptococcus oralis* provides a constant and expanding population for gradual and continuing whitening effects. The hydrogen peroxide metabolites of *Streptococcus oralis* also contribute to the

MOUTHFUL OF ABUSE

The mouth is the gateway to the body, the beginning of digestion, a reflection of our souls, and a harbinger of disease, but even though good health starts in the mouth, we sure don't treat our oral terrain very well. According to the American Dental Association, tooth decay is the most common chronic infectious disease in the world. Five billion people in the world—out of the 7.8 billion currently inhabiting Earth—are affected by tooth decay ranging from cavities to gum disease. You can blame the sugary foods found in every culture across the globe.

"Tooth decay is what we call a multifactorial disease," said Dr. Hillman. "It's all about food, diet, and bacteria. With daily use of ProBiora3, a growing population of good bacteria builds and wins out over the harmful bacteria for space and nutrients."

breath-freshening features of the ProBiora3 blend by inhibiting the growth of periodontal pathogens.

When do ProBiora3 users begin to observe positive benefits? In clinical trials, young, healthy individuals using ProBiora3 twice daily for a month experienced a significant drop in the numbers of opportunistic bacteria in their mouths. In weeks, you'll notice that your teeth are whiter and your breath is fresher—and less offensive to family members and co-workers.

Dr. Hillman's discovery of three naturally occurring strains of bacteria that are normal residents of healthy mouths is why I'm so excited about ProBiora3. I'm thrilled that we finally have a highly effective natural approach to maintaining the balance of oral microflora, which naturally promotes healthy teeth and gums, fresher breath, and whiter teeth.

With these ProBiora3 mints, you take one in the morning and the other in the late afternoon or evening. Since the natural habitat of *Streptococcus oralis*, *Streptococcus uberis*, and *Streptococcus rattus* is the mouth, they are a locally acting probiotic to the mouth and do not cause any harm when they travel on to the digestive system. "These bacteria do not survive in nature outside of the mouth and so simply pass through the gastrointestinal tract and are excreted," explained Dr. Hillman. "They are not absorbed into the body, nor do they stimulate an immune response."

I asked Dr. Hillman if ProBiora3 is appropriate for use by children. "Certainly, because ProBiora3 is safe for all ages. We have reformulated ProBiora3 into a kid's version because gum health is not an issue for children, but tooth decay certainly is. That's why everybody in my family is using ProBiora3."

So will the Rubin family. I see ProBiora3 as a win-win for the body. Not only does the blend of friendly probiotics keep your oral terrain clean and fresh, but fewer bad organisms make their way to the gut, which shows you that oral probiotics are really the first line of defense.

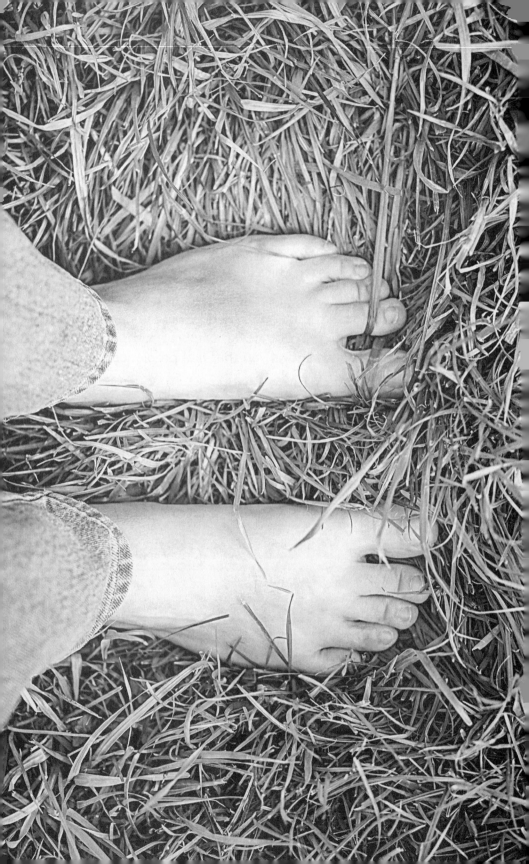

10

IT'S TIME TO EAT DIRT

I didn't know Dr. Josh Axe back when he was helping his mother defeat cancer for the second time, but I was in his life then without me even knowing it. He'd picked up a copy of my book *The Maker's Diet* and was blown away. His mom and he started reading the book and following my advice, and it was amazing what happened in his mom's life after Josh discovered the importance of the gut when it comes to health and healing from the inside out.

For years, he and I have both been striving, searching, and seeking to find the "perfect" probiotic or gut supplement. After trying dozens of different brands of probiotics from around the world, the radical results we wanted never came.

Until, that is, we discovered the power of eating dirt.

Is eating dirt part of your diet? Before you get a bad taste in your mouth, consider this: If you were to take away the water in our bodies, you'd be left with mostly dirt. It's true.

We're made of 60 of the most abundant elements in the Earth's crust, an amalgam of its elements, including oxygen, hydrogen, carbon, nitrogen, calcium and phosphorus, with traces of potassium, sulfur, sodium, iron and magnesium. All of these elements come together to make a living, breathing human being.

Now, when I say "eat dirt," I'm not ordering you to actually scoop up a handful of soil and eat it. (Well, not exactly.) True, ensuring you get daily micro-exposures to soil-based organisms (SBOs) in dirt and other plant life is important for your health. But I urge you to embrace the idea of "eating dirt" as a broader philosophy, an overarching principle my friend Dr. Josh Axe has been teaching for years when he talks about how to treat leaky gut syndrome and transform your health.

Health Benefits of Eating Dirt

Soil-based organisms (SBOs) support gut health and immune response. Why, exactly?

In the plant world, SBOs help plants grow. Without their protection, otherwise healthy plants become malnourished and are susceptible to disease or contamination by fungi, yeasts, molds and candida.

Just as plants grow best in healthy soil teeming with highly active microorganisms, you, too, need these organisms to live a long, healthy life.

More than 800 studies exist in scientific literature that reference soil-based organisms. Their common denominator is that they link SBOs to successfully treating a wide variety of health conditions, including:

- allergies
- asthma
- irritable bowel syndrome
- ulcerative colitis
- flatulence

- nausea
- indigestion
- malabsorption
- nutrient deficiencies
- autoimmune and inflammatory diseases
- bacterial, fungal and viral infections

We now know that SBOs nourish cells in the colon and liver and actually create new compounds, such as B vitamins, vitamin K2, antioxidants and enzymes.

SBOs can destroy or crowd out harmful pathogens, such as candida, fungi and parasites. They also kill off bad bacteria that can bind to or puncture the gut wall. They've been shown to bind to toxins and extract them from the body. SBOs also help regulate the immune system and naturally reduce inflammation in the gut and throughout the entire body.

The idea of eating dirt has also been around a long time, dating back to Hippocrates more than 2,500 years ago. You name the civilized cultures in past millennia and you'll find a record of those people consciously including a bit of dirt in their diets.

Take the era before refrigeration, for example. Back then, it was common to store food by burying it in the ground or storing it in a dirt cellar, which helped keep bad bacteria and yeast at bay because of the lower temperature and microbes in the soil that help preserve the food.

Today's generation is missing out on vitamin dirt in a big way, thanks to our collective obsession with over-sanitizing and anti-bacterial overkill—like sanitizing hand gels, antibacterial soap and germ-killing wipes. Our connection to dirt is dwindling, too.

Decades ago, vegetable gardens and flower beds dotted almost every backyard, putting people in close contact with the earth. Kids played outside in the woods from dawn to dusk, often after taking care of animals on a farm.

We can't reverse time, of course, and we're lucky to be living in an era of such incredible progress. But all that progress comes with a price, and we must be mindful not to get rid of the benefits along with the problems.

We can add facets of that earlier, simpler lifestyle back into our days, and in doing so we will benefit not only physically but also emotionally and spiritually and help heal our ailing guts in the process.

It starts with eating dirt.

From Your Mouth to the Deep South

I'll never forget the moment when I first discovered the power of dirt. I remember it like it was yesterday. I was reading a typewritten page that talked about a dark-colored powder that contained soil-based probiotics you would normally find in healthy food, plants, and in soil. And, unlike the other probiotics that I consumed (which could be called lactic acid bacteria), these probiotics were hardy. They survived extremes in temperature and certainly didn't need refrigeration. Stomach acid didn't destroy them, antibiotics didn't destroy them, caffeine didn't destroy them, and room temperatures didn't destroy them.

They were ultra-hardy, almost as if they had a shield around them naturally.

I also learned that in this powder was a food source for these probiotics called *prebiotics*. The compounds that these probiotics created in fermentation that could now be called *postbiotics* were also there. And despite my disappointments in probiotics previously, I committed to six weeks of consuming this probiotic with soil-based organisms, and my health was transformed.

Of course, this was 20-something years ago now. Since then, neither my nor Josh's family would dream of going a day without our SBOs. They form this army inside that makes us feel comfortable and safe when our families eat at restaurants, travel around the country or around the world, or get exposed to all kinds of people and foods. We know that inside our gut, billions of soil-based organisms are there protecting us.

Josh and I have spent the last few decades telling the world how important digestive health is, how important your gut is to your immune system, how important your gut is to your brain, how important your gut is to every organ and system of the body. And the key to your gut being healthy is the *right* probiotics.

We believe SBOs are the best choice.

Josh and I have often discussed how tragic it is that people believe all probiotics are created equal, when the absolute truth is, most probiotics never survive their journey to your digestive tract. On the other hand, SBO probiotics are so resilient—they actually make it from your mouth all the way through your body to your colon. That's why it is so important when you are buying and using a probiotic that it is a soil-based organism or SBO-based option.

You take typical probiotics out of the refrigerator and they die at room temperature, right? Yet we're supposed to put these into our bodies and expect them to make it all the way to our intestines? That's why I say that taking lactic acid bacteria, an acidophilus or bifidus and expecting it to support your gut is like trying to put out a forest fire with a squirt gun. Soil-based organisms, on the other hand, are able to travel "from your mouth to the deep south."

Still, soil-based organisms have been largely misunderstood, even with all the information available about probiotics at large. They weren't frequently utilized, but all of a sudden, these days we're seeing pizza crust with soil-based organisms, frozen yogurt with soil-based organisms, and most importantly, combination probiotics, such as our Ancient Nutrition SBO Probiotics, with soil-based organisms as well as a beneficial yeast called *Saccharomyces boulardii.*

It's never a bad time to have a strong immune system. I don't care what season it is. And we're talking about not just probiotics but prebiotics and postbiotics, the "gut health trifecta." Together, they work 24/7 creating enzymes and other powerful compounds to help support digestion, healthy immune system function, the reduction of occasional gas, bloating, constipation, and diarrhea.

Super Herbs

I call a good SBO-based probiotic supplement an "internal shield" because those hardy bugs set up shop in your gut and create what science has deemed a "zone of inhibition," which means an environment that is inhospitable to other microorganisms. They create compounds that form an internal shield in your gut and create enzymes around the clock to help you break down your food. I call them "overtime enzymes," or your 24-hour enzyme solution.

You can take them in supplement form, and I recommend doing so! But what if you also had an enzyme factory inside? SBOs last three to seven days in the human body. That means, for optimal health, you should replenish them like our ancestors would have in their diets. That's why, in addition to taking a supplement, eating fermented herbs is a great way to boost SBOs naturally.

- Ginger is the spice of about a thousand different uses. It's known as a stomachic, which is a weird way of saying it's good for your digestion. Ginger is great for supporting and addressing occasional nausea.

- Turmeric is similar to ginger, and together they form a powerful combo.

- Pepper is another great choice. When you consume black or red peppers, you're driving nutrients where they need to go and improving bioavailability. Ayurvedic practitioners knew this. They didn't know the scientific terms, but

PRE AND POST, TOO?!

We've certainly talked a lot about probiotics. But now I've thrown in prebiotics and postbiotics! I know it can get confusing, so I'll simplify it for you.

- **Probiotics**: beneficial bacteria that support gut health, immune health, and so much more.

- **Prebiotics**: fuel for the good bacteria. They are non-digestible fibers that become fermented by the bacteria in the gut—a process that promotes growth of more beneficial microorganisms.

- **Postbiotics**: While probiotics are the live bacteria, postbiotics are the various materials released or secreted by those bacteria. Unlike their probiotic relatives, they are not live. Postbiotics include peptides, as well as short-chain fatty acids such as acetate, butyrate and propionate.

So which ones do you need? The answer is all three! Fortunately, the diet and protocols in this book will provide you with just that.

for thousands of years, people have consumed warming spices with other compounds.

Josh and I hear patients and customers all the time talking about the big difference SBO-based probiotics have made in their lives. Most of the time, these folks have been taking other probiotics in the past and even eaten foods like sauerkraut but hardly noticed the difference. But add in the SBOs and presto! Their gut health was restored after years of dysfunction.

Soil-based organisms such as *Bacillus subtilis, Bacillus clausii, Bacillus coagulans,* and the friendly yeast *Saccharomyces boulardii* support what are known as "immunoglobulins" in the gut. These immunoglobulins are immune proteins that not only promote gut health but also deliver benefits to your entire body.

So if you want a healthy, supported, strong immune system, SBOs may be an answer to prayer.

How to Get "Dirt" into Your Diet

Once you start looking, you'll find countless ways to bring vital practices into your life that will make eating dirt possible. For example, on any given day, do the following:

1. Don't Overclean Your Food.

Our favorite way to eat dirt is through produce. When you purchase a fresh bunch of organically grown carrots at the farmers market, you're going to be far better off simply rinsing the carrots under running water instead of scrubbing them with a brush and some kind of chemical-laden produce wash, because the surface area of every carrot contains beneficial microbes.

When you do a light rinse only before consuming root vegetables like carrots, you can take in an average 500 milligrams of old-fashioned dirt each day, the same amount the average child consumes when playing outdoors.

Five hundred milligrams, essentially the size of an average supplement capsule, may not sound like much, but there are probably more beneficial microbes in that small amount of dirt than there are people living on Earth today.

2. Eat Probiotic Foods Like Kefir, Yogurt and Sauerkraut.

One of the reasons many people today are lactose intolerant (or have an allergy to dairy products) is that pasteurization kills off the beneficial probiotics and enzymes. According to several published medical studies, when someone with lactose intolerance consumes a dairy product that is raw or fermented—which is also higher in probiotics or enzymes—symptoms of lactose intolerance can diminish.

Kefir is especially beneficial, and a study in the *Journal of the American Dietetic Association* showed that kefir improves lactose digestion and tolerance in adults with lactose malabsorption.

3. Consume Raw Honey and Bee Pollen.

Many of us develop seasonal allergies because we don't spend much time outside and only have periodic exposure to pollen. But bee pollen, which worker bees collect on their bodies as they go to and from the hive, is also effective against a wide range of respiratory diseases.

In a study published in the *Journal of Pharmaceutical Biology*, researchers found that a mixture of raw honey and bee pollen showed a significant reduction in inflammation, improvement in immune function, and protection for the liver.

These gradual and natural immunizations from the microbes in the local honey and pollen take up residence in your gut and help modulate your immune system to adjust to the local environment. Honey also provides an excellent source of prebiotics to nourish the gut bugs as it educates them.

4. Get a Dog.

A study published in the medical journal *Clinical and Experimental Allergy* showed that having pets may improve the immune system and reduce allergies in children. The researchers studied 566 children with pets, including dogs and cats, taking blood samples when the children turned 18. They found that children who had cats had a 48 percent decrease in allergies, and those with dogs had a 50 percent decrease in allergies.

The explanation? An animal that plays in the dirt brings diverse microbes into the home, some of which the kids may breathe in and others that enter through the skin from touching their furry friends.

5. Swim in the Ocean.

You've probably heard or experienced for yourself how a cut seems to heal quickly after a dip in the ocean. Part of that is due to the salt content of the water, but the good microbes and bacteriophages present in salt water also have therapeutic merit.

A 2013 study in *Seminars in Arthritis and Rheumatism* found that those who took baths in mineral salts from the Dead Sea had a decrease in skin inflammation, rheumatoid arthritis, and psoriasis.

6. Get Grounded.

Just the simple act of putting your bare feet on the ground can affect your health in several surprising ways. When you stroll barefoot on grass, dirt paths, shoreline sand or even concrete sidewalks after a rainstorm, the soles of your bare feet come into direct contact with the surface of the earth, creating the opportunity for billions of bacteria and other beneficial microbes to catch a ride.

Researchers have become so fascinated with the health benefits of walking barefoot that it's given rise to a whole new field of study on the practice called "earthing" or "grounding."

A study in the *Journal of Environmental and Public Health* found that the earth's negative charges can literally "ground" us, similar to a grounding wire of an electrical tower. The connection between our skin and the earth's surface may help stabilize our internal bioelectrical environment in a way that regulates the normal functioning of our body systems. Researchers believe this exchange of electrical charge may factor into setting the biological clock, regulating circadian rhythms and balancing cortisol levels.

A 2006 study published in the *Journal of European Biology and Bioelectromagnetics* found that after participants engaged in earthing, their cortisol levels reverted to normal levels and rhythms, rising in the morning and falling in the late afternoon.

Just kicking off your shoes and walking on the ground for a few minutes every day could help you absorb this beneficial combination of electrical currents and microbes (or what we like to call "vitamin G").

7. Eat Dirt—Literally.

Perhaps one of the best dirt-based supplements is *shilajit*—pronounced shee-lay-jit—which comes from dense, nutrient- and mineral-rich soil high in the Himalayan mountains bordering India and Tibet.

Shilajit contains at least 85 minerals, including two of our all-time favorites—humic acid and fulvic acid—that are commonly used as a soil supplement in agriculture. Fulvic acid and humic acid help the body transport minerals through thick cell walls and prolong cell life.

Just as plants grow best in healthy soil teeming with highly active microorganisms, you, too, need these organisms to live a long, healthy life. SBOs have been linked to treating conditions like allergies, asthma, IBS, ulcerative colitis, flatulence, nausea, indigestion, malabsorption, nutrient deficiencies, autoimmune and inflammatory diseases, and bacterial, fungal and viral infections.

SBOs also help regulate the immune system and naturally reduce inflammation in the gut and throughout the entire body.

To start eating dirt, don't sanitize your food, eat probiotic foods, consume raw honey and bee pollen, get a dog, swim in the ocean, get grounded, and eat dirt—literally.

Next Up: The Probiotic Diet Eating Plan

We've covered a lot of ground so far, and now I'm ready to introduce the Probiotic Diet Eating Plan, which contains an abundance of probiotic-rich foods as well as a roadmap to following this three-phase, 12-week program.

I understand that this might be the most difficult undertaking that you've ever tried, especially if you're weakened by digestive diseases. If you're dealing with constipation or the bloating side of digestive disorders, then you should consider embarking on a cleanse before commencing with the Probiotic Diet. If you've been regularly afflicted with diarrhea or chronically loose stools, however, then cleansing is not recommended.

A cleanse is a way to "reboot" the digestive system—a chance for the body to restore itself while it purifies, captures, and removes toxins from the body. Cleanses can be done many different ways, but what works for me is spending the first day consuming only homemade chicken soup for breakfast, lunch, and dinner. You can find Grandma Rose's Healing Chicken Soup recipe on page 159.

A cleanse works in harmony with your body to release and remove toxins naturally so that you'll feel like a better you as you begin to follow the Probiotic Diet Eating Plan. If you decide to go longer than one day, then eat bountiful salads with your home-made soup or seasonal fruits. Stay away from anything with starch: breads, rice, pasta, etc. The goal is to leave you feeling lighter on your feet and with a brighter outlook as you begin Phase I of the Probiotic Diet Eating Plan.

All the best!

11

THE PROBIOTIC DIET EATING PLAN

Take a deep breath.

The following chapter—by far the longest one in *The Probiotic Diet*—introduces and outlines the Probiotic Diet Eating Plan. You will see that I have broken down this 12-week program into three phases. Each phase offers approved foods while restricting others, but you should know that the grains, fluid dairy products, sugar, potatoes, and corn curbed in Phase I are done so with an intention of starving the unfriendly microbes currently thriving in your gut.

I'm not going to sugarcoat this—which is an apropos phrase, considering what we must get done—but please listen closely to what I'm about to tell you: Phase I is the most difficult stretch of the Probiotic Diet, a one-month period where the "heavy lifting" gets done. If you follow Phase I to the best of your abilities, however, you should receive excellent results and feel much better digestively. Even if you quit after finishing Phase I, you've accomplished the Probiotic Diet in my book.

I highly recommend that you keep a daily chart or journal of your progress, especially after any of your digestive issues clears up. You want to get a real sense of what foods work for you and what foods react unfavorably in your gut. In our experience—speaking for Dr. Brasco—nearly 95 percent of individuals respond positively and experience improvement within the first month of the diet. The key to success is to adhere to the program with **radical fanaticism.**

Yes, I just put those two words in boldface italics, just like what Elaine Gottschall did in *Food and the Gut Reaction* and later in *Breaking the Vicious Cycle*. But if you follow the Probiotic Diet program to a T and don't experience any improvements in digestive and overall health after completing the first month, you probably should look for another approach, which was Mrs. Gottschall's advice regarding the Specific Carbohydrate Diet.

Once you get through Phase I, you'll find Phase II to be progressively easier as certain foods are reintroduced to your diet. Phase III, simply put, is the "lifestyle phase." I recommend that you start with Phase I, but I've known people who've taken "baby steps" by starting with Phase II or Phase III. If you feel that Phase I would be too difficult, then start with Phase II or Phase III. The way I view things, this approach will be better than nothing.

Dr. Brasco and I salute you for trying the Probiotic Diet Eating Plan and incorporating probiotic-rich foods, beverages, and supplements into your diet.

Phase I (Week 1–Week 4)

The Probiotic Diet 12-week program begins with Phase I, or what I call the "healing stage." This first phase is the most rigorous because you must be very careful about the carbohydrates that you eat. By definition, carbohydrates are the sugars and starches contained in plant foods, and while they are a necessary part of a well-rounded diet, our modern-day diet revolves around sweetened or sugared foods such as breakfast cereals, blueberry muffins, cookies, ice cream, and mocha-flavored coffees. With so many excess carbohydrates piling on, so to speak, too many carbohydrates go undigested and unassimilated by the body, resulting in unfriendly microbes in your terrain.

The predominant form of carbohydrates contained in grains, fluid dairy products, sugar, potatoes, and corn are known as disaccharides, as I outlined in Chapter 6. A disaccharide is a "double sugar" that is composed of two molecules of single molecules (monosaccharides) linked to each other. When you consume too much refined white sugar and other disaccharide-rich foods, you're feeding the "bad" microorganisms and upsetting the balance of the intestinal flora—prompting digestive problems to strike.

During Phase I of the Probiotic Diet, you should avoid eating sugar unnecessarily and cut back on your starches considerably. I know that avoiding sugar and its sweet relatives—high fructose corn syrup, sucrose, molasses, and maple syrup—is easier said than done, but all those sweets can turn your health sour!

The carbohydrates you want to consume are low glycemic, high nutrient, low sugar, and high in monosaccharides. These would be most high-fiber fruits, especially berries, vegetables, nuts, seeds, and some legumes. Eating unrefined carbohydrate foods introduces fiber-rich foods into your body. Fiber is the indigestible remnants of plant cells found in vegetables, fruits, whole grains, nuts, seeds, and beans. Fiber-rich foods take longer to break down and are partially indigestible, which means that as these foods work their way through the digestive tract, they absorb water and increase the elimination of fecal waste in the large intestine.

Good sources of fiber are berries, fruits with edible skins (apples, pears, and grapes), citrus fruits, whole non-gluten grains (quinoa, millet, amaranth, and buckwheat) that are allowed in Phase III, green peas, carrots, cucumbers, zucchini, and tomatoes. Green leafy vegetables such as spinach are also fiber rich. Eating foods high in fiber and low in starches will immediately improve your digestion as you begin to "starve off" the harmful microorganisms in your gut.

You'll see in the approved foods lists that white sugar, artificial sweeteners, and preservatives are forbidden. Not eating these foods often causes temporary withdrawal-type symptoms such as headaches, carbohydrate cravings, less energy, mood swings, or even changes in your bowel habits. These "detox" reactions are indications that the program is working as the body works to cleanse toxins from the system. When you have the blahs, increase water intake and rest.

Phase I is designed to reduce the levels of unhealthy microbes (bacteria, yeast, viruses, and parasites) in your intestines and stabilize blood sugar levels, reduce inflammation, enhance digestion, and balance hormone levels in the body. This phase restricts disaccharide-heavy carbohydrate foods such as pastas and breads but makes up for it in the variety of delicious, filling foods you can enjoy. You are likely to see weight loss during this initial four-week period due to consuming carbohydrate-restrictive foods. There is also the added benefit of improved digestion, smoother skin, and increased energy levels.

During Phase I, you will also have to pay attention to the amount of water that you're drinking. The goal is a half-ounce of water for every pound you weigh, so someone weighing 150 pounds should drink 75 ounces of water daily, which is a little more than a half-gallon. In addition, stay away from any alcohol—wine, beer, or mixed drinks—during Phase I. They can be reintroduced in Phase III.

Phase I Foods

Legend: Approved ✔ Avoid ✗

Meat (grass-fed/organic is best)

✔ Bone broth protein

✔ Bone broth collagen

✔ beef

✔ veal

✔ lamb

✔ buffalo

✔ venison

✔ elk

✔ goat

✔ bone soup/stock

✔ liver and heart (must be organic)

✔ beef or buffalo sausage (no pork casing—natural and nitrite/nitrate-free is best)

✔ beef or buffalo hot dogs (no pork casing—natural and nitrite/nitrate-free is best)

✔ liver and heart (must be organic or grass-fed)

✗ pork

✗ ham

✗ bacon

✗ sausage (pork)

✗ imitation meat product (soy)

✗ ostrich

✗ veggie burgers

✗ emu

✗ frog

✗ turtle

✗ alligator

Fish (wild freshwater/ocean-caught fish is best; make sure it has fins and scales)

✔ salmon

✔ halibut

✔ tuna

✔ cod

- ✔ scrod
- ✔ grouper
- ✔ haddock
- ✔ mahi mahi
- ✔ pompano
- ✔ wahoo
- ✔ trout
- ✔ tilapia
- ✔ orange roughy
- ✔ sea bass
- ✔ snapper
- ✔ mackerel
- ✔ herring
- ✔ sole
- ✔ whitefish
- ✔ fish bone soup/stock
- ✔ tuna (canned in spring water)
- ✔ salmon (canned in spring water)
- ✔ sardines (canned in water or olive oil only)
- ✘ fried, breaded fish
- ✘ catfish
- ✘ eel
- ✘ squid
- ✘ shark
- ✘ avoid all shellfish, including crab, clams, oyster, mussels, lobster, shrimp, scallops, and crawfish

Poultry (pastured/organic is best)

- ✔ chicken
- ✔ Cornish game hen
- ✔ Guinea fowl
- ✔ turkey
- ✔ duck
- ✔ bone soup/stock
- ✔ natural chicken or turkey hot dogs (no pork casing—organic and nitrite/nitrate-free is best)
- ✔ chicken or turkey bacon (no pork casing—organic and nitrite/nitrate-free is best)
- ✔ natural deli meats, including chicken, turkey, and roast beef
- ✔ chicken or turkey sausage (no pork casing—natural and nitrite/nitrate-free is best, and use sparingly in Phase I)

- ✔ liver and heart (must be organic or grass-fed)
- ✘ fried, breaded chicken

- ✘ avoid processed lunch meats, especially ham

Eggs (high omega-3/DHA or organic is best)

- ✔ chicken eggs (whole with yolk)
- ✔ duck eggs (whole with yolk)

- ✘ imitation eggs (such as Egg Beaters)

Dairy (organic is best in whole form)

- ✔ whole milk plain yogurt (plain)
- ✔ sheep's milk yogurt (plain)
- ✔ goat's milk yogurt (plain)
- ✔ soft goat's, cow's, or sheep's milk cheese
- ✔ sheep's milk hard cheese
- ✔ goat's milk hard cheese
- ✔ feta cheese (sheep's milk or goat's milk)
- ✔ full-fat plain kefir
- ✔ full-fat cottage cheese
- ✔ ricotta cheese
- ✔ full-fat sour cream

- ✔ plain almond milk (unsweetened)
- ✔ cultured buttermilk
- ✔ goat's milk protein powder (for use in smoothies)
- ✘ soy milk
- ✘ rice milk
- ✘ avoid milk, ice cream, processed cheese food
- ✘ flavored, low-fat, or fat-free cheese, yogurt, and kefir
- ✘ dry milk (many processed foods contain this ingredient)

Fats and oils (organic is best)

- ✔ flaxseed oil (not for cooking)
- ✔ butter oil (ghee)
- ✔ hempseed oil (not for cooking)
- ✔ avocado
- ✔ cow's milk butter
- ✔ goat's milk butter
- ✔ expeller-pressed sesame oil
- ✔ coconut milk/cream (canned or fresh)
- ✔ extra-virgin coconut oil (best for cooking)
- ✔ extra-virgin olive oil (not best for cooking)
- ✘ lard
- ✘ margarine
- ✘ shortening
- ✘ soy oil
- ✘ safflower oil
- ✘ canola oil
- ✘ sunflower oil
- ✘ corn oil
- ✘ cottonseed oil
- ✘ any partially hydrogenated oil

Vegetables (organic, fresh or frozen, is best)

- ✔ squash (winter or summer)
- ✔ broccoli
- ✔ asparagus
- ✔ beets
- ✔ cauliflower
- ✔ Brussels sprouts
- ✔ cabbage
- ✔ carrots
- ✔ celery
- ✔ cucumber
- ✔ eggplant
- ✔ pumpkin
- ✔ garlic
- ✔ onion
- ✔ okra
- ✔ mushrooms
- ✔ peas
- ✔ peppers
- ✔ string beans
- ✔ tomatoes

- ✔ lettuce (all varieties)
- ✔ spinach
- ✔ artichokes (French, not Jerusalem)
- ✔ leafy greens (kale, collard, broccoli rabe, mustard greens, etc.)
- ✔ sprouts (broccoli, sunflower, pea shoots, radish, etc.)
- ✔ sea vegetables (kelp, dulse, nori, kombu, hijiki, etc.)
- ✔ raw, fermented vegetables (lacto-fermented only, no vinegar)
- ✘ corn
- ✘ sweet potatoes
- ✘ white potatoes

Beans and legumes (soaked or fermented is best)

- ✔ lentils
- ✔ small amounts of fermented soybean paste (miso) as a broth
- ✘ soybeans
- ✘ tofu
- ✘ tempeh (fermented soybean loaf)
- ✘ black beans
- ✘ kidney beans
- ✘ navy beans
- ✘ white beans
- ✘ garbanzo beans
- ✘ lima beans
- ✘ pinto beans
- ✘ red beans
- ✘ split beans
- ✘ broad beans
- ✘ black-eyed peas

Nuts, seeds and their butters (e.g., almond butter organic, raw, or soaked is best; chew well)

- ✔ almonds
- ✔ pumpkinseeds
- ✔ hempseed
- ✔ flaxseed
- ✔ sunflower seeds
- ✔ almond butter

- ✔ hempseed butter
- ✔ sunflower butter
- ✔ tahini, sesame butter
- ✔ pumpkinseed butter
- ✔ macadamia nuts
- ✔ hazelnuts
- ✔ pecans
- ✔ walnuts
- ✔ Brazil nuts
- ✔ chia seeds
- ✔ tempeh
- ✘ honey-roasted nuts
- ✘ peanuts
- ✘ peanut butter
- ✘ cashews

Condiments, spices, seasonings, cooking ingredients, and salad dressings (organic is best)

- ✔ ketchup (natural or organic)
- ✔ hot sauce (preservative-free)
- ✔ salsa (fresh or canned, organic)
- ✔ guacamole (fresh)
- ✔ tomato sauce (no added sugar)
- ✔ apple cider vinegar
- ✔ soy sauce (wheat-free), tamari
- ✔ mustard
- ✔ Herbamare seasoning
- ✔ Celtic sea salt
- ✔ omega-mayonnaise
- ✔ umeboshi paste
- ✔ Bragg brand salad dressings
- ✔ Bragg Liquid Aminos
- ✔ balsamic vinegar
- ✔ red wine vinegar
- ✔ herbs and spices (no added stabilizers)
- ✔ pickled ginger (preservative- and color-free)
- ✔ wasabi (preservative- and color-free)
- ✔ capers
- ✔ cooking wine (organic red and white)

- ✔ homemade salad dressings and marinades using Phase I-allowable ingredients
- ✔ organic flavoring extracts (alcohol-based, no sugar added, vanilla, almond, etc.)
- ✘ all spices that contain added sugar
- ✘ commercial ketchup with sugar
- ✘ commercial barbecue sauce with sugar
- ✘ white vinegar

Fruits (organic, fresh or frozen, is best)

- ✔ blueberries
- ✔ strawberries
- ✔ blackberries
- ✔ raspberries
- ✔ cherries
- ✔ grapefruit
- ✔ lemon
- ✔ lime
- ✔ pomegranate
- ✔ cranberries (not dried)
- ✔ apples (with skin)
- ✔ olives
- ✔ melons
- ✔ apricots (not dried)
- ✔ peaches
- ✔ grapes
- ✔ orange
- ✔ pears
- ✔ papaya
- ✔ kiwi
- ✔ nectarines
- ✔ pineapple
- ✔ plums
- ✔ fresh figs
- ✘ bananas
- ✘ mangoes
- ✘ dried fruit
- ✘ canned fruit

Beverages

- ✔ bone broth
- ✔ purified, non-chlorinated water

- ✔ natural sparkling water, no carbonation added (such as Voss or Gherolsteiner)
- ✔ herbal teas (preferably organic)—unsweetened or with a small amount of honey or Stevia
- ✔ raw vegetable juice (beet or carrot juice—maximum 25 percent of total)
- ✔ lacto-fermented beverages (kombucha, kvass)
- ✔ certified organic coffee—buy whole beans, freeze them, and grind yourself when desired; flavor only with organic cream and a small amount of honey
- ✘ alcoholic beverages of any kind
- ✘ fruit juices
- ✘ pre-ground commercial coffee
- ✘ chlorinated tap water
- ✘ sodas

Sweeteners

- ✔ honey in very small amounts (2 tablespoons per day maximum, unheated and raw is best)
- ✘ Stevia
- ✘ Lo Han Guo
- ✘ sugar (all-natural cane sugar, and organic brown sugar, including organic sugars)
- ✘ maple syrup
- ✘ fructose or corn syrup
- ✘ all artificial sweeteners, including aspartame, sucralose, and acesulfame K
- ✘ sugar alcohol, including sorbitol and malitol, xylitol (in small quantities or in mints and gum)

Snacks/Miscellaneous

- ✔ goat's milk protein powder
- ✘ rice protein powder
- ✘ milk or whey protein powder from cow's milk

Grains and Starchy Carbohydrates

- ✗ arrowroot powder (as a substitute for cornstarch)
- ✗ avoid all grains and starchy foods
- ✗ bread
- ✗ pasta
- ✗ cereal
- ✗ rice
- ✗ oatmeal
- ✗ pastries
- ✗ baked goods
- ✗ corn tortillas

THE PROBIOTIC DIET: PHASE I

Sample 7-Day Eating Plan

Day 1

Upon waking

Probiotic supplement: consume a probiotic supplement containing *Bacillus subtilis, Bacillus coagulans,* and *Saccharomyces boulardii* (visit your local health food store for recommended brands).

Breakfast

Make a probiotic smoothie in a blender with the following ingredients:

> 1 cup plain yogurt or kefir (sheep's or goat's milk is best)
> 1 Tbsp. organic flaxseed oil
> 1 Tbsp. organic raw honey
> 1 cup of organic fruit (berries, peaches, pineapple, etc.)
> 2 Tbsp. multi collagen or bone broth protein powder
> Dash of vanilla extract (optional)

Oral probiotic supplement: after breakfast, consume a probiotic mint containing three probiotic strains clinically proven to improve oral health (visit your local health food store for recommended brands).

Lunch

Before eating, drink 8 ounces of water.

Probiotic beverage: 8 ounces of raw kombucha, kvass, kefir, or other lacto-fermented beverage.

Toss a green salad with mixed greens, tomatoes, avocado, carrots, cucumbers, celery, red cabbage, red peppers, red onions, and sprouts with three hard-boiled omega-3 pasture-raised eggs. **Caution**: if you suffer from frequent diarrhea, too much salad is irritating to your condition. You may consume steamed veggies instead. If you do consume salad, make sure you chew very well and eliminate the cabbage, peppers, and onions.

For the salad dressing, mix extra-virgin olive oil, apple cider vinegar or lemon juice, Celtic sea salt, herbs, and spices, or you may mix 1 tablespoon of extra-virgin olive oil with 1 tablespoon of a healthy store-bought dressing.

One apple with skin

Dinner

Before eating, drink 8 ounces of water.

Probiotic beverage: 8 ounces of raw kombucha, kvass, kefir, or other lacto-fermented beverage

Baked, poached, or grilled wild-caught salmon

Steamed broccoli

Toss a green salad with mixed greens, tomatoes, avocado, carrots, cucumbers, celery, red cabbage, red peppers, red onions, and sprouts.

For the salad dressing, mix extra-virgin olive oil, apple cider vinegar or lemon juice, Celtic sea salt, herbs, and spices, or you may mix 1 tablespoon of extra-virgin olive oil with 1 tablespoon of a healthy store-bought dressing.

Probiotic condiment: 2-4 ounces of cultured veggies, *kimchi*, or sauerkraut.

Oral probiotic supplement: after dinner, consume a probiotic mint containing three probiotic strains clinically proven to improve oral health (visit your local health food store for recommended brands).

Probiotic snacks

Raw almonds and a couple of ounces of raw cheese

Drink 8 ounces of water.

Before bed

Probiotic supplement: consume a probiotic supplement containing *Bacillus subtilis, Bacillus coagulans*, and *Saccharomyces boulardii* or an SBO probiotic.

Day 2

Upon waking

Probiotic supplement: consume a probiotic supplement containing *Bacillus subtilis, Bacillus coagulans,* and *Saccharomyces boulardii* (visit your local health food store for recommended brands).

Breakfast

Two or three pasture-raised eggs any style, cooked in one tablespoon of extra-virgin coconut oil

Stir-fried onions, mushrooms, and peppers

Probiotic beverage: 8 ounces of raw kombucha, kvass, kefir, or other lacto-fermented beverage

Oral probiotic supplement: after breakfast, consume a probiotic mint containing three probiotic strains clinically proven to improve oral health (visit your local health food store for recommended brands).

Lunch

Before eating, drink 8 ounces of water.

During lunch, drink 8 ounces of water or hot tea with honey.

Toss a green salad with mixed greens, tomatoes, avocado, carrots, cucumbers, celery, red cabbage, red peppers, red onions, and sprouts with 3 ounces of tuna. **Caution**: if you suffer from frequent diarrhea, too much salad is irritating to your condition. You may consume steamed veggies instead. If you do consume salad, make sure you chew very well and eliminate the cabbage, peppers, and onions.

For the salad dressing, mix extra-virgin olive oil, apple cider vinegar or lemon juice, Celtic sea salt, herbs, and spices, or you may mix 1 tablespoon of extra-virgin olive oil with 1 tablespoon of a healthy store-bought dressing.

One bunch of organic grapes

Probiotic beverage: 8 ounces of raw kombucha, kvass, kefir, or other lacto-fermented beverage

Dinner

Before eating, drink 8 ounces of water.

Roasted organic chicken

Cooked vegetables (carrots, onions, peas, etc.)

Toss a green salad with mixed greens, tomatoes, avocado, carrots, cucumbers, celery, red cabbage, red peppers, red onions, and sprouts.

For the salad dressing, mix extra-virgin olive oil, apple cider vinegar or lemon juice, Celtic sea salt, herbs, and spices, or you may mix 1 tablespoon of extra-virgin olive oil with 1 tablespoon of a healthy store-bought dressing.

Probiotic beverage: 8 ounces of raw kombucha, kvass, kefir, or other lacto-fermented beverage

Probiotic condiment: one unpasteurized pickled cucumber

Oral probiotic supplement: after dinner, consume a probiotic mint containing three probiotic strains clinically proven to improve oral health (visit your local health food store for recommended brands).

Probiotic snacks

4-6 ounces of whole milk yogurt with raw honey and fruit

Drink 8 ounces of water.

Before bed

Probiotic supplement: consume a probiotic supplement containing *Bacillus subtilis, Bacillus coagulans*, and *Saccharomyces boulardii.*

Day 3

Upon waking

Probiotic supplement: consume a probiotic supplement containing *Bacillus subtilis, Bacillus coagulans*, and *Saccharomyces boulardii.*

Breakfast

Four to eight ounces of organic whole milk yogurt with fruit (pineapple, peaches, or berries), honey, and a dash of vanilla extract

Handful of raw almonds

Oral probiotic supplement: after breakfast, consume a probiotic mint containing three probiotic strains clinically proven to improve oral health (visit your local health food store for recommended brands).

Lunch

Before eating, drink 8 ounces of water.

Toss a green salad with mixed greens, tomatoes, avocado, carrots, cucumbers, celery, red cabbage, red peppers, red onions, and sprouts with three hard-boiled omega-3 pasture-raised eggs.

For the salad dressing, mix extra-virgin olive oil, apple cider vinegar or lemon juice, Celtic sea salt, herbs, and spices, or you may mix 1 tablespoon of extra-virgin olive oil with 1 tablespoon of a healthy store-bought dressing.

One piece of fruit in season

Probiotic beverage: 8 ounces of raw kombucha, kvass, kefir, or other lacto-fermented beverage

Dinner

Before eating, drink 8 ounces of water.

> Red meat steak (beef, buffalo, or venison)
>
> Steamed broccoli
>
> Baked sweet potato with butter

Toss a green salad with mixed greens, tomatoes, avocado, carrots, cucumbers, celery, red cabbage, red peppers, red onions, and sprouts.

For the salad dressing, mix extra-virgin olive oil, apple cider vinegar or lemon juice, Celtic sea salt, herbs, and spices, or you may mix 1 tablespoon of extra-virgin olive oil with 1 tablespoon of a healthy store-bought dressing.

Probiotic condiment: 1-4 ounces of lacto-fermented raw salsa

Probiotic beverage: 8 ounces of raw kombucha, kvass, kefir, or other lacto-fermented beverage

Oral probiotic supplement: after dinner, consume a probiotic mint containing three probiotic strains clinically proven to improve oral health (visit your local health food store for recommended brands).

Probiotic snacks

> Four ounces of whole milk yogurt with fruit, honey, and a few almonds
>
> Drink 8 ounces of water.

Before bed

Probiotic supplement: consume a probiotic supplement containing *Bacillus subtilis*, *Bacillus coagulans*, and *Saccharomyces boulardii*.

Day 4

Upon waking

Probiotic supplement: consume a probiotic supplement containing *Bacillus subtilis, Bacillus coagulans*, and *Saccharomyces boulardii*.

Breakfast

Two or three soft-boiled or poached pasture-raised eggs

One grapefruit or orange

Probiotic beverage: 8 ounces of raw kombucha, kvass, kefir, or other lacto-fermented beverage

Oral probiotic supplement: after breakfast, consume a probiotic mint containing three probiotic strains clinically proven to improve oral health (visit your local health food store for recommended brands).

Lunch

Before eating, drink 8 ounces of water.

Toss a green salad with mixed greens, tomatoes, avocado, carrots, cucumbers, celery, red cabbage, red peppers, red onions, and sprouts with 3 ounces of tuna.

For the salad dressing, mix extra-virgin olive oil, apple cider vinegar or lemon juice, Celtic sea salt, herbs, and spices, or you may mix 1 tablespoon of extra-virgin olive oil with 1 tablespoon of a healthy store-bought dressing.

One bunch of grapes with seeds

Probiotic beverage: 8 ounces of raw kombucha, kvass, kefir, or other lacto-fermented beverage

Dinner

Before eating, drink 8 ounces of water.

Grilled chicken breast

Steamed veggies

Toss a green salad with mixed greens, tomatoes, avocado, carrots, cucumbers, celery, red cabbage, red peppers, red onions, and sprouts.

For the salad dressing, mix extra-virgin olive oil, apple cider vinegar or lemon juice, Celtic sea salt, herbs, and spices, or you may mix 1 tablespoon of extra-virgin olive oil with 1 tablespoon of a healthy store-bought dressing.

Probiotic condiment: 1-4 ounces of cultured veggies

Probiotic beverage: 8 ounces of raw kombucha, kvass, kefir, or other lacto-fermented beverage

Oral probiotic supplement: after dinner, consume a probiotic mint containing three probiotic strains clinically proven to improve oral health (visit your local health food store for recommended brands).

Probiotic snacks

Raw apple with skin and a couple ounces of raw cheese

Drink 8 ounces of water.

Before bed

Probiotic supplement: consume a probiotic supplement containing *Bacillus subtilis, Bacillus coagulans*, and *Saccharomyces boulardii*.

Day 5

Upon waking

Probiotic supplement: consume a probiotic supplement containing *Bacillus subtilis, Bacillus coagulans*, and *Saccharomyces boulardii*.

Breakfast

Two or three soft-boiled or poached pasture-raised eggs

One grapefruit

Probiotic beverage: 8 ounces of raw kombucha, kvass, kefir, or other lacto-fermented beverage

Oral probiotic supplement: after breakfast, consume a probiotic mint containing three probiotic strains clinically proven to improve oral health (visit your local health food store for recommended brands).

Lunch

Before eating, drink 8 ounces of water.

Toss a green salad with mixed greens, tomatoes, avocado, carrots, cucumbers, celery, red cabbage, red peppers, red onions, and sprouts with 3 ounces of tuna.

For the salad dressing, mix extra-virgin olive oil, apple cider vinegar or lemon juice, Celtic sea salt, herbs, and spices, or you may mix 1 tablespoon of extra-virgin olive oil with 1 tablespoon of a healthy store-bought dressing.

One bunch of grapes with seeds

Probiotic beverage: 8 ounces of raw kombucha, kvass, kefir, or other lacto-fermented beverage

Dinner

Before eating, drink 8 ounces of water.

Chicken Soup (see page 159 for the recipe)

Toss a green salad with mixed greens, tomatoes, avocado, carrots, cucumbers, celery, red cabbage, red peppers, red onions, and sprouts.

For the salad dressing, mix extra-virgin olive oil, apple cider vinegar or lemon juice, Celtic sea salt, herbs, and spices, or you may mix 1 tablespoon of extra-virgin olive oil with 1 tablespoon of a healthy store-bought dressing.

Probiotic condiment: 1-4 ounces of cultured veggies

Probiotic beverage: 8 ounces of raw kombucha, kvass, kefir, or other lacto-fermented beverage

Oral probiotic supplement: after dinner, consume a probiotic mint containing three probiotic strains clinically proven to improve oral health (visit your local health food store for recommended brands).

Probiotic snacks

Four ounces of whole milk yogurt with fruit, honey, and a few almonds

Drink 8 ounces of water.

Before bed

Probiotic supplement: consume a probiotic supplement containing *Bacillus subtilis, Bacillus coagulans*, and *Saccharomyces boulardii.*

Day 6

Upon waking

Probiotic supplement: consume a probiotic supplement containing *Bacillus subtilis, Bacillus coagulans*, and *Saccharomyces boulardii*.

Breakfast

> Two or three pasture-raised eggs cooked any style in one tablespoon of extra-virgin coconut oil
>
> One grapefruit or orange
>
> Handful of almonds

Probiotic beverage: 8 ounces of raw kombucha, kvass, kefir, or other lacto-fermented beverage

Oral probiotic supplement: after breakfast, consume a probiotic mint containing three probiotic strains clinically proven to improve oral health (visit your local health food store for recommended brands).

Lunch

Before eating, drink 8 ounces of water.

Toss a green salad with mixed greens, tomatoes, avocado, carrots, cucumbers, celery, red cabbage, red peppers, red onions, and sprouts with 3 ounces of tuna.

For the salad dressing, mix extra-virgin olive oil, apple cider vinegar or lemon juice, Celtic sea salt, herbs, and spices, or you may mix 1 tablespoon of extra-virgin olive oil with 1 tablespoon of a healthy store-bought dressing.

> One organic apple with the skin

Probiotic beverage: 8 ounces of raw kombucha, kvass, kefir, or other lacto-fermented beverage

Dinner

Before eating, drink 8 ounces of water.

> Roasted organic chicken
>
> Cooked vegetables (carrots, onions, peas, etc.)

Toss a green salad with mixed greens, tomatoes, avocado, carrots, cucumbers, celery, red cabbage, red peppers, red onions, and sprouts.

For the salad dressing, mix extra-virgin olive oil, apple cider vinegar or lemon juice, Celtic sea salt, herbs, and spices, or you may mix 1 tablespoon of extra-virgin olive oil with 1 tablespoon of a healthy store-bought dressing.

Probiotic condiment: 1-4 ounces of cultured veggies

Probiotic beverage: 8 ounces of raw kombucha, kvass, kefir, or other lacto-fermented beverage

Oral probiotic supplement: after dinner, consume a probiotic mint containing three probiotic strains clinically proven to improve oral health (visit your local health food store for recommended brands).

Probiotic snacks

> 4-6 ounces of whole milk yogurt with raw honey and vanilla
>
> Drink 8 ounces of water.

Before bed

Probiotic supplement: consume a probiotic supplement containing *Bacillus subtilis*, *Bacillus coagulans*, and *Saccharomyces boulardii.*

Day 7

Upon waking

Probiotic supplement: consume a probiotic supplement containing *Bacillus subtilis, Bacillus coagulans*, and *Saccharomyces boulardii*.

Breakfast

Make a probiotic smoothie in a blender with the following ingredients:

- 1 cup plain yogurt or kefir (sheep's or goat's milk is best)
- 1 Tbsp. organic flaxseed oil
- 1 Tbsp. organic raw honey
- 1 cup of organic fruit (berries, peaches, pineapple, etc.)
- 2 Tbsp. multi collagen or bone broth protein powder
- Dash of vanilla extract (optional)

Oral probiotic supplement: after breakfast, consume a probiotic mint containing three probiotic strains clinically proven to improve oral health (visit your local health food store for recommended brands).

Lunch

Before eating, drink 8 ounces of water.

Toss a green salad with mixed greens, tomatoes, avocado, carrots, cucumbers, celery, red cabbage, red peppers, red onions, and sprouts with 3 ounces of cold, poached, or canned wild-caught salmon.

For the salad dressing, mix extra-virgin olive oil, apple cider vinegar or lemon juice, Celtic sea salt, herbs, and spices, or you

may mix 1 tablespoon of extra-virgin olive oil with 1 tablespoon of a healthy store-bought dressing.

One piece of fruit in season

Probiotic beverage: 8 ounces of raw kombucha, kvass, kefir, or other lacto-fermented beverage

Dinner

Before eating, drink 8 ounces of water.

Baked or grilled fish of your choice

Steamed broccoli

Toss a green salad with mixed greens, tomatoes, avocado, carrots, cucumbers, celery, red cabbage, red peppers, red onions, and sprouts with three hard-boiled omega-3 pasture-raised eggs.

For the salad dressing, mix extra-virgin olive oil, apple cider vinegar or lemon juice, Celtic sea salt, herbs, and spices, or you may mix 1 tablespoon of extra-virgin olive oil with 1 tablespoon of a healthy store-bought dressing.

Probiotic condiment: 1-2 tablespoons of unpasteurized miso paste mixed in warm water to create a broth

Probiotic beverage: 8 ounces of raw kombucha, kvass, kefir, or other lacto-fermented beverage

Oral probiotic supplement: after dinner, consume a probiotic mint containing three probiotic strains clinically proven to improve oral health (visit your local health food store for recommended brands).

Probiotic snacks

Raw almonds and a couple of ounces of raw cheese

Drink 8 ounces of water.

Before bed

Probiotic supplement: consume a probiotic supplement containing *Bacillus subtilis, Bacillus coagulans,* and *Saccharomyces boulardii.*

NEED RECIPES?

You'll find some Probiotic Diet-friendly recipes involving fermented foods, sprouted grains, and dairy-rich smoothies in Chapter 14, "The Probiotic Diet Recipes." You'll also encounter some cleansing recipes made from delicious raw foods. You can also visit DrAxe.com for hundreds of healthy, gut-friendly recipes.

PHASE II (WEEK 5–WEEK 8)

Phase II allows for a greater variety of foods, which are listed below, but grains are still restricted. If you are still suffering painful symptoms in the gut, or you feel like you've gotten off track, you should implement Phase I again.

Phase II Food Additions and Subtractions from Phase I

Legend: Approved ✔ Avoid ✗

Dairy

✔ cow's-milk feta cheese

✔ blue cheese

✔ parmesan cheese

Eggs (high omega-3/DHA or organic is best)

✔ fish roe or caviar (fresh, not preserved)

Fats and oils (organic is best)

✔ expeller-pressed peanut oil (good for cooking)

Vegetables (organic, fresh or frozen, is best)

- ✔ sweet potatoes
- ✔ yams
- ✘ white potatoes
- ✘ corn

Beans and legumes (soaked or fermented is best)

- ✔ tempeh (fermented soybean loaf)
- ✔ black beans
- ✔ kidney beans
- ✔ navy beans
- ✔ white beans
- ✔ garbanzo beans
- ✔ lima beans
- ✔ pinto beans
- ✔ red beans
- ✔ split beans
- ✔ broad beans
- ✔ black-eyed peas
- ✘ tofu
- ✘ soybeans (edamame)

Nuts and seeds (organic, raw, or soaked is best)

- ✔ peanuts
- ✔ peanut butter
- ✔ cashews
- ✘ honey-roasted nuts
- ✘ nuts or seeds roasted in oil

Condiments, spices, seasonings (organic is best)

- ✔ healthy salad dressings (no canola oil, no fat-free dressings, no dressings with chemicals)

Fruits (organic, fresh or frozen, is best)

- ✔ bananas
- ✔ mangoes

- ✔ dates
- ✔ dried figs
- ✘ canned fruit

- ✔ dried fruits, including raisins, prunes, bananas, mango, and papaya

Beverages

- ✔ raw vegetable juice (beet or carrot—maximum 50 percent of total)

- ✔ coconut water

Sweeteners

- ✔ honey (no limitation on amount)
- ✔ Stevia in small quantities
- ✔ Lo Han Guo in small quantities

- ✔ xylitol in small quantities or in mints and gum
- ✔ erythritol in small quantities

Grains and starchy carbohydrates

- ✔ arrowroot powder (as a substitute for cornstarch)

The Probiotic Diet: Phase II

Sample 7-Day Eating Plan

Day 1

Upon waking

Probiotic supplement: consume a probiotic supplement containing *Bacillus subtilis*, *Bacillus coagulans*, and *Saccharomyces boulardii*.

Breakfast

Make a probiotic smoothie in a blender with the following ingredients:

- 1 cup plain yogurt or kefir (sheep's or goat's milk is best)
- 1 Tbsp. organic flaxseed oil
- 1 Tbsp. organic raw honey
- 1 cup of organic fruit (berries, peaches, pineapple, etc.)
- 2 Tbsp. multi collagen or bone broth protein powder
- Dash of vanilla extract (optional)

Oral probiotic supplement: after breakfast, consume a probiotic mint containing three probiotic strains clinically proven to improve oral health (visit your local health food store for recommended brands).

Lunch

Before eating, drink 8 ounces of water.

Probiotic beverage: 8 ounces of raw kombucha, kvass, kefir, or other lacto-fermented beverage.

Toss a green salad with mixed greens, tomatoes, avocado, carrots, cucumbers, celery, red cabbage, red peppers, red onions, and sprouts with three hard-boiled omega-3 pasture-raised eggs. Caution: if you suffer from frequent diarrhea, too much salad is irritating to your condition. You may consume steamed veggies instead. If you do consume salad, make sure you chew very well and eliminate the cabbage, peppers, and onions.

For the salad dressing, mix extra-virgin olive oil, apple cider vinegar or lemon juice, Celtic sea salt, herbs, and spices, or you may mix 1 tablespoon of extra-virgin olive oil with 1 tablespoon of a healthy store-bought dressing.

One apple with skin

Dinner

Before eating, drink 8 ounces of water.

Probiotic beverage: 8 ounces of raw kombucha, kvass, kefir, or other lacto-fermented beverage

Baked, poached, or grilled wild-caught salmon

Steamed broccoli

Toss a green salad with mixed greens, tomatoes, avocado, carrots, cucumbers, celery, red cabbage, red peppers, red onions, and sprouts.

For the salad dressing, mix extra-virgin olive oil, apple cider vinegar or lemon juice, Celtic sea salt, herbs, and spices, or you may mix 1 tablespoon of extra-virgin olive oil with 1 tablespoon of a healthy store-bought dressing.

Probiotic condiment: 2-4 ounces of cultured veggies, *kimchi*, or sauerkraut.

Oral probiotic supplement: after dinner, consume a probiotic mint containing three probiotic strains clinically proven to improve oral health (visit your local health food store for recommended brands).

Probiotic snacks

Raw almonds and a couple of ounces of raw cheese

Drink 8 ounces of water.

Before bed

Probiotic supplement: consume a probiotic supplement containing *Bacillus subtilis*, *Bacillus coagulans*, and *Saccharomyces boulardii*.

Day 2

Upon waking

Probiotic supplement: consume a probiotic supplement containing *Bacillus subtilis*, *Bacillus coagulans*, and *Saccharomyces boulardii*.

Breakfast

Two or three pasture-raised eggs any style, cooked in one tablespoon of extra-virgin coconut oil

Stir-fried onions, mushrooms, and peppers

Probiotic beverage: 8 ounces of raw kombucha, kvass, kefir, or other lacto-fermented beverage

Oral probiotic supplement: after breakfast, consume a probiotic mint containing three probiotic strains clinically proven to improve oral health (visit your local health food store for recommended brands).

Lunch

Before eating, drink 8 ounces of water.

During lunch, drink 8 ounces of water or hot tea with honey.

Toss a green salad with mixed greens, tomatoes, avocado, carrots, cucumbers, celery, red cabbage, red peppers, red onions, and sprouts with 3 ounces of tuna.

For the salad dressing, mix extra-virgin olive oil, apple cider vinegar or lemon juice, Celtic sea salt, herbs, and spices, or you may mix 1 tablespoon of extra-virgin olive oil with 1 tablespoon of a healthy store-bought dressing.

One bunch of organic grapes

Probiotic beverage: 8 ounces of raw kombucha, kvass, kefir, or other lacto-fermented beverage

Dinner

Before eating, drink 8 ounces of water.

Roasted organic chicken

Cooked vegetables (carrots, onions, peas, etc.)

Toss a green salad with mixed greens, tomatoes, avocado, carrots, cucumbers, celery, red cabbage, red peppers, red onions, and sprouts. Caution: if you suffer from frequent diarrhea, too much salad is irritating to your condition. You may consume steamed veggies instead. If you do consume salad, make sure you chew very well and eliminate the cabbage, peppers, and onions.

For the salad dressing, mix extra-virgin olive oil, apple cider vinegar or lemon juice, Celtic sea salt, herbs, and spices, or you

may mix 1 tablespoon of extra-virgin olive oil with 1 tablespoon of a healthy store-bought dressing.

Probiotic beverage: 8 ounces of raw kombucha, kvass, kefir, or other lacto-fermented beverage

Probiotic condiment: one unpasteurized pickled cucumber

Oral probiotic supplement: after dinner, consume a probiotic mint containing three probiotic strains clinically proven to improve oral health (visit your local health food store for recommended brands).

Probiotic snacks

4 to 6 ounces of whole milk yogurt with raw honey and fruit

Drink 8 ounces of water.

Before bed

Probiotic supplement: consume a probiotic supplement containing *Bacillus subtilis, Bacillus coagulans,* and *Saccharomyces boulardii.*

Day 3

Upon waking

Probiotic supplement: consume a probiotic supplement containing *Bacillus subtilis, Bacillus coagulans,* and *Saccharomyces boulardii.*

Breakfast

4 to 8 ounces of organic whole milk yogurt or cottage cheese with fruit (pineapple, peaches, or berries), honey, and a dash of vanilla extract

Handful of raw almonds

Oral probiotic supplement: after breakfast, consume a probiotic mint containing three probiotic strains clinically proven to improve oral health (visit your local health food store for recommended brands).

Lunch

Before eating, drink 8 ounces of water.

Toss a green salad with mixed greens, tomatoes, avocado, carrots, cucumbers, celery, red cabbage, red peppers, red onions, and sprouts with three hard-boiled omega-3 pasture-raised eggs.

For the salad dressing, mix extra-virgin olive oil, apple cider vinegar or lemon juice, Celtic sea salt, herbs, and spices, or you may mix 1 tablespoon of extra-virgin olive oil with 1 tablespoon of a healthy store-bought dressing.

One piece of fruit in season

Probiotic beverage: 8 ounces of raw kombucha, kvass, kefir, or other lacto-fermented beverage

Dinner

Before eating, drink 8 ounces of water.

Red meat steak (beef, buffalo, or venison)

Steamed broccoli

Baked sweet potato with butter

Toss a green salad with mixed greens, tomatoes, avocado, carrots, cucumbers, celery, red cabbage, red peppers, red onions, and sprouts.

For the salad dressing, mix extra-virgin olive oil, apple cider vinegar or lemon juice, Celtic sea salt, herbs, and spices, or you may mix 1 tablespoon of extra-virgin olive oil with 1 tablespoon of a healthy store-bought dressing.

Probiotic condiment: 1-4 ounces of lacto-fermented raw salsa

Probiotic beverage: 8 ounces of raw kombucha, kvass, kefir, or other lacto-fermented beverage

Oral probiotic supplement: after dinner, consume a probiotic mint containing three probiotic strains clinically proven to improve oral health (visit your local health food store for recommended brands).

Probiotic Snacks

4 to 6 ounces of whole milk yogurt with fruit, honey, and a few almonds

Drink 8 ounces of water.

Before bed

Probiotic supplement: consume a probiotic supplement containing *Bacillus subtilis, Bacillus coagulans*, and *Saccharomyces boulardii.*

Day 4

Upon waking

Probiotic supplement: consume a probiotic supplement containing *Bacillus subtilis, Bacillus coagulans*, and *Saccharomyces boulardii.*

Breakfast

Two or three soft-boiled or poached pasture-raised eggs

Probiotic beverage: 8 ounces of raw kombucha, kvass, kefir, or other lacto-fermented beverage

Oral probiotic supplement: after breakfast, consume a probiotic mint containing three probiotic strains clinically proven to improve oral health (visit your local health food store for recommended brands).

Lunch

Before eating, drink 8 ounces of water.

Toss a green salad with mixed greens, tomatoes, avocado, carrots, cucumbers, celery, red cabbage, red peppers, red onions, and sprouts with 3 ounces of tuna.

For the salad dressing, mix extra-virgin olive oil, apple cider vinegar or lemon juice, Celtic sea salt, herbs, and spices, or you may mix 1 tablespoon of extra-virgin olive oil with 1 tablespoon of a healthy store-bought dressing.

One bunch of grapes with seeds

Probiotic beverage: 8 ounces of raw kombucha, kvass, kefir, or other lacto-fermented beverage

Dinner

Before eating, drink 8 ounces of water.

   Grilled chicken breast

   Steamed veggies

   Roasted potatoes, carrots, and peas

Probiotic condiment: 1-4 ounces of cultured veggies

Probiotic beverage: 8 ounces of raw kombucha, kvass, kefir, or other lacto-fermented beverage

Oral probiotic supplement: after dinner, consume a probiotic mint containing three probiotic strains clinically proven to improve oral health (visit your local health food store for recommended brands).

Probiotic snacks

   One raw apple with skin and a couple of ounces of raw cheese

   Drink 8 ounces of water.

Before bed

Probiotic supplement: consume a probiotic supplement containing *Bacillus subtilis, Bacillus coagulans,* and *Saccharomyces boulardii.*

Day 5

Upon waking

Probiotic supplement: consume a probiotic supplement containing *Bacillus subtilis*, *Bacillus coagulans*, and *Saccharomyces boulardii*.

Breakfast

Two or three soft-boiled or poached pasture-raised eggs

One grapefruit

Probiotic beverage: 8 ounces of raw kombucha, kvass, kefir, or other lacto-fermented beverage

Oral probiotic supplement: after breakfast, consume a probiotic mint containing three probiotic strains clinically proven to improve oral health (visit your local health food store for recommended brands).

Lunch

Before eating, drink 8 ounces of water.

Toss a green salad with mixed greens, tomatoes, avocado, carrots, cucumbers, celery, red cabbage, red peppers, red onions, and sprouts with 3 ounces of tuna.

For the salad dressing, mix extra-virgin olive oil, apple cider vinegar or lemon juice, Celtic sea salt, herbs, and spices, or you may mix 1 tablespoon of extra-virgin olive oil with 1 tablespoon of a healthy store-bought dressing.

One bunch of grapes with seeds

Probiotic beverage: 8 ounces of raw kombucha, kvass, kefir, or other lacto-fermented beverage

Dinner

Before eating, drink 8 ounces of water.

Chicken Soup (see page 159 for the recipe)

Toss a green salad with mixed greens, tomatoes, avocado, carrots, cucumbers, celery, red cabbage, red peppers, red onions, and sprouts.

For the salad dressing, mix extra-virgin olive oil, apple cider vinegar or lemon juice, Celtic sea salt, herbs, and spices, or you may mix 1 tablespoon of extra-virgin olive oil with 1 tablespoon of a healthy store-bought dressing.

Probiotic condiment: 1-4 ounces of cultured veggies

Probiotic beverage: 8 ounces of raw kombucha, kvass, kefir, or other lacto-fermented beverage

Oral probiotic supplement: after dinner, consume a probiotic mint containing three probiotic strains clinically proven to improve oral health (visit your local health food store for recommended brands).

Probiotic snacks

4 to 6 ounces of whole milk cottage cheese, raw honey, and half a banana

Drink 8 ounces of water.

Before bed

Probiotic supplement: consume a probiotic supplement containing *Bacillus subtilis, Bacillus coagulans*, and *Saccharomyces boulardii*.

Day 6

Upon waking

Probiotic supplement: consume a probiotic supplement containing *Bacillus subtilis*, *Bacillus coagulans*, and *Saccharomyces boulardii*.

Breakfast

2 or 3 pasture-raised eggs cooked any style in 1 tablespoon of extra-virgin coconut oil

One grapefruit or orange

Handful of almonds

Probiotic beverage: 8 ounces of raw kombucha, kvass, kefir, or other lacto-fermented beverage

Oral probiotic supplement: after breakfast, consume a probiotic mint containing three probiotic strains clinically proven to improve oral health (visit your local health food store for recommended brands).

Lunch

Before eating, drink 8 ounces of water.

Toss a green salad with mixed greens, tomatoes, avocado, carrots, cucumbers, celery, red cabbage, red peppers, red onions, and sprouts with 3 ounces of tuna.

For the salad dressing, mix extra-virgin olive oil, apple cider vinegar or lemon juice, Celtic sea salt, herbs, and spices, or you may mix 1 tablespoon of extra-virgin olive oil with 1 tablespoon of a healthy store-bought dressing.

One organic apple with the skin

Probiotic beverage: 8 ounces of raw kombucha, kvass, kefir, or other lacto-fermented beverage

Dinner

Before eating, drink 8 ounces of water.

> **Roasted organic chicken**
>
> **Cooked vegetables (carrots, onions, peas, etc.)**

Toss a green salad with mixed greens, tomatoes, avocado, carrots, cucumbers, celery, red cabbage, red peppers, red onions, and sprouts.

For the salad dressing, mix extra-virgin olive oil, apple cider vinegar or lemon juice, Celtic sea salt, herbs, and spices, or you may mix 1 tablespoon of extra-virgin olive oil with 1 tablespoon of a healthy store-bought dressing.

Probiotic condiment: 1-4 ounces of cultured veggies

Probiotic beverage: 8 ounces of raw kombucha, kvass, kefir, or other lacto-fermented beverage

Oral probiotic supplement: after dinner, consume a probiotic mint containing three probiotic strains clinically proven to improve oral health (visit your local health food store for recommended brands).

Probiotic snacks

> 4 to 6 ounces of whole milk yogurt, raw honey, and vanilla
>
> Drink 8 ounces of water.

Before bed

Probiotic supplement: consume a probiotic supplement containing *Bacillus subtilis*, *Bacillus coagulans*, and *Saccharomyces boulardii*.

Day 7

Upon waking

Probiotic supplement: consume a probiotic supplement containing *Bacillus subtilis*, *Bacillus coagulans*, and *Saccharomyces boulardii*.

Breakfast

Make a probiotic smoothie in a blender with the following ingredients:

- 1 cup plain yogurt or kefir (sheep's or goat's milk is best)
- 1 Tbsp. organic flaxseed oil
- 1 Tbsp. organic raw honey
- 1 cup of organic fruit (berries, peaches, pineapple, etc.)
- 2 Tbsp. multi collagen or bone broth protein powder
- Dash of vanilla extract (optional)

Oral probiotic supplement: after breakfast, consume a probiotic mint containing three probiotic strains clinically proven to improve oral health (visit your local health food store for recommended brands).

Lunch

Before eating, drink 8 ounces of water.

Toss a green salad with mixed greens, tomatoes, avocado, carrots, cucumbers, celery, red cabbage, red peppers, red onions, and sprouts with 3 ounces of cold, poached, or canned wild-caught salmon.

For the salad dressing, mix extra-virgin olive oil, apple cider vinegar or lemon juice, Celtic sea salt, herbs, and spices, or you may mix 1 tablespoon of extra-virgin olive oil with 1 tablespoon of a healthy store-bought dressing.

One piece of fruit in season

Probiotic beverage: 8 ounces of raw kombucha, kvass, kefir, or other lacto-fermented beverage

Dinner

Before eating, drink 8 ounces of water.

Baked or grilled fish of your choice

Steamed broccoli

Sweet potato with butter

Toss a green salad with mixed greens, tomatoes, avocado, carrots, cucumbers, celery, red cabbage, red peppers, red onions, and sprouts with 3 ounces of cold, poached, or canned wild-caught salmon.

For the salad dressing, mix extra-virgin olive oil, apple cider vinegar or lemon juice, Celtic sea salt, herbs, and spices, or you may mix 1 tablespoon of extra-virgin olive oil with 1 tablespoon of a healthy store-bought dressing.

Probiotic condiment: 1-2 tablespoons of unpasteurized miso paste mixed in warm water to create a broth

Probiotic beverage: 8 ounces of raw kombucha, kvass, kefir, or other lacto-fermented beverage

Oral probiotic supplement: after dinner, consume a probiotic mint containing three probiotic strains clinically proven to improve oral health (visit your local health food store for recommended brands).

Probiotic snacks

Raw flaxseed crackers with soft or hard raw cheese

Drink 8 ounces of water.

Before bed

Probiotic supplement: consume a probiotic supplement containing *Bacillus subtilis, Bacillus coagulans,* and *Saccharomyces boulardii.*

PHASE III (WEEK 9–WEEK 12)

Phase III is the "lifestyle" phase that you can adopt to maintain your improved digestive health. If you're feeling great and feeling like you've turned a corner with your digestive issues, then continue on this life-style phase. If you are still suffering painful symptoms in the gut, or feel

NEED RECIPES?

You'll find some Probiotic Diet-friendly recipes involving fermented foods, sprouted grains, and dairy-rich smoothies in Chapter 14, "The Probiotic Diet Recipes." You'll also encounter some cleansing recipes made from delicious raw foods. You can also visit DrAxe.com for hundreds of healthy, gut-friendly recipes.

like you've gotten off track, then use this time period to implement Phase I or Phase II again.

You're cleared to resume eating grains like quinoa, buckwheat, and brown rice as well as corn grits and corn tortillas. Cereal and breads that use sprouted grains are acceptable as well. While alcohol is discouraged, you're allowed to drink alcohol in moderate amounts with unpasteurized organic wine and beer being the best choice.

Remember: organic red wine is best, followed by organic white wine and unpasteurized beer. Skip the Cosmopolitans and other mixed drinks that use hard spirits. Don't forget that alcohol has twice as many calories per gram as protein or carbohydrates. Cheat meals should be a thing of the past, as well as your cravings for junk food.

Eat meals balanced with whole foods and healthy proteins and fats, watch your portion size, continue to eliminate refined foods, and maintain regular exercise in your week.

Phase III Food Additions and Subtractions from Phase II

Legend: Approved ✔ Avoid ✗

Dairy

✔ raw goat's, sheep's or cow's milk

✗ rice milk

✗ soy milk

✗ processed cheese food or singles

✗ all homogenized commercial dairy products, including milk and ice cream

Vegetables (organic, fresh or frozen, is best)

✔ white potatoes

✔ corn (only organic)

Nuts and seeds (organic, raw, or soaked is best)

✘ honey-roasted nuts

✘ nuts roasted in oil

Fruits (organic, fresh or frozen, is best)

✔ canned fruit (in its own juices)

✔ dried fruit (no sugar or sulfites): raisins, prunes, pineapple, papaya, peaches, apples, and cranberries

✘ canned fruits in syrup

Beverages

✔ raw, unpasteurized vegetable juice

✔ raw, unpasteurized fruit juice

✘ pasteurized fruit and vegetable juices

Grains and starchy carbohydrates (organic, soaked is best)

✔ quinoa

✔ amaranth

✔ buckwheat

✔ millet

✔ brown rice

✔ sprouted cereal

✔ sprouted, Ezekiel-type bread

✔ sprouted Essence bread

✔ corn grits (organic only)

✔ corn tortillas (organic only)

- ✔ whole-grain yeast-free bread

Grains such as wheat, kamut, spelt, oats, barley, and rye contain gluten but may be consumed in yeast-free whole-grain breads.

- ✔ oats
- ✘ kamut
- ✘ spelt
- ✘ barley
- ✘ pastries
- ✘ baked goods
- ✘ white rice
- ✘ dried cereal
- ✘ instant oatmeal
- ✘ bread (except sprouted or sourdough)
- ✘ pastas (except whole-grain kamut or spelt)

Sweeteners

- ✔ Sucanat
- ✔ Rapadura
- ✔ agave nectar
- ✔ unrefined maple syrup
- ✔ fructose or corn syrup
- ✔ sugar (all-natural cane sugar, and organic brown sugar, including organic sugars)

Snacks/Miscellaneous

- ✔ healthy trail mix
- ✔ organic chocolate spreads
- ✔ cocoa powder
- ✔ carob powder
- ✔ healthy popcorn
- ✔ macaroons (made with simple ingredients and naturally sweetened)
- ✔ cacao, naturally sweetened
- ✘ milk or whey protein powder (byproduct of cheese manufacturing, denatured)
- ✘ soy protein powder
- ✘ rice protein powder

THE PROBIOTIC DIET: PHASE III

Sample 7-Day Eating Plan

Day 1

Upon waking

Probiotic supplement: consume a probiotic supplement containing *Bacillus subtilis, Bacillus coagulans,* and *Saccharomyces boulardii* (visit your local health food store for recommended brands).

Breakfast

Make a probiotic smoothie in a blender with the following ingredients:

- 1 cup plain yogurt or kefir (sheep's or goat's milk is best)
- 1 Tbsp. organic flaxseed oil
- 1 Tbsp. organic raw honey
- 1 cup of organic fruit (berries, peaches, pineapple, etc.)
- 2 Tbsp. multi collagen or bone broth protein powder
- Dash of vanilla extract (optional)

Oral probiotic supplement: after breakfast, consume a probiotic mint containing three probiotic strains clinically proven to improve oral health (visit your local health food store for recommended brands).

Lunch

Before eating, drink 8 ounces of water.

Probiotic beverage: 8 ounces of raw kombucha, kvass, kefir, or other lacto-fermented beverage.

Toss a green salad with mixed greens, tomatoes, avocado, carrots, cucumbers, celery, red cabbage, red peppers, red onions, and sprouts with three hard-boiled omega-3 pasture-raised eggs. Caution: if you suffer from frequent diarrhea, too much salad is irritating to your condition. You may consume steamed veggies instead. If you do consume salad, make sure you chew very well and eliminate the cabbage, peppers, and onions.

For the salad dressing, mix extra-virgin olive oil, apple cider vinegar or lemon juice, Celtic sea salt, herbs, and spices, or you may mix 1 tablespoon of extra-virgin olive oil with 1 tablespoon of a healthy store-bought dressing.

One apple with skin

Dinner

Before eating, drink 8 ounces of water.

Probiotic beverage: 8 ounces of raw kombucha, kvass, kefir, or other lacto-fermented beverage

Baked, poached, or grilled wild-caught salmon

Steamed broccoli

Toss a green salad with mixed greens, tomatoes, avocado, carrots, cucumbers, celery, red cabbage, red peppers, red onions, and sprouts.

For the salad dressing, mix extra-virgin olive oil, apple cider vinegar or lemon juice, Celtic sea salt, herbs, and spices, or you may mix 1 tablespoon of extra-virgin olive oil with 1 tablespoon of a healthy store-bought dressing.

Probiotic condiment: 2-4 ounces of cultured veggies, *kimchi*, or sauerkraut.

Oral probiotic supplement: after dinner, consume a probiotic mint containing three probiotic strains clinically proven to improve oral health (visit your local health food store for recommended brands).

Probiotic snacks

Raw almonds and a couple of ounces of raw cheese

Drink 8 ounces of water.

Before bed

Probiotic supplement: consume a probiotic supplement containing *Bacillus subtilis, Bacillus coagulans*, and *Saccharomyces boulardii.*

Day 2

Upon waking

Probiotic supplement: consume a probiotic supplement containing *Bacillus subtilis, Bacillus coagulans*, and *Saccharomyces boulardii.*

Breakfast

Two or three pasture-raised eggs any style, cooked in one tablespoon of extra-virgin coconut oil

Stir-fried onions, mushrooms, and peppers

Probiotic beverage: 8 ounces of raw kombucha, kvass, kefir, or other lacto-fermented beverage

Oral probiotic supplement: after breakfast, consume a probiotic mint containing three probiotic strains clinically proven to improve oral health (visit your local health food store for recommended brands).

Lunch

Before eating, drink 8 ounces of water.

During lunch, drink 8 ounces of water or hot tea with honey.

Toss a green salad with mixed greens, tomatoes, avocado, carrots, cucumbers, celery, red cabbage, red peppers, red onions, and sprouts with 3 ounces of tuna.

For the salad dressing, mix extra-virgin olive oil, apple cider vinegar or lemon juice, Celtic sea salt, herbs, and spices, or you may mix 1 tablespoon of extra-virgin olive oil with 1 tablespoon of a healthy store-bought dressing.

One bunch of organic grapes

Probiotic beverage: 8 ounces of raw kombucha, kvass, kefir, or other lacto-fermented beverage

Dinner

Before eating, drink 8 ounces of water.

Roasted organic chicken

Cooked vegetables (carrots, onions, peas, etc.)

Toss a green salad with mixed greens, tomatoes, avocado, carrots, cucumbers, celery, red cabbage, red peppers, red onions, and sprouts.

For the salad dressing, mix extra-virgin olive oil, apple cider vinegar or lemon juice, Celtic sea salt, herbs, and spices, or you

may mix 1 tablespoon of extra-virgin olive oil with 1 tablespoon of a healthy store-bought dressing.

Probiotic beverage: 8 ounces of raw kombucha, kvass, kefir, or other lacto-fermented beverage

Probiotic condiment: one unpasteurized pickled cucumber

Oral probiotic supplement: after dinner, consume a probiotic mint containing three probiotic strains clinically proven to improve oral health (visit your local health food store for recommended brands).

Probiotic snacks

4 to 6 ounces of whole milk yogurt with raw honey and fruit

Drink 8 ounces of water.

Before bed

Probiotic supplement: consume a probiotic supplement containing *Bacillus subtilis, Bacillus coagulans*, and *Saccharomyces boulardii.*

Day 3

Upon waking

Probiotic supplement: consume a probiotic supplement containing *Bacillus subtilis, Bacillus coagulans*, and *Saccharomyces boulardii.*

Breakfast

4 to 8 ounces of organic whole milk yogurt or cottage cheese with fruit (pineapple, peaches, or berries), honey, and a dash of vanilla extract

Handful of raw almonds

Oral probiotic supplement: after breakfast, consume a probiotic mint containing three probiotic strains clinically proven to improve oral health (visit your local health food store for recommended brands).

Lunch

Before eating, drink 8 ounces of water.

Toss a green salad with mixed greens, tomatoes, avocado, carrots, cucumbers, celery, red cabbage, red peppers, red onions, and sprouts with three hard-boiled pasture-raised eggs.

For the salad dressing, mix extra-virgin olive oil, apple cider vinegar or lemon juice, Celtic sea salt, herbs, and spices, or you may mix 1 tablespoon of extra-virgin olive oil with 1 tablespoon of a healthy store-bought dressing.

One piece of fruit in season

Probiotic beverage: 8 ounces of raw kombucha, kvass, kefir, or other lacto-fermented beverage

Dinner

Before eating, drink 8 ounces of water.

Red meat steak (beef, buffalo, or venison)

Steamed broccoli

Baked sweet potato with butter

Toss a green salad with mixed greens, tomatoes, avocado, carrots, cucumbers, celery, red cabbage, red peppers, red onions, and sprouts.

For the salad dressing, mix extra-virgin olive oil, apple cider vinegar or lemon juice, Celtic sea salt, herbs, and spices, or you may mix 1 tablespoon of extra-virgin olive oil with 1 tablespoon of a healthy store-bought dressing.

Probiotic condiment: 1-4 ounces of lacto-fermented raw salsa

Probiotic beverage: 8 ounces of raw kombucha, kvass, kefir, or other lacto-fermented beverage

Oral probiotic supplement: after dinner, consume a probiotic mint containing three probiotic strains clinically proven to improve oral health (visit your local health food store for recommended brands).

Probiotic snacks

4 to 6 ounces of whole milk yogurt with fruit, honey, and a few almonds

Drink 8 ounces of water.

Before bed

Probiotic supplement: consume a probiotic supplement containing *Bacillus subtilis, Bacillus coagulans*, and *Saccharomyces boulardii.*

Day 4

Upon waking

Probiotic supplement: consume a probiotic supplement containing *Bacillus subtilis, Bacillus coagulans*, and *Saccharomyces boulardii*.

Breakfast

Two or three soft-boiled or poached pasture-raised eggs

Four ounces of sprouted whole grain cereal with 2 ounces of whole milk yogurt.

Probiotic beverage: 8 ounces of raw kombucha, kvass, kefir, or other lacto-fermented beverage

Oral probiotic supplement: after breakfast, consume a probiotic mint containing three probiotic strains clinically proven to improve oral health (visit your local health food store for recommended brands).

Lunch

Before eating, drink 8 ounces of water.

Toss a green salad with mixed greens, tomatoes, avocado, carrots, cucumbers, celery, red cabbage, red peppers, red onions, and sprouts with 3 ounces of tuna.

For the salad dressing, mix extra-virgin olive oil, apple cider vinegar or lemon juice, Celtic sea salt, herbs, and spices, or you may mix 1 tablespoon of extra-virgin olive oil with 1 tablespoon of a healthy store-bought dressing.

One bunch of grapes with seeds

Probiotic beverage: 8 ounces of raw kombucha, kvass, kefir, or other lacto-fermented beverage

Dinner

Before eating, drink 8 ounces of water.

Grilled chicken breast

Steamed veggies

Small portion of cooked non-gluten whole grain (quinoa, amaranth, millet, or buckwheat) cooked with one tablespoon of extra-virgin coconut oil

Toss a green salad with mixed greens, tomatoes, avocado, carrots, cucumbers, celery, red cabbage, red peppers, red onions, and sprouts.

For the salad dressing, mix extra-virgin olive oil, apple cider vinegar or lemon juice, Celtic sea salt, herbs, and spices, or you may mix 1 tablespoon of extra-virgin olive oil with 1 tablespoon of a healthy store-bought dressing.

Probiotic condiment: 1-4 ounces of cultured veggies

Probiotic beverage: 8 ounces of raw kombucha, kvass, kefir, or other lacto-fermented beverage

Oral probiotic supplement: after dinner, consume a probiotic mint containing three probiotic strains clinically proven to improve oral health (visit your local health food store for recommended brands).

Probiotic snacks

One raw apple with skin and a couple of ounces of raw cheese

Drink 8 ounces of water.

Before bed

Probiotic supplement: consume a probiotic supplement containing *Bacillus subtilis, Bacillus coagulans*, and *Saccharomyces boulardii.*

Day 5

Upon waking

Probiotic supplement: consume a probiotic supplement containing *Bacillus subtilis, Bacillus coagulans*, and *Saccharomyces boulardii.*

Breakfast

Two or three soft-boiled or poached pasture-raised eggs

One grapefruit

Probiotic beverage: 8 ounces of raw kombucha, kvass, kefir, or other lacto-fermented beverage

Oral probiotic supplement: after breakfast, consume a probiotic mint containing three probiotic strains clinically proven to improve oral health (visit your local health food store for recommended brands).

Lunch

Before eating, drink 8 ounces of water.

Toss a green salad with mixed greens, tomatoes, avocado, carrots, cucumbers, celery, red cabbage, red peppers, red onions, and sprouts with 3 ounces of tuna.

For the salad dressing, mix extra-virgin olive oil, apple cider vinegar or lemon juice, Celtic sea salt, herbs, and spices, or you

may mix 1 tablespoon of extra-virgin olive oil with 1 tablespoon of a healthy store-bought dressing.

One bunch of grapes with seeds

Probiotic beverage: 8 ounces of raw kombucha, kvass, kefir, or other lacto-fermented beverage

Dinner

Before eating, drink 8 ounces of water.

Chicken Soup (see page 159 for the recipe)

Toss a green salad with mixed greens, tomatoes, avocado, carrots, cucumbers, celery, red cabbage, red peppers, red onions, and sprouts.

For the salad dressing, mix extra-virgin olive oil, apple cider vinegar or lemon juice, Celtic sea salt, herbs, and spices, or you may mix 1 tablespoon of extra-virgin olive oil with 1 tablespoon of a healthy store-bought dressing.

Probiotic condiment: 1-4 ounces of cultured veggies

Probiotic beverage: 8 ounces of raw kombucha, kvass, kefir, or other lacto-fermented beverage

Oral probiotic supplement: after dinner, consume a probiotic mint containing three probiotic strains clinically proven to improve oral health (visit your local health food store for recommended brands).

Probiotic snacks

4 to 6 ounces of whole milk yogurt with fruit, honey, and a few almonds

Drink 8 ounces of water.

Before bed

Probiotic supplement: consume a probiotic supplement containing *Bacillus subtilis*, *Bacillus coagulans*, and *Saccharomyces boulardii*.

Day 6

Upon waking

Probiotic supplement: consume a probiotic supplement containing *Bacillus subtilis*, *Bacillus coagulans*, and *Saccharomyces boulardii*.

Breakfast

Two or three pasture-raised eggs cooked any style in one tablespoon of extra-virgin coconut oil

One grapefruit or orange

Handful of almonds

Probiotic beverage: 8 ounces of raw kombucha, kvass, kefir, or other lacto-fermented beverage

Oral probiotic supplement: after breakfast, consume a probiotic mint containing three probiotic strains clinically proven to improve oral health (visit your local health food store for recommended brands).

Lunch

Before eating, drink 8 ounces of water.

Toss a green salad with mixed greens, tomatoes, avocado, carrots, cucumbers, celery, red cabbage, red peppers, red onions, and sprouts with 3 ounces of tuna.

For the salad dressing, mix extra-virgin olive oil, apple cider vinegar or lemon juice, Celtic sea salt, herbs, and spices, or you may mix 1 tablespoon of extra-virgin olive oil with 1 tablespoon of a healthy store-bought dressing.

One organic apple with the skin

Probiotic beverage: 8 ounces of raw kombucha, kvass, kefir, or other lacto-fermented beverage

Dinner

Before eating, drink 8 ounces of water.

Roasted organic chicken

Cooked vegetables (carrots, onions, peas, etc.)

Toss a green salad with mixed greens, tomatoes, avocado, carrots, cucumbers, celery, red cabbage, red peppers, red onions, and sprouts.

For the salad dressing, mix extra-virgin olive oil, apple cider vinegar or lemon juice, Celtic sea salt, herbs, and spices, or you may mix 1 tablespoon of extra-virgin olive oil with 1 tablespoon of a healthy store-bought dressing.

Probiotic condiment: 1-4 ounces of cultured veggies

Probiotic beverage: 8 ounces of raw kombucha, kvass, kefir, or other lacto-fermented beverage

Oral probiotic supplement: after dinner, consume a probiotic mint containing three probiotic strains clinically proven to improve oral health (visit your local health food store for recommended brands).

Probiotic snacks

4 to 6 ounces of whole milk yogurt, raw honey, and vanilla

Drink 8 ounces of water.

Before bed

Probiotic supplement: consume a probiotic supplement containing *Bacillus subtilis, Bacillus coagulans*, and *Saccharomyces boulardii.*

Day 7

Upon waking

Probiotic supplement: consume a probiotic supplement containing *Bacillus subtilis, Bacillus coagulans*, and *Saccharomyces boulardii.*

Breakfast

Make a probiotic smoothie in a blender with the following ingredients:

1 cup plain yogurt or kefir (sheep's or goat's milk is best)

1 Tbsp. organic flaxseed oil

1 Tbsp. organic raw honey

1 cup of organic fruit (berries, peaches, pineapple, etc.)

2 Tbsp. multi collagen or bone broth protein powder (visit your local health food store for recommended brands or go to AncientNutrition.com)

Dash of vanilla extract (optional)

Oral probiotic supplement: after breakfast, consume a probiotic mint containing three probiotic strains clinically proven to improve oral health (visit your local health food store for recommended brands).

Lunch

Before eating, drink 8 ounces of water.

Toss a green salad with mixed greens, tomatoes, avocado, carrots, cucumbers, celery, red cabbage, red peppers, red onions, and sprouts with 3 ounces of cold, poached, or canned wild-caught salmon.

For the salad dressing, mix extra-virgin olive oil, apple cider vinegar or lemon juice, Celtic sea salt, herbs, and spices, or you may mix 1 tablespoon of extra-virgin olive oil with 1 tablespoon of a healthy store-bought dressing.

One piece of fruit in season

Probiotic beverage: 8 ounces of raw kombucha, kvass, kefir, or other lacto-fermented beverage

Dinner

Before eating, drink 8 ounces of water.

Baked or grilled fish of your choice

Steamed broccoli

Toss a green salad with mixed greens, tomatoes, avocado, carrots, cucumbers, celery, red cabbage, red peppers, red onions, and sprouts.

For the salad dressing, mix extra-virgin olive oil, apple cider vinegar or lemon juice, Celtic sea salt, herbs, and spices, or you

NEED RECIPES?

You'll find some Probiotic Diet-friendly recipes involving fermented foods, sprouted grains, and dairy-rich multi collagen and bone broth smoothies in Chapter 14, "The Probiotic Diet Recipes." You'll also encounter some cleansing recipes made from delicious raw foods. You can also visit DrAxe.com for hundreds of healthy, gut-friendly recipes.

may mix 1 tablespoon of extra-virgin olive oil with 1 tablespoon of a healthy store-bought dressing.

Probiotic condiment: 1-2 tablespoons of unpasteurized miso paste mixed in warm water to create a broth

Probiotic beverage: 8 ounces of raw kombucha, kvass, kefir, or other lacto-fermented beverage

Oral probiotic supplement: after dinner, consume a probiotic mint containing three probiotic strains clinically proven to improve oral health (visit your local health food store for recommended brands).

Probiotic snacks

Raw almonds and a couple of ounces of raw cheese

Drink 8 ounces of water.

Before bed

Probiotic supplement: consume a probiotic supplement containing *Bacillus subtilis, Bacillus coagulans,* and *Saccharomyces boulardii.*

Shopping Tips for the Probiotic Diet

When it comes to following the Probiotic Diet, changing the way you shop for foods will change the way you eat. For many of you, this will mean doing your grocery shopping in health food stores and natural food stores instead of large-chain supermarkets.

I wouldn't blame you if you walked into your local health food store...and felt totally confused. You have no idea where to begin, you don't know how to read the food labels, you don't really know what the word "organic" means, and you're not even sure everything in the store is truly healthy for you. Don't worry. I have some advice for you.

First, I highly suggest you ask the staff members at your local health food store for advice and assistance. They are almost always informed, friendly, and eager to help.

Second, after reading this section of *The Probiotic Diet* book, you'll become much more comfortable and prepared to visit a health food store or natural grocer in your area. Remember, your guiding principle is shopping for fresh, organic fruits and vegetables, properly raised meat and poultry, and wild-caught fish. These have been, and still are, the best choices for ensuring optimal digestive health today.

Our terrains were not designed to operate at optimum levels on all the junk food, fast food, prepackaged food, or any of the genetically modified, antibiotic, and growth hormone-laden foods that most Americans eat today. Yes, organic products do cost more, but organic foods give you a higher percentage of nutrients, no residual pesticides, no antibiotics, no growth hormones, no genetic modification, no potential long-term health effects, or no negative environmental effects. Any extra money you do spend is well worth it. Don't you want to feel better?

If you can't afford or can't find organic produce, however, the next best thing to organic is to apply a veggie wash to your conventionally grown vegetables and fruits. Keep in mind that it's much better to consume fruits and vegetables than not to, even if they are not organic. That said, many regular grocery stores are now carrying certified organic produce.

Fruits and Vegetables

Certified organic fruits and vegetables have an incredible amount of nutrients—vitamins, minerals, live enzymes, antioxidants, and many other healthy compounds. Depending on what season it is, there are different fruits and vegetables available, but every fruit and vegetable has something unique to offer.

Berries

These are some of the most important fruits you can consume. Strawberries, blueberries, blackberries, and raspberries are all high in antioxidants. Antioxidants are nutrients found naturally in the body and in plants such as fruits and vegetables—especially berries. As cells function normally in the body, they produce damaged molecules; these are called free radicals. Free radicals are highly unstable and steal components from other cells, including DNA, thereby spreading the damage. This damage continues in a chain reaction, and entire cells soon become damaged and die off. This process can be beneficial because it helps the body destroy cells that have outlived their usefulness, and it kills germs and parasites. When left unchecked, though, this process can destroy or damage healthy cells. Eating high-antioxidant foods can help the body produce healthy cells.

Of course, buying your berries fresh is best. That way, the most amounts of nutrients are preserved. Be aware that:

- Blueberries are prized as a high source of antioxidants, anti-aging, and many disease prevention properties.

- Cranberries, usually consumed seasonally, are another great source of antioxidants. They are excellent for urinary tract health and come to a harvest peak in November; thus their association with Thanksgiving.

- Raspberries contain ellagic acid, which is an antioxidant with anti-cancer properties and possesses excellent benefits for female health. They are also high in pectin, which makes them an excellent thickener in homemade jellies and jams.

- Pineapple has something called bromalein, an enzyme that aids indigestion and causes fruit salads to get soggy after only a short period of time. Eat pineapple fresh, not canned.

So for your fruits, focus on strawberries, raspberries, blueberries and blackberries, cherries, lemons, limes, and grapefruit.

If you eat dried fruits, avoid the kind with sulfate or sulfite preservatives. Sulfites, or sulfur-based preservatives, are artificial chemicals added to hundreds of foods to stop spoilage, but these chemicals can be toxic to the human body. Some studies have shown sulfur additives may contribute to chronic inflammatory diseases such as ulcerative colitis, Crohn's disease, as well as irritable bowel syndrome. So choose your pineapple and all other dried fruits sulfite- and preservative-free.

Avocado

This much-maligned food is a fruit, not a vegetable. Avocados contain high-quality fats as well as vitamin E and are a great source of fiber and other minerals. Avocados are 75 percent water and contain good fats, similar to olive oil.

Lettuce

There are several varieties of lettuce, which is high in fiber. It is difficult to know which ones to choose. We are used to consuming iceberg lettuce, but today there are many great brands of mixed salad blends. These mixed blends contain things like organic baby lettuces, including green oak leaf, organic baby spinach, red and green chard, and arugula. They're popular, they're pre-washed, and they're easy for people who don't have a lot of time on their hands. These greens contain virtually every mineral and trace element and large amounts of beta-carotene, which fits into the nutritional category of carotenoids, a class of very important antioxidants that give fruit and vegetables their bright colors.

Cabbage is excellent for the digestive tract, particularly when cooked or juiced. It contains something called vitamin U, which is the anti-ulcer vitamin. Cabbage is also extremely effective in its cultured or fermented form, making it very bio-available.

One of the important aspects to the Probiotic Diet is adding raw fermented vegetables like cultured veggies, *kimchi*, natto, and sauerkraut to your shopping list. Very few Americans eat any fermented vegetables, which is a shame since they are one of the healthiest types of food available for those with digestive issues. Other examples of raw fermented vegetables include pickled carrots and fermented beets. These probiotic-rich cultured foods possess a phenomenal source of vitamins, minerals, and live enzymes as well as beneficial microorganisms.

Mushrooms

These are high in nutrients, particularly the mineral selenium, which works with vitamin E as an antioxidant and binds with toxins in the body, rendering them harmless. Mushrooms are over 90 percent water and are high in biotin, one of the B-complex vitamins.

Mushrooms are one of those foods that should be eaten organically because of where they are grown. Mushrooms pick up many nutrients from the soil and the trees they are grown on. If they are grown in a non-organic environment, many times they are high in heavy metals, so you want to be careful about eating non-organic mushrooms. Despite what you hear, eating mushrooms does not contribute to yeast overgrowth in the body. Some people who are yeast sensitive, however, have cross-sensitivities to mushrooms.

Peppers

These are rich in antioxidants, which clean up and prevent cell damage. Green peppers may be more difficult to digest than other colored peppers, so if you have complicated digestive problems, you should eat yellow, orange, or red peppers. The different colors are rich in different nutrients as well. Red peppers are substantially higher in vitamins C and A than green peppers.

Sweet potatoes

These vegetables are one of the highest sources of beta-carotene. Studies have linked the high intake of foods rich in beta-carotene to a reduced risk of cancer, particularly lung cancer. Sweet potatoes also contain vitamin C, calcium, potassium, carbohydrates, and fiber.

Green drinks

In addition to your daily supply of fruits and vegetables, green drinks are another way to supplement your diet with whole food nutritional supplements. The best are made with nutrient-rich grasses, which are a "super food." Cereal grasses are the only foods in the vegetable kingdom that, even if consumed alone, enable animals to continually maintain weight, strength, and optimal health. Grass is richer in nutrients than spinach, broccoli, eggs, and chicken in virtually all categories, including protein.

They abound in unidentified growth factors, powerful antioxidants, immune boosters, and many other health-supporting nutrients.

Another benefit of having a green drink during the day is convenience. It's so easy to just mix and drink, and you've just consumed the recommended amount of vegetables for that day—and more! In today's hectic lifestyle, it's nearly impossible to eat enough vegetables, especially greens, to satisfy our body's needs. Because of this, we are depriving ourselves of nature's ultimate insurance policy. Green drinks were created to meet the demands of our fast-paced lives by supplying every nutrient our body requires to sustain optimal levels of health.

Dairy Products

Dairy

When purchasing dairy products, there are several grades and categories of dairy. The superior dairy products are unpasteurized, cultured dairy products, which are very hard to find. The best way to purchase organic, grass-fed, raw cultured dairy products is by special ordering from your health food store or by ordering directly from a supplier.

Generally speaking, you want to consume whole milk organic cultured dairy products made from cow's, sheep's, and goat's milk. Purchasing "plain" dairy will help you avoid various sugars, especially table sugar and corn syrup. To enhance flavor, just add your own raw honey and fruit.

I recommend goat's milk because the smaller molecules in goat's milk are closer in size and composition to human milk, making it easier to digest. Goat's milk is also substantially less allergenic than cow's milk in susceptible individuals, and it's the dairy of choice when trying to cleanse your body of toxins and allergens.

Be aware of the difference between dairy from grass-fed cows vs. grain-fed cows. Grass-fed is extremely important as cows are designed to live on grass, not grain. Grass-fed animals produce healthier milk and higher nutrients, such as vitamins A, D, and E, and conjugated linoleic acid, more commonly known as CLA, which is a naturally occurring fatty acid found mainly in milk fat and meat and something the body cannot produce.

A few years ago, CLA, or conjugated linoleic acid, received media attention when it was identified as a component of red meat that actually prevents cancer. CLA, a polyunsaturated fat, is a potent anti-cancer agent, an immune-stimulating agent, and a fat-burning agent. CLA is found in meat and milk, but it's most highly concentrated in milk fat. So forget about skim or low fat—you need that full fat found in dairy. Furthermore, full fat or whole milk products from grass-fed cows contain as much as five times more CLA than milk from standard grain-fed cows.

Remember, raw—meaning not cooked or processed—cow's and goat's milk, hard cheeses, butter, and cream are best. Always buy whole fat, organic dairy products instead of skim or 2-percent dairy products, which have undergone processing that removes beneficial enzymes.

Cheese

There are many different varieties of cheese to choose from, but if you can find cheeses made from raw milk, you'll be far better off. Besides raw cow's milk cheese, goat's milk and sheep's milk cheese are widely available.

Look for the raw designation on the label. Raw means the enzymes are intact, it's easier to digest, and the calcium and other nutrients are in their best available form.

There are also soft cheeses like ricotta or cottage cheese. These can be good for us, but many people are allergic to cow's milk, especially when it's pasteurized. When choosing a ricotta or a cottage cheese, make sure it's a brand that is certified organic. That ensures no pesticides, hormones, or antibiotics were used.

Yogurt and kefir

I've already had a great deal to say about the benefits of yogurt and kefir. The naturally occurring bacteria and yeast in yogurt and kefir provide superior health benefits. These cultured or fermented foods are extremely healthy because they are partially predigested, enhancing the absorption and bio-availability of its nutrients.

During the fermentation process, many digestive enzymes are created that aid in the assimilation of food nutrients. This makes it some of the highest quality protein available. When purchasing any dairy product—milk, cheese, yogurt, or kefir—choose the full-fat version because the fat in dairy is crucial for calcium absorption.

Eggs

Eggs contain all the known nutrients except for vitamin C. They are good sources of the fat-soluble vitamins A and D as well as certain carotenoids that guard against free radical damage to the body. They also contain lutein, which has been shown to prevent age-related macular degeneration, the leading cause of blindness in America. But note, when it comes to healthy kinds of eggs, not just any old egg will do.

What kind of eggs should you look for in your health food store? Organic free-range, high omega-3, pasture-raised eggs. These are nature's perfect food. When possible, try to buy eggs from farms where the chickens are allowed to roam free (that's what pasture-raised entails) and eat their natural diet. Eggs produced from chickens in their natural environment contain a healthy balance of omega-3 to omega-6 fatty acids and DHA, which is good for the brain and eyes. High omega-3/DHA or organic eggs have six times the vitamin E and nine times the omega-3 fatty acids as regular store-purchased eggs.

You have heard that you should watch how many eggs you eat because they are high in cholesterol. The myths about cholesterol are completely unfounded. Eggs can be a healthy addition to anyone's diet and actually help reduce the risk of both heart disease and cancer. They can be consumed in a variety of ways: fried, hard-boiled, soft-boiled, and poached. Eggs can be used in baking and can even be added to the smoothie recipes found in the Probiotic Diet Eating Plan.

Meat, Poultry, and Fish

Meat

The Probiotic Diet recommends the consumption of natural, organic, and grass-fed beef, but shopping for this type of meat can be confusing because these terms do not mean the same thing. Here's a glossary:

- **Natural** simply means the meat contains no artificial ingredients and is minimally processed, but that doesn't tell you a thing about how the cattle are raised.

- **Organic** may mean the cattle are raised on organic grain like corn or soy, which are not what cattle are meant to graze on. This can wreak havoc on their digestive systems, causing sickness. On the good side, organic cows are raised without hormones, chemical additives, or antibiotics.

- **Grass-fed**, also known as **pasture-fed** or **grass-fin-ished**, means the cattle are free to roam around under the open skies. They are not crowded in small pens inside commercial feedlots, and they eat only what they were meant to—grass.

I recommend organic, grass-fed, or natural meat such as beef, lamb, chicken, turkey, and duck. Other meat choices include wild game like venison, goat, buffalo, and elk. If grass-fed meat is not available, the next best choice is certified organic meat. The major benefit of eating grass-fed meats is that you will receive between two to six times more omega-3 fatty acids than grain-fed meat. When the animals graze on their natural diet of greens, their diet is automatically rich in these essential fats.

You must avoid certain meats such as breakfast links, bacon, lunchmeats, ham, hot dogs, bratwurst, and other sausages. Strik-ing pork and shellfish from menus is recommended because of the toxins found in their flesh and because of what they eat to sustain themselves. Pigs will eat anything thrust their way, including excrement, and hard-shelled crustaceans such as lob-ster, crabs, shrimp, and clams are "bottom feeders," content to sustain themselves on excrement from other fish.

Fish

For seafood, eat only fish with fins and scales caught in the ocean or freshwater, not farm-raised, fish. Salmon, halibut, tuna, cod, sea bass, and sardines are highly recommended, but don't eat shellfish and crustaceans, because they contain abundant toxins from their water-bound scavenging habits. In fact, scien-tists gauge the contaminant levels of our oceans, bays, and rivers by measuring the biological toxin levels in the flesh of crabs, oys-ters, clams, and lobsters.

Believe it or not, some of the healthiest seafood you can find is canned. The big key is whether the can is marked "wild caught" rather than "farm raised." You want to choose the former. The good news is that when you are looking for salmon, sardines, and even herring, canned is almost always going to be wild.

High-quality sardines are one of the world's greatest foods, although many people hold their nose just thinking about them. Whole, canned sardines are an extremely rich source of omega-3 fats and contain as much calcium as a glass of milk. Make sure to obtain sardines that contain edible soft bones and organs of the fish, which make it a total package.

I also recommend wild-caught canned tuna, but it would be wise to restrict canned tuna to one or two cans a week based upon the possible contamination of heavy metals and PCBs. Research shows chunk light tuna contains less mercury than other types because the natural oils contained in fish are detoxifiers of heavy metals. So, when consuming tuna, try to eat chunk light. The advantage of buying tuna in a health food store is that the product doesn't contain additives or preservatives. The fewer ingredients, the better the tuna.

Omega-3 fatty acids—the fats we lack the most in our diet— are critical in negating the effects of the overabundance of omega-6 fatty acids and hydrogenated fats found in the standard American diet. The ratio of omega-3 to omega-6 fatty acids can be balanced by consuming more omega-3 foods such as ocean-caught fish with fins and scales (salmon, tuna, and sardines) and cod liver oil and omega-3 eggs.

Grains (Phase III only)

During Phase I and Phase II of the Probiotic Diet, you shouldn't be eating grains such as breads, pastas, and cereals. During Phase III, you can include grains like quinoa, buckwheat, brown rice, and cereal and breads that use sprouted grains. Feel free to enjoy whole organic grain products in your diet as long as they have been properly treated through soaking, sprouting, or fermenting.

When choosing bread, look for the term "sprouted" on the label. Brands such as Ezekiel bread, Essence bread, and fermented whole-grain sourdough bread are labeled "whole-grain yeast-free bread." When you buy bread made from sprouted organic grains, you can be assured that you're getting the highest-quality products.

Most breads you find in the grocery store have been treated with pesticides and other sprays that inhibit mold. White bread is totally devoid of any nutritional properties and should never be eaten—never. In fact, a diet high in white bread, white rice, and white potatoes puts women at much higher risk of pancreatic cancer, especially if they are overweight and don't get adequate exercise, according to a National Cancer Institute report from 2002.

Whole-grain sourdough and sprouted breads and cereals are healthy grains. Before the advent of modern food processing technology, it was common for our ancient ancestors to soak their grains overnight and then allow them to dry in the open air until they sprouted. Many times, they allowed their grains to go through an ancient leavening process that resulted in whole-grain sourdough bread.

Be aware that white rice is just like white bread, meaning that it is a high-glycemic carbohydrate that is absorbed quickly into the bloodstream and can raise insulin levels rapidly. As a result, white rice causes a spike of blood sugar and a surge of insulin. Instead, try whole-grain brown rice, quinoa, amaranth, buckwheat, or oats soaked overnight. Instant oatmeal is processed and refined and is much less healthy than slowly cooked whole oats. Puffed or flaked wheat, oats, and rice have been processed by high heat and pressure. They also shoot your insulin levels way up.

Some of the largest sources of mineral-depleting nutrients are contained in the sugary breakfast cereals lining the shelves of America's grocery stores. Studies show these cereals can have even more detrimental effects on blood sugar than refined sugar and white flour. As a healthier alternative, I recommend hot cereals made from soaked or sprouted whole grains during Phase III. They are not processed and do not have preservatives, artificial flavors, added colors, added synthetic vitamins, hidden sugars, or artificial sweeteners.

Oils, Spices, Condiments, and Salt

Oils

When it comes to oils, I suggest cooking and baking with saturated fats, which are stable, healthy fats. The two best fats to cook with are extra-virgin coconut oil and organic butter from grass-fed animals. These fats can withstand high heat without oxidizing. Coconut oil has antiviral and antifungal properties and supports healthy digestion, enhances metabolism, and improves thyroid and immune system function. High-quality extra-virgin coconut oil produced through natural fermentation should have the aroma of a fresh coconut.

Margarine is a man-made fat produced using bleaching agents, deodorization, and high heat, destroying nearly all of its nutrients. Margarine contains harmful hydrogenated oils. These hydrogenated oils contain trans fatty acids and are the real culprits behind many of our nation's health problems.

Olive oil is extremely healthy, but olive oil should only be used on food and never heated. Look for certified organic extra-virgin olive oil in a dark bottle since light coming into clear bottles can decrease some of the important health properties of the oil as well as its freshness. Extra-virgin olive oil is produced from the first cold pressing of the olives, and that's where you'll get the most antioxidants and other nutrients. Choose a colorful oil with a rich aroma. Stay away from the hydrogenated vegetable oils and polyunsaturated oils, especially when cooked, as well as soy, sunflower, canola, or safflower oils.

So, when choosing cooking oil, your first choice should be extra-virgin coconut oil or organic, raw butter. Extra-virgin olive oil, a popular cooking oil, is not as stable under heat as coconut oil or butter and is best used in salad dressings. Polyunsaturated, hydrogenated oils are unstable fats that should not be used as cooking oils. These include canola oil, sunflower oil, corn oil, safflower oil, soybean oil, and cottonseed oil.

Read the labels of the food you buy because oils are frequently key ingredients in packaged or canned foods. Many contain artificially processed fats and oils called hydrogenated and partially hydrogenated trans-fatty acids. The processing they undergo makes them more stable, enabling them to sit on a shelf for weeks or even years at a time, but this artificial processing also makes them a foreign and indigestible substance in our bodies, which is tough on the digestive system.

Spices

The best spices are organic spices because they don't contain caking agents and other preservatives that you may find in non-organic spices. Flavored spices are combination seasonings with a variety of organic herbs and spices. Some other favorite seasonings include unrefined sea salt. You can use them in cooking and add them to your favorite foods.

Condiments

Cultured veggies and spicy *kimchi* are condiments *par excellence*. Be brave and give them a try.

This would be a good time to clear your refrigerator and pantry of any commercial ketchup, mustard, mayonnaise, pickled relish, or other common condiments. Organic versions of these popular condiments are readily available these days, even in supermarkets. They come without refined sugar and unhealthy preservatives.

Salt

Regular table salt is highly refined with chemical and high temperature processes. These processes remove many of the valuable minerals, use harmful and potentially toxic additives, and employ bleaching agents to make the salt pristine white. Unrefined sea salt, however, still has all the important minerals, and is actually slightly gray in color. Celtic Sea Salt and RealSalt are recommended brands.

Sweeteners

We've all seen the pink, blue, and yellow packets on restaurant tables. Stay away from those artificial sweeteners! Aspartame, saccharin, sucralose, and their sweet cousins are made from chemicals that have sparked debate for decades. Though the Food and Drug Administration has approved the use of artificial sweeteners in drinks and food, these chemical additives may prove to be detrimental to your health in the long term. The fear is that these highly addictive artificial sweeteners can cross the blood-brain barrier, causing neurological problems.

The best sweetener you should be using is raw, unheated honey. Raw honey means it is unheated, preserving its rich store-house of naturally occurring enzymes and bee pollen.

Snacks from Nuts and Seeds

Snacks

The good news is that snacks have a place in the Probiotic Diet. The bad news is that when blood sugar levels fall, many reach for a candy bar or soda for a quick pick-me-up. These commercially produced snack foods are loaded with sugar, preservatives, and artificial ingredients that can rob your health.

Some of the most convenient and healthiest snacks are nuts and seeds, which are great sources of fiber, healthy fats, and nutrients. If properly prepared, they are extremely nutritious. "Properly prepared" means raw, soaked, or dry-roasted nuts and seeds not roasted in vegetable oil. Just make sure they are organic. Try almonds, walnuts, pecans, pumpkin seeds, and sunflower seeds, or make your own healthy trail mix.

Raw nut butters, made from almonds, cashews, and sunflower seeds, are something worth checking out. They're special because when they're raw (not roasted or heated), they're easy to digest and still have their vitamins, minerals, and enzymes. Nut butters can be used as a veggie dip or spread onto sprouted bread or fresh fruit. Organic peanut butter is also recommended and can even be found in warehouse clubs these days, but don't forget that peanut butter is stricken from Phase I of the Probiotic Diet Eating Plan.

It is worthy to note that the phytates found on the covering of grains and seeds "grab" minerals in the intestinal tract and block their absorption. The sprouting process effectively removes these phytates from the outer covering of the natural grain. Germination initiates a chemical transformation in the seed grains that neutralizes the phytates, causing them to come alive, making all of the nutrition within the seed available for digestion.

Beverages

If you're used to drinking sports drinks, sodas, sweet teas, and fruit juices, you may be in for a rude awakening because I'm asking you to drink a lot of water during the Probiotic Diet. The water I want you to hydrate with is purified or filtered and non-carbonated. Steer away from plain tap water since most municipal water supplies are contaminated by potentially harmful chemicals and treated with chlorine.

You can purchase purified water at the store or have a filtering system hooked up to your sink and shower. Why the shower? Because chlorine is absorbed through the skin when you take a shower. As for drinking household water, chlorine found in tap water kills both friendly and unfriendly bacteria. It also eats through lead pipes, corrodes most metals, and harms cells and DNA strands in virtually every living thing it touches. Chlorine also introduces to our water supplies some highly carcinogenic chemicals call trihalomethanes (THMs). Studies show a strong link between chlorinated water supplies with elevated THM levels and cancers of the bladder, kidney, liver, pancreas, GI tract, urinary tract, colon, and brain.

It is risky enough to drink chlorinated tap water, but the mass exposure created by swimming in a chlorinated pool or taking extended hot showers in heavily chlorinated water isn't very healthy at all. That's because the heat opens skin pores and increases the already high absorption rate of chlorine through the skin.

As for fruit juices, most juices are full of concentrated sugars with a loss of nutrients from pasteurization and concentration, often making it as nutritionally void as refined white flour. If you do purchase bottled juice, look at the label. You want to find the words "Not from concentrate." You may want to dilute the juice with purified or naturally carbonated mineral water so you don't ingest more fruit sugar than you would normally get by eating a piece of fruit.

This is the time to be brave and try some of those lacto-fermented beverages that I've been telling you about, like kombucha, a fermented mushroom tea. If kombucha is too fizzy for you, you can always sip on herbal teas. Studies are revealing many beneficial effects of tea on the heart and cardiovascular systems, particularly green tea, which has been found to lower the risk of heart disease, reduce cholesterol levels, and may even help prevent cancer. Many of these teas are well studied for their antioxidant effects that retard hardening of the arteries. Make sure to drink only organic herbal teas that are unsweetened, but you can add a small amount of raw honey.

DINING OUT TIPS

While the Probiotic Diet Shopping Guide assists you in preparing foods at home, I'd like to also offer you some tips when you eat out:

1. Opt for water as your beverage of choice, preferably filtered or bottled (not chlorinated). Avoid alcohol, coffee, tea, juice, and soda, although in Phase III, you're allowed to imbibe wine.

2. Don't reach for the bread or chips at the table. This includes dinner rolls, bread sticks, sliced bread, muffins, and tortilla chips.

3. Avoid appetizers as much as possible. Eat your soup (grain-, flour-, and dairy-free) or salad before eating your entrée.

4. When ordering soup, make sure no sugar is added. Avoid the use of toppings such as crackers, bacon, cream cheese, or cheese.

5. Choose the house salad over the Caesar salad or other salads with numerous ingredients and toppings. The plainer the salad, the better.

6. Salad dressing is simple: balsamic vinegar and/or olive oil. Other dressings are full of hydrogenated oils and sugars. It is safer to just order the balsamic vinaigrette as the waiter may not know exactly what is in the other dressings. Also, avoid the croutons.

7. Ask your server how the food is prepared. To avoid some hidden traps in your meal, inquire about the butter, margarine, cream, or oil that may be used in

preparing that item. Have your meal cooked in butter or olive oil only.

8. Request that your food be cooked without MSG or sugar.

9. Avoid entrees with a lot of ingredients. Avoid foods that have the following descriptions: fried, buttery, creamy, rich, au gratin, scalloped, béarnaise, Newburg, BBQ, sweet and sour, teriyaki, or breaded.

10. Choose a simply prepared solid piece of steak, lamb, duck, veal, venison, fish, or poultry. Look for the words grilled, poached, baked, roasted, or broiled on the menu. This is the No. 1 rule to remember when dining out. If all else fails, you can always find a simple piece of meat with vegetables as your side and a salad.

11. Don't be afraid to make special requests. Most restaurants are willing to accommodate your dietary needs when possible. Order steamed vegetables instead of mashed potatoes, French fries, or coleslaw.

12. There is no need to dress your food up with salt. Most foods already have salt added to them while being cooked.

13. Breakfast can be simple if you focus on eggs as your main dish. Mix it up a little by requesting diced tomatoes, peppers, and onions—but no ham, please.

14. If you are eating a light dinner, try a salad with grilled fish, chicken, or steak with balsamic vinegar and/or olive oil for the dressing.

11

THE PROBIOTIC Q & A

When beginning the Probiotic Diet program, will I experience any adverse symptoms?

You may experience what is known as a period of "detoxification." This is when the body rids itself of stored toxins because of the major changes in your diet, and this may cause short-term constipation or diarrhea. The increased catabolic (breakdown) activity and the release of metabolic debris into the circulation at an accelerated rate are responsible for this. The symptoms one may experience are fatigue, headaches, diarrhea or constipation, gas and bloating, skin outbreaks, flu-like symptoms, depression, anxiety, restlessness, or joint and muscle aching. Allergic reactions, withdrawal reactions, toxic reactions, and increased disease processes cause similar symptoms, so it is important to monitor such symptoms. Please note, not everyone experiences detoxification. The detox process can be compared to doing some house cleaning and stirring up the dust.

You may also experience something known as the "Herxheimer Reaction," which happens when your symptoms of distress increase at first. This is the "die-off" effect that many people experience when they dramatically improve their diet and lifestyles, and it's a response to the toxic byproducts produced when the body's pH is changed for the better. During detoxification, large numbers of dangerous bacteria and yeast organisms die and leave the body. Throughout this period, your body is responding to the positive dietary and lifestyle changes you have made. After this initial detoxification period, you should see significant improvement of your symptoms.

Why can't I start with the easiest phase (Phase III) and ease into dietary changes?

To get the greatest benefit from this 12-week experience, a clean break from a previous lifestyle and diet is required. Your best chance for success is to break free from food addictions and cut out specific foods as planned in each phase. In fact, many people say that their favorite phase is Phase I because it provides the best results for digestive health.

Why is the program so restrictive at the start with grains?

All grains are high in disaccharide sugars, which feed harmful microorganisms in the gut that can cause digestive upset. Foods from Phase I help balance essential fats with quality proteins. The low glycemic carbohydrates suggested in Phase I enable the body to balance glucose and insulin in the blood. Sprouted, gluten-free grains are added in Phase III.

Is it normal to have cravings while going through this program?

Cravings are part of any drastic change in your diet. If you're craving sweets, then a teaspoon of unheated, raw honey may help reduce that craving. If you're craving fats, then a tablespoon of coconut oil will help. Caffeine is another common craving. Body movement, exercise, or refreshing yourself with a face wash may be used as substitutes for the stimulation one normally expects from caffeine.

What are the symptoms of artificial sweetener withdrawal?

Typical withdrawal symptoms from eliminating an addictive substance may include irritability, jitters, nervousness, sleeplessness, anxiety, mild depression, and excessive thirst.

What is the recommended ratio for daily consumption of proteins, carbohydrates, and fats?

For participants on Phase III of the Probiotic Diet (the lifestyle phase), the following range for macronutrients is recommended:

- protein: 25-35 percent
- carbohydrates: 30-50 percent
- fat: 25-40 percent

This ratio will not apply for participants of the Probiotic Diet during Phases I and II.

Without chips, crackers, and bread, how can I satisfy cravings during Phase I? Any suggestions?

Buy raw sprouted crackers, which are grain-free and made with Phase I-approved ingredients. Visit www.itsalivefood.com, which offers products like dill garlic crackers or thaichi crackers.

What happens if a recipe calls for ingredients that aren't allowed?

You should seek out a substitute for the ingredient that's not allowed.

What are foods that I should absolutely not eat?

We call them the "Dirty Dozen." The following 12 foods (or food components) are some of the most popular but least healthy things you can put into your mouth:

1. pork products
2. shellfish and fish without fins and scales (catfish, shark, eel)

3. hydrogenated oils (margarine, shortening, etc.)

4. artificial sweeteners (aspartame, saccharine, sucralose, etc.)

5. white flour

6. white sugar

7. soft drinks

8. pasteurized, homogenized skim milk

9. corn syrup (high fructose corn syrup)

10. hydrolyzed soy protein (imitation meat products)

11. artificial flavors and colors

12. excessive amounts of alcohol

What are the best dairy products to consume on the Probiotic Diet?

This is how the Probiotic Diet ranks milk or yogurt:

1. cultured sheep's milk (yogurt)

2. cultured goat's milk (yogurt)

3. cultured organic cow's milk (yogurt or kefir)

Is buttermilk fermented?

Yes, but be aware that only *cultured* buttermilk is fermented. You must have a starter culture for this transformation to occur.

How do you make homemade whey?

You can make whey by straining yogurt with a cheese cloth or buying continental liquid acidophilus, which contains whey.

Why does the Probiotic Diet recommend honey over other sugar substitutes?

We recommend raw, unheated honey due to the amount of natural enzymes, vitamins, minerals, and amino acids it contains, as compared to white sugar, which is unhealthy because it is processed and refined with chemical residues void of any vitamins, minerals, or enzymes. We also recommend 100 percent maple syrup as a sweetener in Phase II. If you're looking for a sugar substitute, then you may try Stevia, which is a plant extract shown to actually have some healthy effects.

We also approve of Rapadura or Sucanat, which are natural cane sugars grown organically. If you're looking for a non-chemical/non-artificial sweetener, it would be an acceptable natural choice, although the preference would be honey.

How do you soak grains as part of the fermentation process?

Soaking is a form of culturing the product by soaking it in a special solution to break it down through the addition of beneficial bacteria.

If you are unfamiliar with fermentation, you could purchase Sally Fallon's *Nourishing Traditions* book for specific instructions on culturing or fermenting (see pages 451-495). There are many variables to the process, and this book can be a great assistance if you plan on doing this.

Why does the Probiotic Diet recommend avoiding pork?

Modern science indicates that pork has toxins that are harmful to the body. Pigs have a very elementary digestive system that does a poor job in breaking down their food before it becomes part of their flesh. This poor digestive system, coupled with the fact that pigs eat anything and everything, means that what they eat will become part of their flesh within a four-hour time span. Therefore, if you ingest pork, then you have ingested all that they have eaten.

What's the story on soy? Is it good or bad for you?

The origin of soy-based products is Japan, where it was never intended to be a meat substitute or staple part of their diet. The Japanese have traditionally used soy in small amounts, mostly as a condiment. Here in America, however, false information has been spread to increase the uses of soy. Soy is marketed as a healthy meat substitute and elite health product.

Much information shows the opposite. Soy has high levels of phytic acid, which reduces the assimilation of many minerals and causes growth problems in children. Soy increases the body's needs for vitamins B_{12} and D. The processing of soy protein results in the formation of toxic and carcinogenic substances. Soy also contains high levels of aluminum, which is toxic to the nervous system and kidneys. When eating soy, it's best to eat only fermented soy products in small amounts.

Is that why soy protein powder and soy milk are on the avoid list?

Yes, because soy protein powder and soy milk are processed, difficult-to-digest substances that inhibit iron and zinc absorption in the body.

In addition, soybean lacks the vital sulfur-containing amino acids cystine and methionine, which makes them incomplete proteins. Soy should never be considered as a substitute for animal products like meat or milk. However, traditional fermented soy products such as miso, natto, and tempeh, which are usually made with organically grown soybeans, are beneficial.

12

THE PROBIOTIC DIET PROTOCOLS

r. Brasco, Dr. Axe, and I believe that the Probiotic Diet can help anyone, especially those with a balky digestive system. That said, there are ways to fine-tune the Probiotic Diet that can better target the benefits to those facing different and difficult health challenges.

Please know that anyone with a medical condition should consult a licensed physician prior to starting any aspect of the Probiotic Diet. Before taking any dietary supplement, you should consult with your health-care practitioner before using the product, especially if you are pregnant, nursing, or under medical supervision.

With these medical disclaimers out of the way, we invite you to peruse this chapter for guidance on how the Probiotic Diet, when adapted to your medical condition or that of a child or close family member, can improve your terrain and create a better internal environment.

Developmental Disorders (Autism, Asperger's Syndrome, and Attention Deficit Hyperactivity Disorder)

Description

Developmental disorders are mild-to-serious medical conditions at some stage in a child's development, often stunting his or her development. They may include psychological or physical disorders. The five conditions considered to be pervasive development disorders (PDDs) are autism, Asperger's Syndrome, childhood disintegrative disorder, Rett Syndrome, and PDDNOS, which stands for "pervasive development disorder not otherwise specified."

Attention Deficit Hyperactivity Disorder (ADHD) has been classified as a neurobehavioral developmental disorder that affects an estimated 3 percent to 10 percent of school-aged children and is characterized by a persistent patter of impulsiveness and inattention. ADHD is twice as common in boys as in girls.

Dietary instructions

Follow the basic principles of the Probiotic Diet. You may have to ease your child into this new way of eating by making a slow but steady transition into the Probiotic Diet Eating Plan. Many children with PDDs such as autism do well by completely eliminating grains and cow's milk dairy products for two to four weeks. After two weeks of following Phase I and eliminating grains and cow's milk dairy, you should see dramatic improvements in all aspects of your child's health.

Focus on consuming the following foods and supplements as often as possible, and you could see a health turnaround.

Healing foods

- cold water fish, including wild salmon
- flaxseed and chia seed products, including fresh ground seed and oil
- coconut products, including extra-virgin coconut oil
- raw cultured dairy if available, especially kefir and cream (goat's milk may be more tolerable, but as long as the dairy is raw and comes from grass-fed animals, cow's milk should be fine)

Healing supplements

- SBO probiotic blend containing *Bacillus subtilis, Bacillus coagulans, Bacillus clausii Saccharomyces boulardii,* providing probiotics, prebiotics, parabiotics and postbiotics
- omega-3 fatty acid supplement
- a whole food vitamin/mineral supplement with glandulars
- digestive enzymes (plant-based)

Irritable Bowel Syndrome

Description

Irritable bowel syndrome is not a disease but a painful, life-altering, functional digestive disorder in which the muscular contractions of the digestive tract become irregular and uncoordinated. IBS goes by other names as well: spastic colon, mucus colitis, spastic colitis, nervous stomach, or irritable colon. *The Encyclopedia of Natural Healing* says that in well over 80 percent of cases, tests reveal the presence of an overgrowth of fungi, parasites, or pathogenic bacteria.

In addition, a change in the number and strength of intestinal contractions that push food through the intestine causes IBS. When the waves are faster and stronger, the contractions cause diarrhea; when the waves are slower, constipation follows. Anxiety and emotional tension—those "butterflies in your stomach" or gut feelings—can adversely affect IBS symptoms and bring on an attack. The very nature of IBS symptoms—painful cramps, frequent flatulence, and alternating constipation and diarrhea—makes it difficult to discuss with family members, work colleagues, or strangers.

Dietary instructions

Follow the basic principles of the Probiotic Diet. If diarrhea remains persistent, you should consume only cooked vegetables since raw veggies can aggravate the digestive system. In severe cases, refrain from consuming any dairy products for the first week of the diet. Raw nuts and seeds may be difficult to digest at the onset of the program. Nut and seed butters or soaked nuts and seeds may be a safer choice.

If following Phase I brings about a marked improvement but the introduction of new foods in Phases II and III bring about a return of symptoms, repeat Phase I as many times as necessary. Following Phase I for a year or more is not only acceptable but the first phase of the Probiotic Diet makes for a wonderful long-term eating plan and provides for excellent total body health.

Healing foods

- chicken soup (please see the recipe for Grandma Rose's Healing Chicken Soup on page 159)

- cold water fish, including wild salmon

- flaxseed and chia seed products, which improve elimination when you're feeling constipated and boost energy levels

- coconut products, including extra-virgin coconut oil, up to four tablespoons per day used in cooking, baking, smoothies, or right off the spoon. Coconut products, including coconut oil, can help with all facets of digestion and elimination and have anti-viral and anti-fungal properties.

- raw cultured dairy if available, especially kefir and cream (goat's milk may be more tolerable, but as long as the dairy is raw and comes from grass-fed animals, cow's milk should be fine). Cultured dairy (preferably raw from goat's or cow's milk or pasteurized sheep's milk yogurt) is usually well tolerated, and I recommend consuming as much as one to two quarts per day.

Healing supplements

- SBO probiotic blend containing *Bacillus subtilis, Bacillus coagulans, Bacillus clausii Saccharomyces boulardii,* providing probiotics, prebiotics, parabiotics and postbiotics

- omega-3 fatty acid supplement

- a whole food vitamin/mineral supplement with glandulars

- digestive enzymes (plant-based)

Inflammatory Bowel Disease
(Crohn's disease and ulcerative colitis)

Description

These chronic digestive disorders of the small and large intestines have symptoms that range from mild to severe and life-threatening and include any or all of the following:

- persistent diarrhea
- abdominal pain or cramps
- blood passing through the rectum
- fever and weight loss
- skin or eye irritations
- delayed growth and stunted sexual maturation in children

Surgery is sometimes recommended when medication can no longer control the symptoms, or when there are intestinal obstructions. An estimated two-thirds to three-quarters of persons with Crohn's disease will have one or more operations in the course of their lifetimes. The surgery for Crohn's disease, however, is not considered a permanent cure because the disease frequently returns elsewhere in the gastrointestinal tract. For ulcerative colitis, surgical removal of the entire colon and rectum (colectomy) is a permanent cure. Approximately 25 percent to 40 percent of ulcerative colitis patients will require surgery at some point during their illness.

Dietary instructions

Follow the basic principles of the Probiotic Diet. If diarrhea is persistent, you should consume only cooked vegetables since raw veggies may aggravate the digestive system. In severe cases, you should refrain from consuming any dairy products for the first week of the diet. Raw nuts and seeds may be difficult to digest. Nut and seed butters or soaked nuts and seeds would be a safer choice at the onset of the program.

If following Phase I brings about a marked improvement but the introduction of new foods in Phases II and III bring about a return of symptoms, repeat Phase I as many times as necessary. Following Phase I for a year or more is not only acceptable but it is a wonderful long-term diet and provides for excellent total body health.

Healing foods

- chicken soup (please see the recipe for Grandma Rose's Healing Chicken Soup on page 159)
- cold water fish, including wild salmon
- coconut products, including extra-virgin coconut oil, up to 4 tablespoons per day used in cooking, baking, smoothies, or right off the spoon. Coconut products, including coconut oil, can help add pounds to those who are underweight and have anti-viral and anti-fungal properties.
- raw cultured dairy if available, especially kefir and cream (goat's milk may be more tolerable, but as long as the dairy is raw and comes from grass-fed animals, cow's milk should be fine). Cultured dairy (preferably raw from goat's or cow's milk or pasteurized sheep's milk yogurt) is usually well tolerated, and I recommend consuming as much as one to two quarts per day.

Healing supplements

- SBO probiotic blend containing *Bacillus subtilis, Bacillus coagulans, Bacillus clausii Saccharomyces boulardii,* providing probiotics, prebiotics, parabiotics and postbiotics
- omega-3 fatty acid supplement
- a whole food vitamin/mineral supplement with glandulars
- digestive enzymes (plant-based)
- Montmorillonite clay (an iron-rich healing clay discovered in Montmorillon, France) in powder or liquid form, which is a great way to detoxify the colon and decrease diarrhea

Chronic Fatigue Syndrome and Fibromyalgia

Description

Approximately four million Americans suffer from chronic fatigue syndrome (CFS) and nearly as many deal with fibromyalgia (FM) on a daily basis. CFS and FM are among the most mysterious and controversial maladies of the last 20 years with symptoms such as:

- headaches
- insomnia
- muscle and joint pain

- loss of appetite
- mood swings
- muscle spasms
- night sweats
- swollen lymph nodes

I suffered from symptoms of both afflictions when I faced significant health challenges shortly after my freshman year of college. Chronic fatigue syndrome and fibromyalgia present themselves through persistent, overwhelming symptoms of fatigue and feelings of exhaustion. Today they're viewed as a complex and continual cycle of symptoms that dramatically lower the quality of one's life.

Thankfully, CFS and FM have become better understood in the last decade or so, although as researchers learn more about chronic fatigue syndrome and fibromyalgia, they're discovering significant differences between them. The immune systems behave differently, for instance, meaning that the immune systems of people with chronic fatigue syndrome behave as though they have an important infection to fight, while those with fibromyalgia don't have the same sort of immune response.

Dietary instructions

Follow the basic principles of the Probiotic Diet. Focus on consuming the following foods and supplements as often as possible, and you could see a health turnaround.

Healing foods

- chicken soup (please see the recipe for Grandma Rose's Healing Chicken Soup on page 159)

- apple cider vinegar (unpasteurized), which pro-vides an excellent source of potassium and malic acid, nutrients both known to benefit those with fibromyalgia
- fresh veggie juice high in greens such as celery, parsley, cucumber, and cilantro, which is a wonderful daily detoxification tonic
- avocados, which are a great source of vitamin E and potassium as well as healthy fats and fiber
- flaxseed and chia seed products, including fresh ground seed and oil, which can boost energy levels
- cold water fish, including wild salmon
- coconut products, including extra-virgin coconut oil, up to four tablespoons per day used in cooking, baking, smoothies, or right off the spoon
- raw cultured dairy if available, especially kefir and cream (goat's milk may be more tolerable, but as long as the dairy is raw and comes from grass-fed animals, cow's milk should be fine)

Healing supplements

- SBO probiotic blend containing *Bacillus subtilis, Bacillus coagulans, Bacillus clausii Saccharomyces boulardii,* providing probiotics, prebiotics, parabiotics and postbiotics
- omega-3 fatty acid supplement
- a whole food vitamin/mineral supplement with glandulars
- digestive enzymes (plant-based)

Heartburn, Acid Reflux, and GERD

Description

According to the latest government statistics, 25 million people suffer from heartburn daily, while more than 60 million American adults endure occasional occurrences of heartburn. Heartburn lowers quality of life, while long-term acid reflux can cause scarring and narrowing of the esophagus. This can lead to swallowing difficulties and even prevent food and liquid from reaching the stomach.

The stomach acids that cause heartburn and acid reflux are also known as hydrochloric acid. To help digest food, the stomach produces about a quart of hydrochloric acid a day to aid in the digestion process. Usually, the acid doesn't present a problem because the gastrointestinal tract is coated with a protective mucous lining. When that hydrochloric acid moves up the esophagus, however, watch out. The delicate tissue of the esophagus doesn't have a protective lining like the stomach, which means that the corrosive nature of the hydrochloric acid produces the burning sensation known around the world as heartburn.

When acid reflux, the more severe form of indigestion, hits those pain buttons, it becomes a medical condition known as GERD, an acronym for "gastroesophageal reflux disease." Normally, during the act of swallowing, the muscle at the bottom of the esophagus—the lower esophageal sphincter—cooperates by opening up and allowing food into the stomach. With age, stress, or poor physical condition, however, the lower esophageal sphincter can weaken, allowing food and acid to go back up the hatch. Left untreated, GERD can lead to ulcers and bleeding of the esophagus as well as increasing the risk of developing cancer of the esophagus.

Dietary instructions

Follow the basic principles of the Probiotic Diet. In severe cases, it may be best to refrain from consuming any dairy products for the first week of the diet. Raw nuts and seeds are usually difficult to digest.

If following Phase I brings about a marked improvement but the introduction of new foods in Phases II and III bring about a return of symptoms or a worsening, repeat Phase I as many times as necessary. Following Phase I for a year or more is not only acceptable but the first phase of the Probiotic Diet makes for a wonderful long-term eating plan and provides for excellent total body health.

Healing foods

- chicken soup (please see the recipe for Grandma Rose's Healing Chicken Soup on page 159)

- cold water fish, including wild salmon

- coconut products, including extra-virgin coconut oil, up to two to four tablespoons per day used in cooking, baking, smoothies, or right off the spoon. Coconut products have anti-viral and anti-fungal properties.

- raw cultured dairy if available, especially kefir and cream (goat's milk may be more tolerable, but as long as the dairy is raw and comes from grass-fed animals, cow's milk should be fine). Cultured dairy (preferably raw from goat's or cow's milk or pasteurized sheep's milk yogurt) is usually well tolerated, and I recommend consuming as much as one to two quarts per day, especially if you're underweight.

- cultured raw veggies (sauerkraut) are wonderful for those battling upper GI diseases. Cabbage contains vitamin U, a sulfur compound known as an anti-ulcer vitamin. Drinking the juice of fresh cabbage, up to 16 ounces per day, mixed with a small amount of carrot juice, has been reported to greatly improve this condition.

Healing supplements

- SBO probiotic blend containing *Bacillus subtilis, Bacillus coagulans, Bacillus clausii Saccharomyces boulardii,* providing probiotics, prebiotics, parabiotics and postbiotics
- omega-3 fatty acid supplement
- a whole food vitamin/mineral supplement with glandulars
- digestive enzymes (plant-based)

Ulcers

Description

Ulcers are sores on the lining of your digestive tract, and they are often quite painful. Most ulcers are located in the duodenum, the part of the intestinal tract that links the stomach and the small intestine. Ulcers located in the stomach are called gastric ulcers.

Ulcers occur when the lining of the esophagus, stomach, or duodenum is corroded by acidic digestive juices secreted by stomach cells. For many years, excess acid was believed to be the major cause of ulcers, but medical researchers today believe that the leading cause of ulcer disease is an infection of the stomach caused by a bacteria called *Helicobacter pyloridus*, or *H. pylori*, which points more to the need for the Probiotic Diet and the introduction of beneficial organisms to the gut.

Dietary instructions

Follow the basic principles of the Probiotic Diet. In severe cases, it may be best to refrain from consuming any dairy products for the first week of the diet. Raw nuts and seeds are usually difficult to digest.

If following Phase I brings about a marked improvement but the introduction of new foods in Phases II and III bring about a return of symptoms or a worsening, repeat Phase I as many times as necessary. Following Phase I for a year or more is not only acceptable but the first phase of the Probiotic Diet makes for a wonderful long-term eating plan and provides for excellent total body health.

Healing foods

- chicken soup (please see the recipe for Grandma Rose's Healing Chicken Soup on page 159)
- cold water fish, including wild salmon
- coconut products, including extra-virgin coconut oil, up to two to four tablespoons per day used in cooking, baking, smoothies, or right off the spoon. Coconut products have anti-viral and anti-fungal properties.
- raw cultured dairy if available, especially kefir and cream (goat's milk may be more tolerable, but as long

as the dairy is raw and comes from grass-fed animals, cow's milk should be fine). Cultured dairy (preferably raw from goat's or cow's milk or pasteurized sheep's milk yogurt) is usually well tolerated, and I recommend consuming as much as one to two quarts per day, especially if you're underweight.

- cultured raw veggies (sauerkraut) are wonderful for those battling upper GI diseases like peptic ulcers. Cabbage contains vitamin U, a sulfur compound known as an anti-ulcer vitamin. Drinking the juice of fresh cabbage, up to 16 ounces per day, mixed with a small amount of carrot juice, has been reported to greatly improve this condition.

Healing supplements

- SBO probiotic blend containing *Bacillus subtilis, Bacillus coagulans, Bacillus clausii Saccharomyces boulardii,* providing probiotics, prebiotics, parabiotics and postbiotics
- omega-3 fatty acid supplement
- a whole food vitamin/mineral supplement with glandulars
- digestive enzymes (plant-based)

Gas and Bloating

Description

We all chuckle and make jokes about flatulence—also known as an anal salute, backfire, a butt burp, and passing wind—but there's no doubt that "cutting the cheese" at a dinner party is one of the most embarrassing social faux pas that can happen to you.

And that's no laughing matter.

Bloating, belching, and passing gas are natural, but when their occurrence happens repeatedly throughout the day, that may be an indication of something more serious happening in your gastrointestinal tract. Bloating is the common term for gas buildup in the stomach and intestines. It's often accompanied by sharp abdominal pains, although passing gas or having a bowel movement may relieve the symptoms.

Dietary instructions

Follow the basic principles of the Probiotic Diet. Avoid or reduce any foods that are known to cause discomfort. These include broccoli, baked beans, Brussels sprouts, cabbage, cauliflower, carbonated drinks (you shouldn't be drinking sodas anyway), lettuce, and fruits such as apples, peaches, and pears.

When you start Phase I, gas and bloating usually improve dramatically within the first few days. Focus on consuming the following foods and supplements as often as possible, and you could see a health turnaround.

Healing foods

- chicken soup (please see the recipe for Grandma Rose's Healing Chicken Soup on page 159)

- cold water fish, including wild salmon

- coconut products, including extra-virgin coconut oil, up to two to four tablespoons per day used in cooking, baking, smoothies, or right off the spoon. Coconut products, including coconut oil, have anti-viral and anti-fungal properties.

- raw cultured dairy if available, especially kefir and cream (goat's milk may be more tolerable, but as long as the dairy is raw and comes from grass-fed animals, cow's milk should be fine)

Healing supplements

- SBO probiotic blend containing *Bacillus subtilis, Bacillus coagulans, Bacillus clausii Saccharomyces boulardii,* providing probiotics, prebiotics, parabiotics and postbiotics

- omega-3 fatty acid supplement

- a whole food vitamin/mineral supplement with glandulars

- digestive enzymes (plant-based)

Skin Disorders (acne, eczema, psoriasis)

Description

I mentioned in Chapter 3 how our son Samuel developed a nasty case of eczema while he was in foster care until the adoption process could be finalized. Skin disorders like eczema as well as acne and psoriasis often reflect an unhealthy internal environment. That's why one of the first things I did when we brought Samuel home after the adoption was to feed him a probiotic-rich infant formula that delivered healthy microorganisms into his tiny terrain.

Samuel's inflamed and irritated skin eventually cleared up, but for many infants and young children, eczema remains a troubling skin condition. The exact cause of eczema is unknown, but medical researchers believe the itchy skin condition can be linked to an overactive response by the body's immune system to a bacterium.

Acne, as any parent of teenagers knows, is often the bane of adolescence. Pimples and blackheads occur due to an overproduction of oil by the skin's oil glands. Acne is often treated with antibiotics, which is robbing Peter to pay Paul because killing the surface bacteria aggravates the skin and compromises gut and immune function by killing all the good bacteria in the terrain.

Dietary instructions

Follow the basic principles of the Probiotic Diet. People with severe skin conditions such as cystic acne should eliminate all dairy products for the first week of the diet to see if improvement is dramatic. If the reintroduction of dairy causes symptoms to reappear, eliminating dairy for an entire month may be indicated.

Focus on consuming the following foods and supplements as often as possible, and you could see a health turnaround.

Healing foods

- chicken soup (please see the recipe for Grandma Rose's Healing Chicken Soup on page 159)
- flaxseed and chia seed products, including fresh ground seed and oil
- cold water fish, including wild salmon
- coconut products, including extra-virgin coconut oil, up to two to four tablespoons per day used in cooking, baking, smoothies, or right off the spoon
- fresh carrot juice mixed with green juice such as celery and parsley is wonderful for most skin conditions, especially acne
- raw cultured dairy if available, especially kefir and cream (goat's milk may be more tolerable, but as long as the dairy is raw and comes from grass-fed animals, cow's milk should be fine). Cultured dairy (preferably raw from goat's or cow's milk or pasteurized sheep's milk yogurt) is usually well tolerated, and I recommend consuming one quart per day.

Healing supplements

- SBO probiotic blend containing *Bacillus subtilis, Bacillus coagulans, Bacillus clausii Saccharomyces boulardii,* providing probiotics, prebiotics, parabiotics and postbiotics
- omega-3 fatty acid supplement

- a whole food vitamin/mineral supplement with glandulars
- digestive enzymes (plant-based)

Weight Management

Description

An estimated 65 percent of Americans aged 20 and older are overweight. The problem of childhood obesity is growing exponentially. You probably don't need to be reminded that packing on too many pounds is unhealthy or has become part of the national discussion these days. You'd have to be Stevie Wonder not to notice all the jiggly tummies or padded thighs in the malls these days.

As a culture, we are a little taller but a lot heavier than we were a generation ago; today we weigh 25 pounds more than our grandparents or parents did in the 1960s, with the biggest weight gains attached to men 40 and older. Being overweight is a cause of high blood pressure, high cholesterol, hypertension, type 2 diabetes, and a host of other ailments that shorten one's life span.

The correlation between being overweight—which comes from eating unhealthily—and having an unhealthy terrain is undeniable. Although the Probiotic Diet is not touted as a weight-loss diet plan, I can practically issue a money-back guarantee that you *will* lose weight if you complete all three phases of the 12-week Probiotic Diet. Why's that? Because you will be consuming carbohydrate-restrictive foods.

Dietary instructions

Follow the basic principles of the Probiotic Diet. You will notice the most rapid weight loss in Phase I. If your weight loss slows or you gain some weight back on Phase II or III, return to Phase I and remain there until you reach your ideal weight.

Focus on consuming the following foods and supplements as often as possible, and you could see a health turnaround.

Healing foods

- chicken soup (please see the recipe for Grandma Rose's Healing Chicken Soup on page 159)

- cold water fish, including wild salmon

- flaxseed and chia seed products, including fresh ground seed and oil, boost energy levels when you have the blahs

- berries are a wonderful source of nutrients and fiber and are extremely low in calories

- coconut products, including extra-virgin coconut oil, up to two tablespoons per day used in cooking, baking, smoothies, or right off the spoon. Coconut products, including coconut oil, can help balance the health of the thyroid and ward off infections, leading to improved health.

- raw cultured dairy if available, especially kefir (goat's milk may be more tolerable, but as long as the dairy is raw and comes from grass-fed animals, cow's milk should be fine)

Healing supplements

- SBO probiotic blend containing *Bacillus subtilis, Bacillus coagulans, Bacillus clausii Saccharomyces boulardii,* providing probiotics, prebiotics, parabiotics and postbiotics
- omega-3 fatty acid supplement
- a whole food vitamin/mineral supplement with glandulars
- digestive enzymes (plant-based)

Food Allergies

Description

Food allergies, also known as food sensitivities, are a measurable immune response to a normally harmless food. Symptoms include itchy hives, lip swelling, nausea, vomiting, diarrhea, and difficulty breathing. Common food allergies are to peanuts, wheat, milks, eggs, MSG, and shellfish.

Scientists have yet to pinpoint what exactly causes food allergies. There is evidence that some allergies are the result of exposure to a certain food or foods early in life before the immune system has fully developed. Many infants who are given cow's milk instead of breast milk in the first month develop an allergic reaction. At any rate, food allergies and sensitivities can sometimes be difficult to identify, which means that you'll have to employ some trial-and-error testing of the Probiotic Diet.[1]

Dietary instructions

Follow the basic principles of the Probiotic Diet. If you have suspected allergies to dairy, it's best to avoid all dairy products for the first week. Many people with food allergies do better on goat's or sheep's milk dairy products. Avoid any known allergens while following the diet.

Healing foods

- chicken soup (please see the recipe for Grandma Rose's Healing Chicken Soup on page 159)
- flaxseed and chia seed products, including fresh ground seed and oil
- cold water fish, including wild salmon
- coconut products, including extra-virgin coconut oil, up to four tablespoons per day used in cooking, baking, smoothies, or right off the spoon. Coconut products, including coconut oil, have anti-viral and anti-fungal properties.
- raw cultured dairy if available, especially kefir (goat's milk may be more tolerable, but as long as the dairy is raw and comes from grass-fed animals, cow's milk should be fine). Cultured dairy (preferably raw from goat's or cow's milk or pasteurized sheep's milk yogurt) is usually well tolerated, and I recommend consuming as much as one quart per day.

Healing supplements

- SBO probiotic blend containing *Bacillus subtilis, Bacillus coagulans, Bacillus clausii Saccharomyces boulardii,* providing probiotics, prebiotics, parabiotics and postbiotics

- omega-3 fatty acid supplement
- a whole food vitamin/mineral supplement with glandulars
- digestive enzymes (plant-based)

Candida Yeast Infections

Description

Candida albicans are a form of yeast normally found in the lower bowel and vagina. Normally the presence of friendly bacteria like *Lactobacillus acidophilus* and *Bifidobacteria bifidum* provide a natural control mechanism to prevent the overgrowth of *candida albicans.*

As long as your immune system is healthy and strong, *candida albicans* growth is regulated and kept under control. The insidious candida yeast infection can morph from the normally innocent *Candida albicans* when you take antibiotics, acne medications, or birth control pills, providing an opportunity for a yeast infection to take hold. When this happens—and it can quite often—the candida albicans yeast cells have an open opportunity to overpopulate the terrain and infect other body organs and tissues.

Dietary instructions

Follow the basic principles of the Probiotic Diet. Stay on Phase I of the diet as long as desired. If you proceed to Phase II and notice yeast infection symptoms returning, start Phase I again and remain there for twice the amount of time as previously before moving to Phase II.

Healing foods

- chicken soup (please see the recipe for Grandma Rose's Healing Chicken Soup on page 159)
- cold water fish, including wild salmon
- flaxseed and chia seed products, including fresh ground seed and oil
- coconut products, including extra-virgin coconut oil, up to four tablespoons per day used in cooking, baking, smoothies, or right off the spoon. Coconut products, including coconut oil, have amazing anti-viral and anti-fungal properties.
- raw cultured dairy if available, especially kefir and cream (goat's milk may be more tolerable, but as long as the dairy is raw and comes from grass-fed animals, cow's milk should be fine). Cultured dairy (preferably raw from goat's or cow's milk or pasteurized sheep's milk yogurt) is usually well tolerated, and I recommend consuming as much as one to two quarts per day to support immune system and digestive health.

Healing supplements

- SBO probiotic blend containing *Bacillus subtilis, Bacillus coagulans, Bacillus clausii Saccharomyces boulardii,* providing probiotics, prebiotics, parabiotics and postbiotics
- omega-3 fatty acid supplement

- a whole food vitamin/mineral supplement with glandulars
- digestive enzymes (plant-based)

Asthma

Description

Asthma is one of the most common chronic diseases of child-hood and the most common cause of school absenteeism. As a medical condition, asthma is an inflammation of the bronchial tubes that cause airway obstruction, chest tightness, coughing, and wheezing. Since asthma is a chronic disease that affects a child's breathing, you may be wondering, *What does asthma have to do with the digestive issues or the Probiotic Diet?*

Here's your answer: If your infant received several courses of antibiotics before celebrating his or her first birthday, then your child has a significantly higher chance of developing asthma by age seven, according to a study reported in the medical journal *Chest*, which outlines the evidence for an antibiotic-asthma link.[2]

The Probiotic Diet Eating Plan can help your children—or you, if you're an adult asthma sufferer—replenish the friendly micro-flora that the digestive tract needs, which will help the immune system, which, in turn, will help the respiratory system.

Dietary instructions

Follow the basic principles of the Probiotic Diet. Focus on consuming the following foods and supplements as often as possible, and you could see a health turnaround.

Healing foods

- chicken soup (please see the recipe for Grandma Rose's Healing Chicken Soup on page 159)
- cold water fish, including wild salmon
- flaxseed and chia seed products, including fresh ground seed and oil
- coconut products, including extra-virgin coconut oil, up to two tablespoons per day used in cooking, baking, smoothies, or right off the spoon. Coconut products, including coconut oil, have anti-viral and anti-fungal properties.
- raw cultured dairy if available, especially kefir and cream (goat's milk may be more tolerable, but as long as the dairy is raw and comes from grass-fed animals, cow's milk should be fine). Cultured dairy (preferably raw from goat's or cow's milk or pasteurized sheep's milk yogurt) is usually well tolerated, and I recommend consuming as much as one quart per day.

Healing supplements

- SBO probiotic blend containing *Bacillus subtilis, Bacillus coagulans, Bacillus clausii Saccharomyces boulardii,* providing probiotics, prebiotics, parabiotics and postbiotics
- omega-3 fatty acid supplement
- a whole food vitamin/mineral supplement with glandulars
- digestive enzymes (plant-based)

Diarrhea

Description

Let's say that 30 minutes after finishing a meal, a thumping headache bounces around the inside of your skull like a leaded Pachinko ball. Your stomach gurgles like Mount St. Helens, and you know what's coming next: a sprint to the nearest throne before the volcano explodes.

Eat.

Get diarrhea.

Eat.

Get diarrhea.

Eat.

Get diarrhea.

Spot a pattern here?

Perhaps you've always lived with a "touch" of diarrhea, and you've learned how to endure these discomforting episodes. When your stools are continually loose or diarrhea is unremitting, however, that's when you know something is definitely off-kilter in the digestive tract. When it comes to enjoying life, eating is no fun if you're sitting on porcelain half the day.

If you go see your family physician about persistent diarrhea, he or she is apt to write a prescription for an anti-diarrheal like Loperamide, which slows the rate of food traveling through the stomach and intestines. This antimotility drug—Loperamide is not an antibiotic—also acts to increase stool density and reduce the amount of fluid in the stool. Side effects, which are said not to be common, include difficulty breathing, swelling of the lips, tongue, or face, and development of a fever.

Now if you take Loperamide *with* an antibiotic, watch out—or at least know where the nearest bathroom is located. Quick-hitting diarrhea often occurs when antibiotics disturb the natural balance of good and bad bacteria in your intestinal tract, causing harmful bacteria to grow beyond their normal numbers. The result is often frequent, watery bowel movements.

Dietary instructions

Follow the basic principles of the Probiotic Diet. If diarrhea has persisted for more than six weeks, you should begin the diet with a three-day chicken soup cleanse. Follow Grandma Rose's Healing Chicken Soup recipe on page 159 and consume only the contents of the soup and drink pure water for three days. Begin Phase I of the diet, avoiding raw veggies for the first week until bowel movements are formed.

Healing foods

- chicken soup
- cold water fish, including wild salmon
- flaxseed and chia seed products, including fresh ground seeds and oil (two tablespoons per day), which improve regularity and boost energy levels
- coconut products, including extra-virgin coconut oil, up to four tablespoons per day used in cooking, baking, smoothies, or right off the spoon. Coconut products, including coconut oil, have anti-viral and anti-fungal properties and can relieve diarrhea.
- raw cultured dairy if available, especially kefir and cream (goat's milk may be more tolerable, but as long as the dairy is raw and comes from grass-fed animals, cow's milk should be fine). Cultured dairy (preferably

raw from goat's or cow's milk or pasteurized sheep's milk yogurt) is usually well tolerated, and I recommend consuming as much as one to two quarts per day, especially if you're underweight. Eating yogurt is said to relieve symptoms and help prevent antibiotic-associated diarrhea.

Healing supplements

- SBO probiotic blend containing *Bacillus subtilis, Bacillus coagulans, Bacillus clausii Saccharomyces boulardii,* providing probiotics, prebiotics, parabiotics and postbiotics
- omega-3 fatty acid supplement
- a whole food vitamin/mineral supplement with glandulars
- digestive enzymes (plant-based)

Constipation

Description

Constipation is probably the most common gastrointestinal complaint in the U.S., as evidenced by 2.5 million doctor visits each year from people complaining that they hurt from constipation stools that are frequently hard, small in size, and difficult to eliminate. Technically, constipation is defined as having a bowel movement fewer than three times a week, but I think that if you're not going at least once a day, then your digestive system is off track.

Constipation is not a disease but a road sign that your terrain isn't clicking the way it should. Poor diet is typically the cause, as well as not drinking enough water. You also can't ignore the urge to have a bowel movement. When the urge presses, you need to take care of business.

Dietary instructions

Follow the basic principles of the Probiotic Diet. Bowel movements should increase after two weeks on the diet once your bowel begins to adapt to more fiber-rich foods. Be intentional about drinking much more water than you're used to. Keep a glass of water nearby at your place of work or around the house. Try to drink the proverbial eight glasses of water per day.

Healing foods

- chicken soup (please see the recipe for Grandma Rose's Healing Chicken Soup on page 159)
- cold water fish, including wild salmon
- flaxseed and chia seed products, including fresh ground seeds and oil, which improve elimination when you're feeling backed up and boost energy levels
- avocados, which are a wonderful source of vitamins, minerals, healthy fats, and fiber
- coconut products, including extra-virgin coconut oil, up to four tablespoons per day used in cooking, baking, smoothies, or right off the spoon. Coconut products, including coconut oil, can help increase elimination and have anti-viral and anti-fungal properties.

- raw cultured dairy if available, especially kefir and cream (goat's milk may be more tolerable, but as long as the dairy is raw and comes from grass-fed animals, cow's milk should be fine). Cultured dairy (preferably raw from goat's or cow's milk or pasteurized sheep's milk yogurt) is usually well tolerated, and I recommend consuming as much as one to two quarts per day, especially if you're chronically constipated.

Healing supplements

- SBO probiotic blend containing *Bacillus subtilis, Bacillus coagulans, Bacillus clausii Saccharomyces boulardii*, providing probiotics, prebiotics, parabiotics and postbiotics
- omega-3 fatty acid supplement
- a whole food vitamin/mineral supplement with glandulars
- digestive enzymes (plant-based)

Intestinal Parasites

Description

This may make you feel queasy reading this, but parasites live and reproduce in the human intestines, and there is a parasite connection to many health problems facing Americans today. Parasites compete with the digestive system for nutrients, but also—and this part will gross you out—secrete waste products into the gut and bloodstream that can cause various allergic and autoimmune reactions. Parasites typically cause appetite changes, abdominal discomfort, cramping and changes in stool, and diarrhea.[3]

When parasites are in the intestines, they attach to the inside of the intestinal wall, where they can disrupt the normal function of the intestines and jockey for nutrients from food passing through the digestive tract. Giardia is one of the most common parasites found in humans, and it's usually picked up when you drink water in an underdeveloped country or from contaminated rivers and streams here in the United States. Food preparers who do not wash their hands after going to the restroom is another way this fecal-oral condition is spread. A healthy terrain remains your best defense against parasitic infection.

Dietary instructions

Follow the basic principles of the Probiotic Diet. If diarrhea is a main symptom and has persisted for more than six weeks, you should begin the diet with a three-day chicken soup cleanse. Follow Grandma Rose's Healing Chicken Soup recipe on page 159 and consume only the contents of the soup and drink pure water for three days. Begin Phase I of the diet avoiding raw veggies for the first week until bowel movements are formed.

Healing foods

- chicken soup
- cold water fish, including wild salmon
- flaxseed and chia seed products, including fresh ground seeds and oil (two tablespoons per day), which improve elimination and boost energy levels
- coconut products, including extra-virgin coconut oil, up to four tablespoons per day used in cooking,

baking, smoothies, or right off the spoon. Coconut products, including coconut oil, have anti-viral and anti-fungal properties.

- raw cultured dairy if available, especially kefir and cream (goat's milk may be more tolerable, but as long as the dairy is raw and comes from grass-fed animals, cow's milk should be fine). Cultured dairy (preferably raw from goat's or cow's milk or pasteurized sheep's milk yogurt) is usually well tolerated, and I recommend consuming as much as one to two quarts per day, especially if you're underweight.

Healing supplements

- SBO probiotic blend containing *Bacillus subtilis, Bacillus coagulans, Bacillus clausii Saccharomyces boulardii,* providing probiotics, prebiotics, parabiotics and postbiotics
- omega-3 fatty acid supplement
- a whole food vitamin/mineral supplement with glandulars
- digestive enzymes (plant-based)

Celiac Disease/Gluten Intolerance

Description

Celiac disease is a digestive disease that damages the small intestine and interferes with the absorption of nutrients from food. Those suffering from celiac disease cannot tolerate gluten, a protein found in wheat, rye, and barley. Gluten is present in just about every commercially baked product on store shelves.

Remember those hair-like microvilli that line the inside of the small intestine that I told you about in Chapter 6? When people with celiac disease eat foods containing gluten, their immune system responds by damaging or destroying microvilli. Without healthy villi, you become malnourished, no matter how much food you eat.

The only treatment for celiac disease is a gluten-free diet, and to stay well, people with celiac disease must avoid gluten for the rest of their lives. Even a small amount of gluten can do a number on your small intestine. Realize that small amounts of gluten are hidden in additives such as modified food starch, preservatives, and stabilizers made with wheat. Because many corn and rice products are produced in factories that also manufacture wheat products, they may be contaminated with wheat gluten as well.

Dietary instructions

You will have to follow Phase I of the Probiotic Diet closely, which calls for avoiding all grains and starchy foods: no bread, pasta, cereal, baked goods, pastries, or rice. Whatever you eat, double-check to make sure it's gluten-free.

If gas, bloating, and diarrhea are persistent, you should consume only cooked vegetables as raw veggies may aggravate the digestive system. In severe cases of celiac disease, it may be best to refrain from consuming any dairy products for the first week of the diet. Raw nuts and seeds are usually difficult to digest. Nut and seed butters or soaked nuts and seeds may be a safer choice at the onset of the program.

If following Phase I brings about a marked improvement, you may add some of the new foods in Phases II and III, but obviously refrain from any foods that might contain gluten. If your symptoms of celiac disease return, repeat Phase I as many times as necessary. In fact, Phase I makes for a wonderful long-term gluten-free diet and provides for excellent total body health when you're dealing with a lifelong condition like celiac disease.

Healing foods

- chicken soup (please see the recipe for Grandma Rose's Healing Chicken Soup on page 159)

- cold water fish, including wild salmon

- coconut products, including extra-virgin coconut oil, up to four tablespoons per day used in cooking, baking, smoothies, or right off the spoon. Coconut products, including coconut oil, can help add weight to those who are underweight and have anti-viral and anti-fungal properties.

- raw cultured dairy if available, especially kefir and cream (goat's milk may be more tolerable, but as long as the dairy is raw and comes from grass-fed animals, cow's milk should be fine). Cultured dairy (preferably raw from goat's or cow's milk or pasteurized sheep's milk yogurt) is usually well tolerated, and I recommend consuming as much as one to two quarts per day, especially if you're underweight.

Healing supplements

- SBO probiotic blend containing *Bacillus subtilis, Bacillus coagulans, Bacillus clausii Saccharomyces boulardii,* providing probiotics, prebiotics, parabiotics and postbiotics

- omega-3 fatty acid supplement
- a whole food vitamin/mineral supplement with glandulars
- digestive enzymes (plant-based)
- Montmorillonite clay (an iron-rich healing clay discovered in Montmorillon, France) in powder or liquid form, which is a great way to detoxify the colon and decrease diarrhea

Liver and Gallbladder Heath

Description

The liver and gallbladder work as a team to eliminate toxins and other potentially harmful agents taken into the body. The liver does most of the work, while the gallbladder stores the bile that the liver produces and empties the bile into the small intestine, where it's further broken down for absorption.

Since the liver and gallbladder are tied at the hip, so to speak, with your digestive system, following the Probiotic Diet will send fewer toxins to the liver and gallbladder. This will ease the workload on your terrain. Sometimes, however, the bile can harden and form granules—or stones—that result in gallbladder problems. Trying the Probiotic Diet may help you avoid a surgical procedure as well as other symptoms of gallstones, which include abdominal bloating, belching, gas, and indigestion.

Dietary instructions

Follow the basic principles of the Probiotic Diet. Focus on consuming the following foods and supplements as often as possible, and you could see a health turnaround.

Healing foods

- chicken soup (please see the recipe for Grandma Rose's Healing Chicken Soup on page 159)
- cold water fish, including wild salmon
- avocado, which is a wonderful source of vitamins, minerals and healthy fats and is very soothing to the liver
- coconut products, including extra-virgin coconut oil, up to two tablespoons per day used in cooking, baking, smoothies, or right off the spoon. Coconut products, including coconut oil, are easily tolerated by most, but should be consumed with caution by those who have liver or gallbladder issues.
- raw cultured dairy if available, especially kefir and cream (goat's milk may be more tolerable, but as long as the dairy is raw and comes from grass-fed animals, cow's milk should be fine)

Healing supplements

- SBO probiotic blend containing *Bacillus subtilis, Bacillus coagulans, Bacillus clausii Saccharomyces boulardii,* providing probiotics, prebiotics, parabiotics and postbiotics
- omega-3 fatty acid supplement

- a whole food vitamin/mineral supplement with glandulars
- digestive enzymes (plant-based)

Colds and Flu

Description

Colds and flu are viral illnesses that share many of the same symptoms and are caused by the same family of respiratory viruses, although there are some key differences. A cold is an infection of the upper respiratory tract that includes a runny nose, sneezing, and coughing. A flu usually features the same symptoms, only more severe, along with fever, muscle aches, and more persistent coughing.[4]

Flu sufferers will sometimes experience spikes of high fever followed by chills, which can exhaust victims and cause their whole body to feel sore. Here's an amateur, non-medical description of the differences between a cold and the flu: When you have a cold, you can still go to work, do your chores, or carry on with a normal day. When you have the flu, you're down for the count and too weak to get out of bed.

According to the Mayo Clinic, the average American adult contracts between two to four upper respiratory illnesses a year—mostly during the "cold-and-flu season" between October and April. Children, as any parent knows, are more susceptible since they're cooped up with 20 or 30 classmates every day; they average between six to ten colds a year.[5]

Most people, when they see their family physician for a sinus problem or a nasty bronchial infection, walk out of the doctor's office holding a prescription for antibiotics. But as you've learned by now, our society is so intent on destroying bacteria that we've eradicated much of the beneficial bacteria in our bodies and the environment. In fact, I would argue that the lack of probiotics in our diet can be associated with allergies, frequent colds, and the flu.

Dietary instructions

Follow the basic principles of the Probiotic Diet, especially on the consumption of chicken soup. Stay focused on consuming the following foods and supplements as often as possible, and you could see a health turnaround.

Healing foods

- chicken soup (please see the recipe for Grandma Rose's Healing Chicken Soup on page 159)
- coconut products, including extra-virgin coconut oil, up to four tablespoons per day used in cooking, baking, smoothies, or right off the spoon. Coconut products, including coconut oil, have anti-viral and anti-fungal properties.

Healing supplements

- SBO probiotic blend containing *Bacillus subtilis, Bacillus coagulans, Bacillus clausii Saccharomyces boulardii,* providing probiotics, prebiotics, parabiotics and postbiotics
- omega-3 fatty acid supplement

- a whole food vitamin/mineral supplement with glandulars
- digestive enzymes (plant-based)

Urinary Tract Infections

Description

Your urinary system is composed of the kidneys, ureters, bladder, and urethra—the structures that urine passes through before being eliminated from the body. When a bacterial infection affects any part of the urinary tract, then you're dealing with a urinary tract infection. Most infections involve the lower urinary tract—the urethra and the bladder.

Women, as we described in Chapter 8, are at greater risk of developing a urinary tract infection than men because of the terrain of their reproductive systems, which includes the urinary system. Statistics tell us that these infections are much more common in girls and women than in boys and men younger than 50 years of age. About half of all women will have a urinary tract infection at some time in their lives, while many women will have multiple infections throughout their lifetime.[6]

Keep in mind that physicians routinely prescribe antibiotics for a urinary tract infection since bacteria are involved, but that only compounds your compromised terrain.

Dietary instructions

Follow the basic principles of the Probiotic Diet. Focus on consuming the following foods and supplements as often as possible, and you could see a health turnaround.

Healing foods

- chicken soup (please see the recipe for Grandma Rose's Healing Chicken Soup on page 159)
- dark berries such as cranberries and blueberries, which are wonderful for urinary tract health and should be consumed daily. I recommend consuming fresh or frozen blueberries one to two cups per day.
- cold water fish, including wild salmon
- coconut products, including extra-virgin coconut oil, up to four tablespoons per day used in cooking, baking, smoothies, or right off the spoon. Coconut products, including coconut oil, have anti-viral and anti-fungal properties.
- raw cultured dairy if available, especially kefir and cream (goat's milk may be more tolerable, but as long as the dairy is raw and comes from grass-fed animals, cow's milk should be fine)

Healing supplements

- SBO probiotic blend containing *Bacillus subtilis, Bacillus coagulans, Bacillus clausii Saccharomyces boulardii,* providing probiotics, prebiotics, parabiotics and postbiotics
- omega-3 fatty acid supplement

- a whole food vitamin/mineral supplement with glandulars
- digestive enzymes (plant-based)

Tooth and Gum Disease

Description

As Dr. Hillman said in Chapter 9, tooth decay is a major problem in this country and around the world. As anyone who's reclined in a dental chair knows all too well, dental problems are painful, costly, and preventable. Dental caries (cavities) and periodontal disease (gum disease) are the most common oral health problems and are caused by bacteria in the dental plaque that forms on oral surfaces.

Eating probiotic-rich foods builds the body's defenses against oral health disease by reducing the production of plaque biofilm, which is the primary factor associated with periodontal disease. And every adult who ever went trick-or-treating as a kid knows that a surefire way to get cavities is to eat candy for a month. If you follow Phase I of the Probiotic Diet diligently, however, you'll be consuming very little sugar or sweeteners, which will prevent cavities from developing. Brushing your teeth with an electric toothbrush will help as well.

According to a U.S. Surgeon General report on oral health, the mouth can function as an "early warning" system for some diseases and can provide a useful means to understanding organs and systems in other parts of the body.

Dietary instructions

Follow the basic principles of the Probiotic Diet. Focus on consuming the following foods and supplements as often as possible, and you could see a health turnaround.

Healing foods

- chicken soup (please see the recipe for Grandma Rose's Healing Chicken Soup on page 159)
- cold water fish, including wild salmon
- raw cultured dairy if available, especially kefir and cream (goat's milk may be more tolerable, but as long as the dairy is raw and comes from grass-fed animals, cow's milk should be fine)

Healing supplements

- oral probiotic dissolvable mints containing beneficial bacteria
- SBO probiotic blend containing *Bacillus subtilis, Bacillus coagulans, Bacillus clausii Saccharomyces boulardii,* providing probiotics, prebiotics, parabiotics and postbiotics
- omega-3 fatty acid supplement
- a whole food vitamin/mineral supplement with glandulars
- digestive enzymes (plant-based)

High Cholesterol

Description

Too many Americans have too much cholesterol swirling in their bloodstreams. Approximately 37 million adults in this country have high blood cholesterol counts, and 105 million—*half* the U.S. adult population—have cholesterol levels that are higher than desirable, according to the Mayo Clinic.[7]

In medical terms, the genesis of high cholesterol begins when the levels of cholesterol and triglycerides, a blood fat, become too high in your bloodstream. This causes the development of cholesterol-containing fatty deposits—known as plaque—to form and begin traveling through your blood vessels. Over time, plaque can clog your arteries and veins like sludge in a drainpipe.

I believe high cholesterol is highly preventable and even reversible if you take hold of the Probiotic Diet. Many physicians, however, have a way of putting the fear of God into their patients when it comes to what foods they should eat. Doctors will bluntly tell you to lay off barbecued steak, stop eating hamburgers, stay away from deep-dish pizza, shake your salt habit, substitute a "margarine spread" for butter, and say no to nuts.

Some so-called "high fat" foods—steak, eggs, butter, and dairy products, when consumed from free-range and organic sources—actually contain fats that your body needs for optimal health. We *need* these fats to do the following functions: play a vital role in bone health, enhance the immune system, protect the liver from alcohol and other toxins, and guard against harmful microorganisms in the digestive tract.

Dietary instructions

Follow the basic principles of the Probiotic Diet. Focus on consuming the following foods as often as possible, and you could see a health turnaround.

Healing foods

- flaxseed and chia seed, including fresh ground powder and their oils

- avocados, which are an excellent source of vitamins, minerals, and healthy fats

- berries, which are a great source of fiber and antioxidants

- cold water fish, including wild salmon

- coconut products, including extra-virgin coconut oil, up to two tablespoons per day used in cooking, baking, smoothies, or right off the spoon. Coconut products, including coconut oil, support healthy cholesterol levels.

- raw cultured dairy if available, especially kefir and cream (goat's milk may be more tolerable, but as long as the dairy is raw and comes from grass-fed animals, cow's milk should be fine)

Healing supplements

- SBO probiotic blend containing *Bacillus subtilis, Bacillus coagulans, Bacillus clausii Saccharomyces boulardii*, providing probiotics, prebiotics, parabiotics and postbiotics

- omega-3 fatty acid supplement

- a whole food vitamin/mineral supplement with glandulars
- digestive enzymes (plant-based)
- flaxseed-based fiber blend

Cancer

Description

Cancer was never made more personal to me than when I watched bladder cancer emaciate my Grandma Rose the last year of her life. This once-vibrant woman shrank to a skeleton-like 70 pounds as the cancer—like a slow-moving army—invaded her body, plundered her mind, and eventually snuffed out the burning embers of a remarkable life.

Unfortunately, death-by-cancer stories like my Grandma Rose are way too common these days because "The Big C" has made a grim comeback: in 2005, the American Cancer Society announced that cancer had surpassed heart disease as the No. 1 killer of Americans under the age of 85, which comprise 98.4 percent of the population. This development has occurred during the federal government's three-decade-old "War on Cancer," which has poured more than $50 billion into research, on top of the billions more that private industry has kicked in. Despite the concerted scientific effort, about 1.4 million *new* cases of cancer were diagnosed in 2005, and approximately 570,000 died from the lethal disease. While one's eyes tend to glaze over from so many numbers, the stark reality is that half of all American men and one-third of American women will develop some type of cancer during their lifetimes.[8]

Dietary instructions

Follow the basic principles of the Probiotic Diet, but consume as much raw food as possible, which is the key to fighting this dreaded disease. I cannot stress to you enough the importance of avoiding sugar in all its forms. This directive is imperative.

Healing foods

- chicken soup (please see the recipe for Grandma Rose's Healing Chicken Soup on page 159)
- cold water fish, including wild salmon
- dark-colored fruits, including grapes, berries, and plums, which are wonderful sources of antioxidants
- coconut products, including extra-virgin coconut oil, up to four tablespoons per day used in cooking, baking, smoothies, or right off the spoon. Coconut products, including coconut oil, have anti-viral and anti-fungal properties.
- raw cultured dairy if available, especially kefir and cream (goat's milk may be more tolerable, but as long as the dairy is raw and comes from grass-fed animals, cow's milk should be fine)
- avocados, which are a wonderful source of vitamins, minerals, fiber, and healthy fats

Healing supplements

- SBO probiotic blend containing *Bacillus subtilis, Bacillus coagulans, Bacillus clausii Saccharomyces boulardii,* providing probiotics, prebiotics, parabiotics and postbiotics

- omega-3 fatty acid supplement
- a whole food vitamin/mineral supplement with glandulars
- digestive enzymes (plant-based)

Autoimmune Disease

Description

When germs, viruses, and bacteria attack the body, the immune system revs up to protect us from disease and infection. But when you have an autoimmune disease, your immune system attacks itself by mistake, and that's when you get sick. The American Autoimmune Related Diseases Association defines autoimmune disease as a group of more than 80 serious and chronic illnesses that involve nerves, muscles, and the digestive system. Inflammatory bowel disease is considered to be an autoimmune disease, as is multiple sclerosis and rheumatoid arthritis.

Life's no fun when your immune system turns on you and decides to upset the apple cart, so to speak, traveling through your digestive tract. Symptoms vary widely and depend on the specific disease, but most sufferers of an autoimmune disease say they experience dizziness, fatigue, low-grade fever, and a general ill-feeling during their waking hours.

Dietary instructions

Follow the basic principles of the Probiotic Diet. The best results will be achieved by staying on Phase I for two to three months to reduce inflammation. Focus on consuming the following foods as often as possible, and you could see a health turnaround.

Healing foods

- chicken soup (please see the recipe for Grandma Rose's Healing Chicken Soup on page 159)
- cold water fish, including wild salmon
- coconut products, including extra-virgin coconut oil, up to four tablespoons per day used in cooking, baking, smoothies, or right off the spoon. Coconut products, including coconut oil, have anti-viral and anti-fungal properties.
- raw cultured dairy if available, especially kefir and cream (goat's milk may be more tolerable, but as long as the dairy is raw and comes from grass-fed animals, cow's milk should be fine)

Healing supplements

- SBO probiotic blend containing *Bacillus subtilis, Bacillus coagulans, Bacillus clausii Saccharomyces boulardii,* providing probiotics, prebiotics, parabiotics and postbiotics
- omega-3 fatty acid supplement
- a whole food vitamin/mineral supplement with glandulars
- digestive enzymes (plant-based)

13

THE PROBIOTIC PATIENTS

We asked several of Dr. Brasco's patients as well as people who reached out to Dr. Axe and me to share their comeback stories. We hope you will be inspired.

Samantha Credle

Age: 18

Hometown: Chesapeake, Virginia

The hardest part has been sitting on the toilet so much.

There were days I had to go to the bathroom 15 or 20 times. My record was four hours in one sitting.

You see, I became a very sick little girl when I turned 13 years old in 2004. I'll never forget the bike ride I took with Mom and my sisters on Memorial Day that year, and we had to turn around because my bum was bleeding.

The low-grade fevers and feeling fatigued all the time told us that something was terribly wrong with me. My family physician thought I had a virus and told us to keep a temperature diary, which we did for three months. Each month we went back and were told the same thing: I was sick from a virus that had something to do with the onset of puberty.

"But what about her hemorrhoids?" Mom asked.

"Treat her with Tucks pads," the doctor replied, so Mom would fold and compress these hygienic wipes on my inflamed tissues, but the relief was always temporary.

Mom had to give up her job as an interior designer to look after me and drive me to all my doctor visits. For the next few months, we heard a lot of "educated guesses" about what was wrong with me. Anorexia. Leukemia. Addison's disease. Then we saw a gastroenterologist who ordered up a colonoscopy and EGD, the latter involving passing a long, flexible black tube with a light and video camera on one end though the mouth to examine the esophagus, stomach, and the first part of the small intestine called the duodenum. No matter which end got plumbed, those tests were awful.

But we got an answer. I had IBD—inflammatory bowel disease—from Crohn's disease and ulcerative colitis. My hemorrhoids? Those were perianal tags. At least now we knew what we were up against. But we were told there was no cure for IBD— that I would be dealing with it for the rest of my life. To manage these conditions, I began taking medications, but they came with heavy side effects: arthritis, steroid-induced diabetes, and autoimmune hepatitis, just to name a few.

I struggled a lot when I was on meds. Anything I ate felt like I was swallowing rocks. My illnesses affected my entire digestive tract; I had disease from the back of my tongue all the way through the anus. I even had three fissures at the base of my spine to my anus.

Weight practically evaporated off my body. I went from 104 pounds to 61 pounds only two months after my 13th birthday. My mom wasn't aware that I knew she slept each night with her hand on my chest, praying for me to heal. I didn't know what was going to happen to me.

I hated to see all my doctors. Lots of needles. I could recite my symptoms in my sleep: intense abdominal pain, fever spikes, constant diarrhea, and rectal bleeding. At 61 pounds, you could count my ribs and see my hip bones. If you don't believe me, go to my Facebook page.

One of the photos is me with Dr. Joe Brasco. He's done so much to help me. He is the finest doctor I have encountered, and I have seen a bunch of doctors. Jordan Rubin is not only my hero, but he's become a personal friend as well. In late 2004, Mom had volunteered to use her interior design skills and help decorate our church when a lady, Joy Halstead, walked up to Mom and told her she had been praying for me. She went on to ask Mom if she had heard of Jordan Rubin and how he had won his battle with Crohn's disease.

Mom went out and bought *The Maker's Diet* and *Restoring Your Digestive Health* and stayed up three days reading these books and taking notes. Then she read both books to me.

I thought Mom was really "out there" when we started a very strict regimen based on Jordan's writings. We called this version "Eat on Purpose: Nutrition or Nonsense." After eating the foods that Jordan recommended, I really started to feel well for the first time. I began putting on much-needed weight, and not long after that, my Crohn's disease went into a state of complete remission. I was thrilled! I could battle Crohn's and colitis and win!

Mom took Jordan's suggestion about drinking goat's milk seriously. When she couldn't find any goat's milk in the local health food stores, she found a farm with a goat herd, learned how to milk a goat, and then found out how to purchase a goat share.

Mom began working in health food stores to help us afford my food and supplements. Please understand that Mom did this for me and for my three sisters. If this disease could happen to me, it could happen to them as well. Mom always tells me that my struggle with Crohn's has helped save my sisters' health from deteriorating like mine did.

Mom and I met Jordan at a natural health trade show in October 2006, which was fantastic. When Jordan heard my story, he invited Mom and me to go to Florida for Jordan's first "Weekend of Wellness" seminars held in in Jupiter, Florida. Even better, he gave us a scholarship—all expenses paid. I was too scared to fly on a plane, so I asked Mom if Mrs. Joy could go with her since she had been the one to tell Mom about Jordan. They departed in early January to sunny Florida.

One of the speakers at the three-day conference was Dr. Brasco, and Mom really liked what he had to say. She said he was the least pretentious doctor she had ever encountered. Fortunately, she had brought all my medical records with her. Mom had a meeting with Dr. Brasco and asked if he would be willing to take me on as a patient. I was 15 at the time, in remission since February 2005, but my doctor had "fired" Mom because I wanted to continue treating my Crohn's with nutrition and probiotic supplementation, and he wasn't happy that we had weaned me off all meds. We needed a new gastroenterologist, and I wanted to be under Dr. Brasco's care.

"I've never had a patient that young, but I'll take her on," he said. Normally, Dr. Brasco has a four- to five-month wait to see him, but two weeks later, we were in Huntsville, Alabama, for our first visit.

Dr. Brasco was quite impressed with the diet Mom had me on and said it was even stricter than what he would suggest. He told me to stay on the same course and make sure I stayed away from grains. "Don't load the gun with a bullet, if you know it's a bullet," he said. I've since learned to heed that advice because if I do eat a grain product, I'll have a flare-up, and that's *no* fun. If I don't consume raw fermented dairy, then I'm in trouble again.

My weight fluctuates between 90 and 100 pounds these days. Dr. Brasco would like me at 115 pounds, so I'm working my way there. But another great part of my story is that Dr. Brasco, Jordan Rubin, and my mother, Michele, have formed the Guts to Glory Foundation to help other families with IBD. They believe proper nutrition and probiotic supplements are a viable medical protocol, and so do I.

We have support groups and organize benefits and galas to raise money for research. We do a benefit 10k walk each year close to home, and let me tell you: I really appreciate getting out in the fresh air and walking for a worthwhile cause.

Barbara Brown

Age: 73

Hometown: Huntsville, Alabama

I love Southern cooking, and always have. Deep-fried catfish and okra with all the trimmings and pies, cakes, and candy for dessert. I like most anything with chocolate and nuts, and chocolate meringue pies and lemon meringue pies are my favorite desserts. You could say I have a real sweet tooth.

Maybe all that sugar didn't like me. I suffered for years from acid reflux—that burning feeling that comes up in your esophagus. I had a classic case of heartburn.

My brother had colon cancer, and he told me I better do something about my digestive troubles because they could be a sign that I had something worse. I started seeing Dr. Brasco just as he was testing the Probiotic Diet. He asked me if I would like to follow the program and see what happens. I said yes because I just wanted to get healthier.

I knew it was going to be tough, but I wanted to do it. You have to make up your mind that this is something you want to do, not something that someone is going to make you do. That was important for me.

The sugar had to go first, and that was hard. I had to cut out desserts and say no to sweets when they were offered to me in social settings. I would say I did really well, except for the occasions when my 95-year-old mother-in-law, Pauline Brown, tempted me with her delicious banana pudding and chocolate meringue pies. For nearly a year, though, about the only "bad" thing I ate was a piece of cake that my sister-in-law, Alice Counts, made for my husband, Ken, and me. It was our 50th wedding anniversary cake, and how could I resist? But I just had a small piece.

Besides that petite indiscretion, I did everything I was supposed to. I drank apple cider vinegar with my meals. I took the probiotic supplements that Dr. Brasco suggested for me. I learned to drink kefir—something totally new for me. I put good olive oil and ground flaxseed on my salads. I ate salad for lunch instead of a po' boy sandwich. Dinner was salmon, baked sweet potatoes, broccoli, or asparagus. Giving up biscuits and muffins was hard to do, but I did it.

Ken got a little frustrated at times. One time he said, "Can we have something besides salad for lunch?" But even though he didn't follow the Probiotic Diet as closely as I did, he lost a good 15 pounds. As for me, I've lost 20 pounds, going from 145 pounds to 125 pounds on my five-foot, one-inch frame. I lost two dress sizes, and that was fun shopping for new clothes.

Everything has been a pleasant surprise, although some of my friends were concerned because they thought I was losing weight from being sick. I didn't tell them what I was up to, figuring they don't want to hear about my diet, just as I don't want to hear about their diets.

After nearly a year of following the Probiotic Diet, I can unequivocally say that I'm much healthier. The Probiotic Diet took care of my acid reflux. Took care of my triglycerides and cholesterol levels, which were too high. Took care of my food cravings.

I'm pleased with the way things turned out and look forward to spending many more years with Ken and our three grandchildren.

Bryan Ott

Age: 33

Hometown: San Diego, California

You could say I reached my low point in 2006. Miserable does not begin to describe the state of my mental and physical being. I had been coping with Crohn's disease since I was 17 years old, and dealing with the fallout of this disease for 13 long, arduous years had taken a major toll on my body.

I spent many years on virtually every medication available to treat the disease. The protocol of numerous drugs and medications kept me functional at best, yet with a greatly diminished quality of life. Side effects from the drugs initiated the onset of many other conditions, including osteoporosis, which called for further medications and treatments. To this day I am still surprised—and impressed—that I graduated from college with degrees in engineering during a very dark time in my life.

A year before, in 2005, my Crohn's disease had created a fistula—in essence a hole—from my colon to the bladder. Waste from the colon was entering the bladder, creating an infection.

Surgery was required to repair the damage and resulted in the removal of eight inches of my sigmoid colon and two inches of the ileum.

But things turned a lot worse in 2006. I was five months removed from surgery, and for some unknown reason, my colon had ceased to function and was lying dormant, a condition called colonic inertia. This essentially prevented me from having a bowel movement, and if you cannot expel what you eat, you cannot eat. This compounded my digestive disorder and created greater malnutrition and weight loss.

In July, at the age of 30, my doctors told me there was nothing they could do for me. They recommended I have a colectomy, which was the complete removal of my colon. I would be fitted with a permanent external ostomy pouch to collect the waste my body produced for the rest of my life. I had gone from seemingly bad to somewhere so low on the chart that it didn't register.

Knowing my fate was in the hands of modern medicine, it was now up to me to save my own butt (no pun intended). So with nothing but my colon to lose, I turned to alternative methods to prevent such a catastrophic change in my life.

My acupuncturist loaned me one of Jordan Rubin's books, which is how I was introduced to the Maker's Diet and proper nutrition. I committed myself to the Maker's Diet, but I cheated and started on Phase III instead of Phases I and II, which were too intimidating. Within the first week of being on the Maker's Diet, starting at the maintenance Phase III, however, I noticed better bowel function. Shortly thereafter I started to take probiotic nutritional supplements.

A few months later, I was feeling well enough to try surfing again. For my sanity's sake, I needed to get back in the water. Although my condition had greatly improved, I knew I could do better. I was experiencing the power of the Maker's Diet, but I just could not get over the hump. I knew that renewed health was within my grasp, but I did not know how to accomplish it.

By providence, I heard that Jordan Rubin was putting on his first health and wellness seminar in Jupiter, Florida. I booked a flight and flew from San Diego to West Palm Beach. This would have been in January 2007. The three-day seminar gave me an excellent opportunity to learn from Jordan and his team. Plus, I had a personal one-on-one meeting with Jordan to go over my health concerns and tailor-make a diet plan to help improve my health.

I have to say, though, that Jordan gave me a real whopper of a plan that I had to stick to over the next four months, which was basically Phase I of the Maker's Diet. Jordan added special caveats and a longer duration that made the book version look like a walk in the park. But as this was the answer to my prayers, I knew the decision had been made for me and I would complete this new diet.

One of the unique things about my new diet was eating cultured dairy products like kefir and goat's milk yogurt. The tart taste of kefir was fine; the "goaty" taste of goat's milk dairy products took some getting used to, but now I prefer them. What I didn't know at the time was that Jordan was recommending these cultured dairy products as a way to populate my gut with beneficial microorganisms. I think eating fermented foods like you find in the Probiotic Diet, in combination with the dietary changes Jordan recommends in all his books, really helped me feel better than I had in a long, long time.

After a month on my special version of the Maker's Diet, the problems of abdominal distension were gone, my bowel function was vastly improved, and I had increased energy levels. At the end of February 2007, I was due for my bimonthly Remicade infusion. (Remicade is a pharmaceutical drug used to treat Crohn's disease, but side effects include decreasing the body's ability to fight off an infection.) I was feeling so well at this time that I decided to skip it and really give the diet thing its fair chance.

Two months later, I was due for another Remicade infusion, but I decided to skip that one, too. Two months after that, my doctor agreed that I could stop receiving Remicade since I was feeling so well. I was no longer experiencing any of the classic Crohn's disease symptoms—abdominal pain, incontinence, cramping, bloating, fever, chills, and other flu-like symptoms. And my bowel function had been restored. The dreaded colectomy had been averted.

In October 2007 it was time for the next step—stopping all my medication. My doctors greatly admonished this decision, but after several weeks of contemplation and prayer, I felt it was the right thing to do. I was ready to fully trust my health to the Maker's Diet and what I had learned from Jordan. So I stopped all my medications on October 31, 2007.

At the time I am writing this, it's March 2009, and I feel fantastic. I've been off all medications for over one year, using food as my medicine, and I have not had a single flare-up. From diet alone, I was able to greatly transform and regain my health. I had forgotten how it felt to feel well. I am in awe of how just changing my eating habits had such a tremendous effect on my life and wellbeing. I have more energy, my mental outlook and demeanor are very positive, and the constant nagging stomach aches from Crohn's disease that had plagued me for many years are gone.

The way I see things, I have written off my twenties, basically forfeiting a decade of my life as I was so sick and depressed due to problems from Crohn's disease. But my thirties are looking better and better. For the first time since my teenage years, I feel like I am finally living.

Madisson Solid

Age: 15

Hometown: Fayetteville, Tennessee

Maybe it was the chili hot dogs my parents fixed up at my little sister's birthday party during the summer of 2007. All I know is that I felt really, really sick, and I had never felt that poorly before.

Mom thought I had got food poisoning from the canned chili she heated up to pour over the hot dogs. I felt horrible for a week and then got a little better, but by Labor Day weekend, my stomach hurt every time I ate something. I got to the point where I couldn't put anything in my mouth. I would go lie down on my bed and curl up in a fetal position, pulling my knees into my chest. That's when the tears would start.

My doctor kept telling me I had something called gastro-esophageal reflux disease, or GERD, so he put me on Prevacid. I took that prescription drug for three days, but it only made my symptoms worse. Then Mom took me to see a pediatric gastro-enterologist in Huntsville, who did an endoscopic procedure on me. That was no fun. He said I had GERD, too. He wanted me to continue taking the Prevacid, but I didn't want to take that medicine because it made me feel worse. My pediatrics doctor told me that I would just have to ride it out.

Mom didn't like what she was seeing. She sat down at our home computer and starting Googling some keywords like "digestive health" and Jordan Rubin and Dr. Brasco's book *Restoring Your Digestive Health* came up. She had heard of Mr. Rubin because of another book he wrote called *The Maker's Diet*, and Mom liked the book. We had made changes in what the family ate after reading *The Maker's Diet*, but we didn't stick to things real religiously, even though we did eat a lot more raw foods like fruits and vegetables. Anything with sugar in it was reserved for a special treat on Saturday nights. That's when Mom would bake some cookies or brownies, and we'd have some with our ice cream.

Mom purchased a copy of *Restoring Your Digestive Health* after Labor Day in 2007. She loved Dr. Brasco's philosophy of traditional medicine as well as alternative therapy in treating patients. The back of the book said that Dr. Brasco was practicing in Indianapolis, Indiana, but we were so desperate at this point—I was still feeling awful six months after eating those chili dogs—that Mom and Dad were ready to drive me to Indianapolis if that's what it took.

But then Mom did a Google search on Dr. Brasco and found out that he was practicing in Huntsville, just a 45-minute drive from our home. I'll never forget watching Mom blink back tears at the computer when she learned that help could be around the corner.

We got an appointment to see Dr. Brasco within two weeks. He asked some questions and then explained that he wanted to see me every week until we could narrow down what the problem was. Of course, he looked over all my old charts from the previous doctors, but he didn't think I had GERD. The first thing he did was start me on nutritional supplements with probiotics and digestive enzymes. Then he asked me to try sipping raw apple cider vinegar at my next meal. If I had GERD, the apple cider vinegar would help. If it wasn't GERD, then I would feel worse.

Sure enough, the apple cider vinegar burned terribly, so Dr. Brasco was fairly sure I didn't have GERD. Next, he turned his attention toward my gallbladder, and he ordered me to complete some tests. Sure enough, he discovered that I had a low-functioning gallbladder. I'll never forget what he said. "Madisson, I don't want to take out your gallbladder. I think we can fix this. It may take a year, but only if you're willing to work with me and stick to the plan."

"Sure, Dr. Brasco," I said. "Whatever you say."

He asked me to follow a prototype diet he was working on with Jordan Rubin called "The Probiotic Diet." I started eating high omega-3 eggs in the morning. A tuna salad with carrots and celery for lunch along with some fruits. Dad bought half a cow from Peaceful Pastures Co., where they raise only grass-fed meat. That's one of the benefits of living in a farming community like we do. Instead of brownies and ice cream for dessert, I satisfied myself with apples and peanut butter.

I'm amazed at how quickly I started feeling better. I felt so good that I even tried tomatoes, which used to cause my gallbladder to rebel and give me a lot of pain. Not anymore. I could eat tomatoes and tomato sauce.

I gained weight, too. I had gotten down to 104 pounds on my five-foot, six-inch frame. Now I'm 118 pounds. The Probiotic Diet has become a way of life for my family and me, and everyone can feel the difference in our health.

I've started taking horseback riding lessons again, but my real love is sewing costumes. I made my own Regency gown with a long straight skirt and an empire waist for a birthday party I had. For "Reformation Day" at our church, I sewed a Renaissance gown with a long full skirt out of ten yards of decorator's fabric. I had to play the role of Queen Elizabeth I of England. Both dresses had a lot of blood, sweat, and tears over them, but making those gowns myself really helped my sewing skills.

I hope to make many costume dresses in the future, and I think I will, thanks to Dr. Brasco and Jordan Rubin.

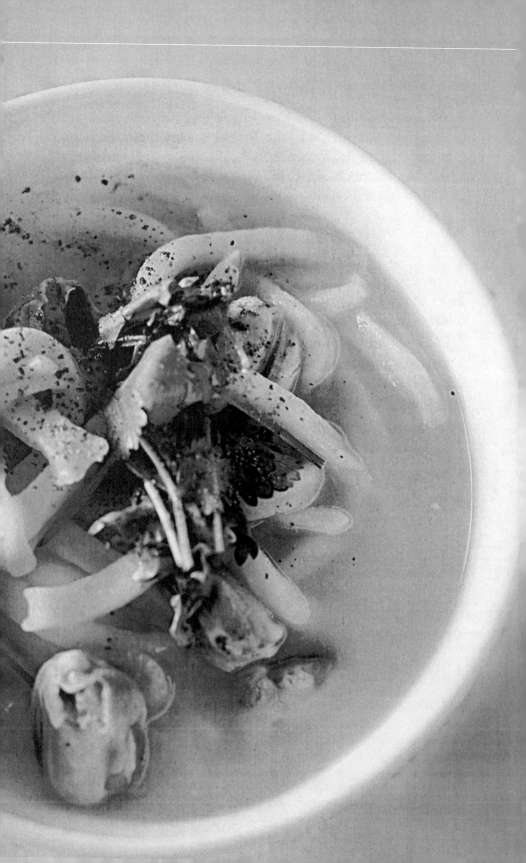

14

THE PROBIOTIC DIET RECIPES

By now, you know how important it is to consume a diet based on natural or whole foods—including healthy carbohydrates, proteins, and fats—for optimal gut health. Foods such as fermented dairy products, soaked or sprouted grains, grass-fed meats, raw foods—including fruits and vegetables—and foods high in omega-3 fatty acids rate high on the list.

Here are some recipes that will not only support gut health but will also satisfy your taste buds.

Fermented Foods Recipes

Did you know that the food of our ancestors, including fermented foods, contained several thousand times more bacteria—mainly the good probiotic bacteria—than our food does today? It's true and explains why our modernized way of eating has dramatically reduced or excluded foods produced by natural fermentation. The lack of good bacteria in our foods can decrease optimal digestion and assimilation of nutrition for gastrointestinal and overall health.

Homemade Kefir

While there are numerous places to get kefir starters or cultured vegetable starters, I recommend Body Ecology (bodyecologydiet.com) for kefir starters and cultured vegetable starters. Once you have your kefir starter, following this recipe:

Ingredients

1 quart raw goat's or cow's milk
1 packet kefir starter

Directions

Pour into quart-sized Mason jar. Add kefir starter. Set in a room temperature area for around 12-24 hours, but no more than 48 hours, then transfer to refrigerator. A cupboard is an ideal place to ferment. The temperature range should be between 70 to 75 degrees. Kefir can last several months in the refrigerator but will become sourer over time.

Source: Jordan Rubin

Cultured Vegetable Juice

Ingredients

- 3 red beets
- 1 carrot
- 2-4 Tbsp. fermented whey or 1 packet cultured vegetable starter
- 1 oz. grated ginger
- 1 tsp. fine Celtic sea salt
- purified water

Directions

Peel and chop beets and carrot; combine with peeled and grated ginger. Place in a 1-2 quart glass container with a seal. Cover with water and add whey and salt. Stir well and cover. Leave at room temperature for 2-3 days, then transfer to the refrigerator.

Source: Jordan Rubin

Five-Grain Porridge

Yield: serves 4

Ingredients

1 cup five-grain cereal mix (or choose any five whole
  grains, such as wheat, barley, spelt, millet, or quinoa)
1 cup water, plus 2 Tbsp. fermented whey or yogurt
½ tsp. Celtic sea salt
1 cup water
1 Tbsp. flaxseeds (optional)

Directions

Mix five-grain mixture and salt with water, add whey or
yogurt, then cover and let stand at room temperature
for at least 7 hours and as long as 24 hours. Bring
additional 1 cup of water to boil. Add soaked cereal,
reduce heat, cover, and simmer several minutes.
Meanwhile, grind flaxseed in a mini grinder. Remove
cereal from heat and stir in flax meal. Serve with butter
or cream thinned with a little water, and an organic
natural sweetener like Sucanat, date sugar, maple syrup,
or raw honey.

Source: Sally Fallon, author of *Nourishing Traditions*

General Recipes

These excellent, all-around recipes are built around foods that are part of the Probiotic Diet Eating Plan and include sprouted grains, smoothies, salads, grass-fed meats, nuts, and seeds. The smoothie recipes are great opportunities to use raw dairy products or kefir, goat's milk yogurt, or sheep's milk yogurt. Feel free to use whatever fresh fruits you would like.

Easy Oatmeal

Yield: serves 2

Ingredients

1 cup of rolled oats
2 cups of water
1 tsp. yogurt
1 Tbsp. extra-virgin coconut oil or butter
honey to taste

Directions

Soak the oats overnight in 1 cup of water with 1 tsp. of yogurt added. In the morning, add remaining water. Bring to a boil, then simmer for 1–2 minutes. Soaked oatmeal cooks very fast. Add the oil or butter and honey.

Easy French Toast

Yield: serves 4

Ingredients

1 cup plain yogurt

½ tsp. honey

2 pasture-raised eggs, slightly beaten

½ tsp. sea salt

8 slices sprouted or sourdough whole grain bread

Directions

Combine eggs, yogurt, honey, and salt in a mixing bowl. Dip each slice of bread quickly into the mixture and brown in extra-virgin coconut oil. Serve with butter and unheated honey, maple syrup, or fresh fruit.

Quick Sprouted Apple Crisp

Yield: serves 4

Ingredients

4 medium baking apples

1 oz. purified water

⅔ cup Ezekiel 4:9 sprouted cereal

1 Tbsp. butter

2 Tbsp. honey, separated

Directions

Preheat oven to 375 degrees. Peel, core, and chop the apples. Place apples in medium–sized pot with water and butter. Cover and cook on medium heat for 15 minutes or until apples can be mashed with a fork to the consistency of apple sauce. Stir in 1 Tbsp. of honey. Pour mixture into a medium–sized baking dish. Pour cereal evenly over apple mixture and press down with a fork. Drizzle with remaining 1 Tbsp. of honey. Bake for 15 minutes. Remove from heat, let cool, and serve.

Easy Whole Grain Waffles

Yield: serves 6

Ingredients

- 1 ⅓ cups whole grain flour (sprouted whole wheat, einkorn or spelt)
- ¾ tsp. sea salt
- 2 tsp. non–aluminum baking powder
- 2 Tbsp. unheated honey
- 1 cup water
- 2 Tbsp. plain yogurt
- 4 Tbsp. extra-virgin coconut oil
- 2 pasture-raised eggs, separated

Directions

Soak the flour in water with 2 Tbsp. of yogurt for at least 7 hours. Separate the eggs. Beat the yolks and add the yogurt and butter. Combine salt, honey, and flour and add this to the first mixture. Beat the egg whites until they form stiff peaks, and then fold them into the mix. Mix in the baking powder quickly. Cook in your waffle iron.

Creamsicle Smoothie

Yield: serves 2

Ingredients

- 6 oz. of yogurt or kefir
- 4 oz. freshly squeezed orange juice
- 1–2 raw omega–3 pasture-raised eggs (optional)
- 1 Tbsp. of flaxseed oil or hemp seed oil
- 1–2 Tbsp. unheated honey
- 1 Tbsp. of multi collagen or bone broth protein powder (optional)
- 1–2 fresh or frozen bananas
- vanilla extract (optional)

Directions

Combine all ingredients in a high-speed blender and blend until desired texture.

Banana Peach Smoothie

Yield: serves 2

Ingredients

- 10 oz. of yogurt, kefir, or coconut milk/cream
- 1-2 raw omega-3 pasture-raised eggs (optional)
- 1 Tbsp. of extra-virgin coconut oil
- 1 Tbsp. of flaxseed oil or hemp seed oil
- 1-2 Tbsp. unheated honey
- 1 Tbsp. of multi collagen or bone broth protein powder (optional)
- ½-1 cup fresh or frozen peaches
- 1 fresh or frozen banana
- ½ tsp. vanilla extract (optional)

Directions

Combine all ingredients in a high-speed blender and blend until desired texture.

Source: Nicki Rubin

Beef and Chicken Fajitas

Yield: serves 4-6

Ingredients

- 2 pounds chicken breast (or beef) cut into strips, about ¼ to ½ inch thick
- 6 Tbsp. extra-virgin olive oil
- ½ cup lemon or lime juice
- ¼ cup pineapple juice (optional)
- 4 garlic cloves, peeled and mashed
- ½ tsp. chili powder
- 1 tsp. dried oregano
- ½ tsp. dried thyme
- 1 red pepper, seeded and cut into julienne strips
- 1 green pepper, seeded and cut into julienne strips
- 2 medium onions, thinly sliced
- extra-virgin olive oil
- 12 sprouted whole wheat tortillas
- melted butter
- crème fraîche or sour cream for garnish
- chismole for garnish
- guacamole for garnish

Directions

Make a mixture of oil, lemon or lime juice, pineapple juice and spices and mix well with the meat. Marinate for several hours. Remove with a slotted spoon to paper towels and pat dry. Using a heavy skillet, sauté the meat, a batch at a time in olive oil, transferring to a heated platter and keeping warm in the oven. Meanwhile, mix vegetables in marinade. Sauté vegetables in batches in olive oil and strew over meat. Heat tortillas briefly in a heavy cast iron skillet and brush with melted butter. Serve meat mixture with tortillas and garnishes.

Source: Sally Fallon, author of *Nourishing Traditions*

Blueberry Muffins

Yield: 12 muffins

Ingredients

- 1¼ cups freshly ground or soaked whole grain flour (sprouted whole wheat, einkorn or spelt)
- ¾ cup water mixed with 1 Tbsp. of yogurt
- 1 cup blueberries, fresh or frozen
- 1 egg, lightly beaten
- ¼ tsp. fine Celtic sea salt
- ½ cup extra-virgin coconut oil
- ⅓ cup honey
- 2 tsp. baking powder
- 1 tsp. vanilla

Directions

Mix flour with water and yogurt and let stand overnight. Mix in remaining ingredients. Pour into well-buttered muffin tin about three quarters full. Place 5-7 blueberries on each muffin. Berries will fall partway into the muffins. Preheat oven to 400 degrees F. Bake for 15-20 minutes. Note: 1 cup buckwheat flour or cornmeal may be used in place of 1 cup spelt, kamut or whole wheat flour.

Source: Sally Fallon, author of *Nourishing Traditions*

Blueberry Pecan Pancakes

Yields: 12 pancakes

Ingredients

1½ cups freshly ground or soaked whole grain flour
(sprouted whole wheat, einkorn or spelt)

¾ cup water mixed with 1 Tbsp. of yogurt

1 egg, lightly beaten

½ cup blueberries (fresh or frozen)

½ cup crispy pecans

¼ tsp. Celtic sea salt

½ cup extra-virgin coconut oil

2 tsp. baking powder

1 tsp. vanilla

Directions

Mix flour with water and yogurt and let stand overnight.
Defrost blueberries in refrigerator if frozen. Mix
ingredients into a bowl. Heat a half-cup of extra-virgin
coconut oil in a skillet or pan over low heat. Increase
temperature to moderate heat. Use about 3 Tbsp. of
batter for each pancake. Serve with honey, maple syrup
and butter.

Source: Sally Fallon, author of *Nourishing Traditions*

Easy Oriental Salmon Salad

Yield: serves 4

Ingredients

3 Tbsp. soy sauce

2 tsp. grated fresh ginger

2 salmon filets

5 cups mixed salad greens

1 cup fresh bean sprouts

1 cup fresh snow pea pods, trimmed

½ green bell pepper, thinly sliced

½ red bell pepper, thinly sliced

1 small or medium cucumber, thinly sliced

1 cup sliced green onions

2 tsp. sesame seeds, toasted

Oriental Salad Dressing (see 410 for recipe)

Spicy Peanut Sauce (see 411 for recipe)

Directions

Combine soy sauce and ginger in a shallow baking dish. Add salmon. Cover and marinate in refrigerator up to 4 hours. Remove salmon from marinade and discard remaining marinade. Cook fish until lightly browned. Combine mixed salad greens and next 6 ingredients. Pour a half-cup Oriental Salad Dressing over salad and toss. Arrange cooked salmon and pour more salad dressing on top. Serve with Spicy Peanut Sauce.

Oriental Salad Dressing

Yield: one cup

Ingredients

4 Tbsp. rice vinegar

2 Tbsp. soy sauce

2 tsp. grated ginger

2 tsp. toasted sesame oil

2 tsp. finely chopped green onion or chives

2 cloves garlic, peeled and mashed

1 tsp. raw honey

⅔ cup extra-virgin olive oil

2 tsp. unrefined flax seed oil

Directions

Place all ingredients in a jar and shake vigorously.

Spicy Peanut Sauce

Yields 1 and ⅓ cups

Ingredients

- ½ cup peanut butter
- ⅓ cup coconut milk
- 2 Tbsp. soy sauce
- 1 Tbsp. grated fresh ginger
- 1 Tbsp. sesame oil
- ¼ tsp. dried crushed red pepper
- ¼ cup chicken broth

Directions

Combine all ingredients in a bowl and mix well.

Source: Nicki Rubin

Marinated Raw Vegetables with Jack Cheese Wrap

Yield: serves 1

Ingredients

marinated raw vegetables

Jack cheese

sprouted grain or sprouted wheat tortilla

Directions

Place ingredients in sprouted grain tortilla. Add and spread mayonnaise, mustard, or hummus. Roll up tortilla.

Source: Sheila Barcelo of Eden's Gourmet in Central Florida

Mocha Swiss Almond Smoothie

Yield: serves 2

Ingredients

- 10 oz. of yogurt, kefir, or coconut milk/cream
- 1-2 raw omega-3 pasture-raised eggs (optional)
- 1 Tbsp. of extra-virgin coconut oil
- 1 Tbsp. of flaxseed oil or hemp seed oil
- 1-2 Tbsp. unheated honey
- 1 Tbsp. of multi collagen or bone broth protein powder (optional)
- 2 Tbsp. cocoa or carob powder and 2 Tbsp. raw almond butter or 4 Tbsp. chocolate almond spread
- 1-2 fresh or frozen bananas
- ½ tsp. vanilla extract

Directions

Combine all ingredients in a high-speed blender and blend until desired texture.

Source: Nicki Rubin

Mushroom, Spinach, and Swiss Cheese Wrap

Yield: single serving

Ingredients

sautéed mushrooms

cooked spinach

Swiss cheese

sprout grain or sprouted wheat tortilla

Directions

Place ingredients in sprouted grain tortilla. Add and spread mayonnaise, mustard, or hummus. Roll up tortilla.

Source: Sheila Barcelo of Eden's Gourmet in Central Florida

Pepitas

Yield: 4 cups

Ingredients

4 cups raw, hulled pumpkin seeds
1 Tbsp. sea salt or Herbamare
1 tsp. cayenne pepper (optional)
filtered water

Directions

This recipe imitates Aztec practices of soaking seeds in brine, then letting them dry in the hot sun. They ate pepitas whole or ground into meal. Dissolve salt in water and add pumpkin seeds and optional cayenne. Soak for at least 7 hours or overnight. Drain in a colander and spread on 2 stainless steel baking pans. Place in a warm oven (no more than 150 degrees) for about 12 hours or overnight, stirring occasionally, until thoroughly dry and crisp. Store in an airtight container.

Source: Sally Fallon, author of *Nourishing Traditions*

Roast Beef with Marinated Cabbage and Provolone Cheese Wrap

Yield: single serving

Ingredients

roast beef

marinated cabbage

Provolone cheese

sprout grain or sprouted wheat tortilla

Directions

Place ingredients in sprouted grain tortilla. Add and spread mayonnaise, mustard, or hummus. Roll up tortilla.

Source: Sheila Barcelo of Eden's Gourmet in Central Florida

Turkey and Goat Cheese Wrap

Yield: single serving

Ingredients

turkey

sprouts

tomatoes

goat cheese

sprouted grain or sprouted wheat tortilla

Directions

Place ingredients in sprouted grain tortilla. Add and spread mayonnaise, mustard, or hummus. Roll up tortilla.

Creamy High Enzyme Dessert

Yield: single serving

Ingredients

4 oz. goat's milk, plain yogurt, or cultured cream
1 Tbsp. raw, unheated honey
1 tsp. flaxseed oil
½ cup fresh or frozen organic berries

Directions

Mix yogurt, honey, and flaxseed oil and top with berries.

Mochaccino Smoothie

Yield: serves 2

Ingredients

10 oz. of yogurt, kefir, or coconut milk or cream
1–2 raw omega-3 pasture-raised eggs (optional)
1 Tbsp. of extra-virgin coconut oil
1 Tbsp. of flaxseed or hemp seed oil
1–2 Tbsp. of unheated honey
1 Tbsp. of multi collagen or bone broth protein powder
(optional)
2 Tbsp. of cocoa or carob powder
1 Tbsp. of organic roasted coffee beans
1–2 fresh or frozen bananas
½ tsp. vanilla extract

Directions

Combine all ingredients in a high–speed blender and
blend until desired texture.

Piña Colada Smoothie

Yield: serves 2

Ingredients

- 10 oz. of coconut milk/cream
- 1–2 raw omega–3 pasture-raised eggs (optional)
- 1 Tbsp. of flaxseed oil or hemp seed oil
- 1–2 Tbsp. unheated honey
- 1 Tbsp. of multi collagen or bone broth protein powder (optional)
- 1 cup fresh or frozen pineapple
- 1 fresh or frozen banana
- ½ tsp. vanilla extract

Directions

Combine all ingredients in a high–speed blender and blend until desired texture.

Berry Smoothie

Yield: serves 2

Ingredients

- 10 oz. of yogurt, kefir, or coconut milk or cream
- 1–2 raw omega–3 pasture-raised eggs (optional)
- 1 Tbsp. of extra-virgin coconut oil
- 1 Tbsp. of flaxseed oil or hemp seed oil
- 1–2 Tbsp. of raw honey
- 1 Tbsp. of multi collagen or bone broth protein powder (optional)
- ½–1 cup of fresh or frozen berries (blueberries, strawberries, raspberries, blackberries)
- vanilla extract (optional)

Directions

Combine all ingredients in a high–speed blender and blend until desired texture.

Crispy Almonds

Yield: 4 cups

Ingredients

4 cups blanched almonds
2 tsp. sea salt or Herbamare
filtered water

Directions

Blanched or skinless almonds will still sprout, an indication that the blanching process has not destroyed the enzymes. (The skins are probably removed by a machine process.) Many people find that almond skins are irritating to the mouth, even when they have been soaked or sprouted. There is still plenty of goodness in skinless almonds. You can use crispy almonds in numerous dessert recipes. Soak almonds in salt and filtered water for at least 7 hours or overnight. Drain in a colander. Spread on two stainless steel baking pans and place in a warm oven (no more than 150 degrees) for 12 to 24 hours, stirring occasionally, until completely dry and crisp. Store in an airtight container.

Omega-3 Recipes

Omega-3 fatty acids, one of four basic types of fat that the body derives from food, are a form of polyunsaturated fats that are increasingly recognized as important to human health. It's important to note, however, that omega-3 fatty acids are not a single nutrient but a collection of several nutrients. The three most important omega-3 fatty acids are eicosapentaenoic acid (EPA), docosahexanoic acid (DHA), and linolenic acid.

Omega-3 fatty acids can be found in salmon, cod, albacore tuna, mackerel, lake trout, herring, high omega-3/DHA pasture-raised eggs, flaxseed oil, fish or cod liver oil, walnuts, as well as some fruits and vegetables.

The following fish and egg recipes have been selected based on their omega-3 content. Take a look at just how packed with these nutritious fats the ingredients are.

Sample Nutritional Values

- Four ounces of salmon provide 87.1 percent of the daily value, or DV, of omega-3 fatty acids.

- Four ounces of cod provide 13.3 percent of DV of omega-3 fatty acids.

- Four ounces of halibut provide 25.8 percent of the DV of omega-3 fatty acids.

- Four ounces of tuna provide 13.8 percent of the DV of omega-3 fatty acids.

Organic pasture-raised eggs from hens allowed to feed on insects and green plants usually contain omega-6 and omega-3 fatty acids in the beneficial ratio of approximately 1:1. Commercial supermarket eggs, however, often contain as much as *19 times* more omega-6 fatty acids than omega-3 fatty acids, so be sure to choose organic.

Cilantro-Lime Marinated Fish Tacos

Yield: serves 4

This simple fish taco recipe yields huge flavor. You can prepare most of this ahead of time, although we recommend that you marinate the fish for only a few hours. You can substitute any white fish; just make sure to use wild-caught, deep-water fish.

Ingredients

1 pound halibut filets
4 limes, juiced
2 Tbsp. extra-virgin olive oil
⅛ tsp. sea salt
⅛ tsp. fresh ground black pepper
sprouted corn tortillas
black bean and corn salsa (see recipe on page 423)

Directions

Cut the fish into 1-inch cubes and place in plastic baggie. In a small bowl, combine the lime juice, olive oil, salt, and pepper and whisk together. Pour marinade into baggie containing fish. Seal and let sit in the refrigerator for 1-2 hours.

Heat 1 Tbsp. of olive oil in a 10-inch non-stick skillet over medium-high heat. Add fish (including marinade) to the pan and cook for 6-8 minutes until just cooked through. In a medium-sized bowl, gently mix the cooked fish and the black bean and corn salsa, being careful not to break up the fish. Serve with warmed sprouted corn tortillas.

Black Bean and Corn Salsa

Ingredients

1 cup black beans, cooked

1 cup corn

¼ cup red onion, diced

3 Tbsp. cilantro, chopped

1 Tbsp. extra-virgin olive oil

1 tsp. lime juice

Sea salt and pepper to taste

Directions

In a small bowl, combine black beans, corn, onions, and cilantro. Mix together olive oil and lime juice, drizzle over salsa, and toss to combine. Season with salt and pepper.

Maple-Crusted Salmon and Mixed Greens

Yield: serves 4

The subtle sweetness imparted by the maple syrup lends sophistication to an otherwise simple meal. Feel free to toss your favorite vegetables (or fruit) into the salad.

Ingredients

1 ½ pounds fresh salmon filets

extra-virgin olive oil

butter

2 Tbsp. maple syrup

6 cups baby lettuces, or mixed greens such as watercress or Mache

1 red pepper, seeded, cut into a julienne, and sautéed in olive oil

1 pound brown mushrooms, washed, dried very well, sliced, and sautéed in butter and olive oil

¾ cup basic salad dressing (see recipe on page 425)

Directions

Preheat oven to 350 degrees. Brush sides and bottom of salmon with olive oil and place on non-stick baking sheet. Brush the top of the salmon with maple syrup and sprinkle with salt and pepper. Bake at 350 degrees for about 10 minutes. Place under broiler for another 2 minutes until just lightly browned.

Meanwhile, mix greens with dressing and divide between four plates. Make a mound of red peppers and mushrooms on each plate. Place a portion of salmon on each mound of greens and pour pan juices over. Serve immediately.

Basic Salad Dressing

Ingredients

1 tsp. Dijon-type mustard, smooth or grainy

2 ½ Tbsp. raw wine vinegar

½ cup extra-virgin olive oil

1 Tbsp. flaxseed oil

Directions

Place the mustard into a small bowl. Add vinegar and mix. Add olive oil in a thin stream, stirring continually with a fork, until the oil is well-mixed. Add flaxseed oil and use immediately.

Tuna Tahini Salad

Yield: serves 6-8

This tuna salad is probably a far cry from the one your mom used to make and pack in your school lunch. For best results, use high-quality canned tuna packed in water.

Ingredients

2 large cans water-packed tuna, drained and flaked

¼ tsp. cayenne pepper

2 cups tahini sauce (see recipe on page 427)

4 medium onions, thinly sliced

melted butter and extra-virgin olive oil

⅓ cup toasted pine nuts

cilantro sprigs for garnish

toasted, sprouted, or sourdough bread or sprouted crackers

Directions

Preheat oven to 375 degrees. Place the onions on an oiled cookie sheet, brush with mixture of melted butter and olive oil, and bake at 375 degrees until crispy.

Mix tuna with cayenne pepper and 1 cup tahini sauce. Mound tuna on a platter. Scatter onions and pine nuts on top. Garnish with cilantro and serve with sprouted whole grain crackers and remaining tahini.

Tahini Sauce

Ingredients

2 cloves garlic, peeled and coarsely chopped

1 tsp. sea salt

½ cup tahini

1 Tbsp. unrefined flaxseed oil

1 cup water

½ cup fresh lemon juice

Directions

Place garlic in food processor with salt. Blend until minced. Add tahini and flaxseed oil and blend. Using an attachment that allows addition of liquids drop by drop, with motor running, add water. When completely blended, add lemon juice all at once and blend until smooth. Sauce should be the consistency of heavy cream. If too thick, add more water and lemon juice.

Seared Tuna with Brown Rice Cakes and Wakame Salad

Yield: serves 4

This meal is as impressive as it is healthy. Wakame is an edible kelp that has been consumed for centuries in Japan. As a bonus, it also contains fucoxanthin!

Ingredients

4 6-ounce tuna steaks

½ cup sake

½ cup soy sauce

1 tsp. ginger, grated

2 Tbsp. cilantro, chopped

4 Tbsp. clarified butter

1 medium onion, diced

1 clove garlic, chopped

1 jalapeño, seeded and chopped

1 cup shiitake mushrooms, chopped

3 cups brown rice, cooked

½ cup vegetable or fish stock

4 Tbsp. butter

1 ounce dried wakame

Directions

Mix together the sake, soy sauce, ginger and cilantro and marinate tuna steaks for 1-2 hours. Place tuna steaks in a hot pan with 2 Tbsp. of clarified butter sear to desired doneness.

In a 12-inch skillet over medium heat, melt 2 Tbsp. of butter. Add onions and garlic and sauté for 4-5 minutes. Add jalapeño and mushrooms and cook for another 6-8 minutes. Take 1 cup of cooked brown rice and place in food processor and pulse until coarsely ground. Put the ground rice and whole rice in a bowl, season with salt and pepper, and add sautéed vegetables. Mix well. Form rice into cakes. Heat 12-inch skillet over medium-high heat and add remaining 2 Tbsp. of clarified butter. Sear rice cakes for about 2 minutes per side.

In a medium saucepan, warm ½ cup fish or vegetable stock. Add 2 Tbsp. of cold unsalted butter and melt. Remove from heat and add wakame. To serve, place wakame (with sauce) on the plate, top with rice cake and then tuna steak.

Miso Soup

Yield: serves 6-8

Taking the time to make your own fish stock will greatly enhance the flavor of this healthy and hearty soup that originated in Japan. You can find miso paste in most health food stores or high-end grocery stores. For an added kick, you can always add edible kelp in the form of dried kombu.

Ingredients

1 ½ quarts homemade fish stock (see recipe on page 430)
4 Tbsp. soy sauce
3–4 Tbsp. miso
1 onion, sliced
½ green or Chinese cabbage, coarsely shredded
2 Tbsp. fish sauce (optional)

Directions

Bring stock to a boil, skim, and whisk in miso. Add remaining ingredients and simmer gently until vegetables are soft.

Fish Stock

Ingredients

3 or 4 whole fish carcasses, including heads (make sure to use wild-caught, deep-water fish)

2 Tbsp. extra-virgin coconut oil or butter

2 onions, coarsely chopped

1 carrot, coarsely chopped

several sprigs of fresh thyme

several sprigs of parsley

1 bay leaf

1 cup dry white wine

1 Tbsp. cider vinegar

Directions

Melt coconut oil in a large stainless-steel pot. Add the vegetables and cook gently for about 30 minutes, until soft. Add wine and bring to boil. Add fish carcasses and cover with cold filtered water. Add vinegar and bring back to boil. Add thyme, parsley, and bay leaf and simmer for four hours. Remove carcasses with slotted spoon and strain the liquid prior to use.

Basic Omelet

An omelet is a great way to start the morning and empty out your fridge of leftovers. Below you will find the basic recipe and some fun variations. To get the most nutrition out of your omelet, make sure you choose pasture-raised eggs that are high in omega-3 content.

Ingredients

4 fresh pasture-raised eggs, at room temperature

3 Tbsp. extra-virgin coconut oil or butter

pinch of sea salt

Directions

Crack eggs into a bowl. Add water and sea salt, and blend with a wire whisk. (Do not over-whisk or the omelet will be tough.) Melt coconut oil or butter in a well-seasoned cast iron skillet or frying pan. When foam subsides, add egg mixture. Tip pan to allow egg to cover the entire pan. Cook several minutes over medium heat until underside is lightly browned. Lift up one side with a spatula and fold omelet in half. Reduce heat and cook another 30 seconds or so—this will allow the egg on the inside to cook. Slide omelet onto a heated platter and serve.

Omelet Variations to Suit Your Taste

- **Mexican Omelet:** Add salsa, avocado, sour cream, and jack cheese to omelet just before folding.

- **Onion, Pepper, and Goat Cheese Omelet:** Sauté 1 small onion, thinly sliced, and ½ red pepper, cut into julienne strips, in a little extra-virgin coconut oil or butter until tender. Strew this evenly over the egg mixture as it begins to cook, along with 2 oz. of goat's milk, cheddar, or feta cheese.

- **Garden Herb Omelet:** Scatter 1 Tbsp. parsley, finely chopped, 1 Tbsp. chives, finely chopped, and 1 Tbsp. thyme or other garden herb, finely chopped, over omelet as it begins to cook.

- **Mushroom Swiss Omelet:** Sauté ½ pound fresh mushrooms, washed, well-dried, and thinly-sliced, in extra-virgin coconut oil or butter and olive oil. Scatter mushrooms and grated Swiss cheese over the omelet as it begins to cook.

Cleansing Recipes

Wanting to do some digestive cleansing—allowing your body to take a break from excess calories, starches, and heavy processed foods? If so, here are some recipes for you.

Everyone can benefit from a good dietary cleansing to help sweep away unwanted toxins and perhaps unwanted fat. Toxins, which enter our systems through our food, air and water, and the accumulation of toxins in the environment, need to be cleansed or "detoxified" from our bodies.

The following recipes call for foods (including an abundance of high-fiber, antioxidant-packed vegetables and fruits) that support a cleaner you.

Taco Lettuce Wraps

Yield: serves 8

This recipe calls for a host of healthy ingredients, including tomatoes and walnuts. Tomatoes are carotenoids—a type of antioxidant that supports heart health and helps to support a strong immune system. Walnuts are one of the best sources of protein and omega-3 fatty acids—rich in fiber, B vitamins, magnesium, and antioxidants such as vitamin E. Walnuts also help support already healthy levels of cholesterol.

Taco "Meat" Ingredients

2 cups walnuts, soaked
⅓ cup wheat-free tamari soy sauce
1 bunch cilantro
1 Tbsp. cumin powder
½ Tbsp. coriander powder

Taco wraps and toppings:

1 head romaine lettuce
3 tomatoes, sliced
3 avocados, sliced
Celtic sea salt to taste
Equipment needed: food processor

Directions

In the afternoon of the day before, soak walnuts overnight in filtered water. Process taco "meat" ingredients in a food processor until the mixture resembles ground taco meat. Stop to scrape sides. Remove and set aside. Wash and choose from crispy lettuce leaves for taco wraps. Prepare avocados and tomatoes. Fill lettuce cavities with taco "meat" and top with toppings. Serve two tacos on a white salad plate with a favorite Mexican seasoning on top.

Salmon Sushi

Yield: serves 8

Included in this recipe are alfalfa sprouts—among some of the highest antioxidant foods. Carrots are included, too, and are carotenoids, a type of antioxidant that lowers the risk of heart disease and some types of cancer and helps to strengthen the immune system. The Salmon Pâté recipe calls for flaxseeds, which provide fiber and help support healthy estrogen metabolism and breast health in women and supports prostate health in men.

Ingredients for the Rolls:

2 cups Salmon Pâté (see recipe on page 436)
2 carrots, shredded or julienned
2 avocados, julienned
2 cucumbers, seeded and thinly sliced
2 red bell peppers, julienned
2 cups alfalfa sprouts or any variety
2 mangos, julienned
8 Nori seaweed sheets

Condiments:

wheat-free tamari
wasabi
pickled ginger

Equipment needed: food processor

Directions

Prepare ingredients. To assemble rolls, lay one sheet of Nori shiny side down. Layer ingredients stacked atop 2-3 rows, on one-third of the Nori sheet closest to you. To roll the sushi, grip the edge of the Nori sheet with your thumbs and forefingers. Press the filling back with your other fingers. Roll the front end of the Nori over the filling. Pull the Nori back with your fingers, giving the roll a tight squeeze, and continue rolling. Seal the edge with water and set seam side down. Cut the roll into 8 pieces with a sharp knife. Serve sushi with condiments for a satisfying light meal.

Salmon Pâté

Yield: serves 8

Ingredients for Flaxnaise:

- ¼ cup golden flaxseeds, soaked
- 1 cup filtered water
- 2 tsp. ground mustard powder
- ¼ cup lemon juice
- 1 Tbsp. raw honey
- ½ tsp. Celtic sea salt

Pâté:

- 1 and ½ cups carrot pulp
- ¾ cup minced onion
- 2 Tbsp. minced garlic
- ¾ cup Flaxnaise (from recipe)
- 1 cup chopped dill
- 1 Tbsp. dulse

Directions

To make Flaxnaise, crush flaxseeds to meal. Blend soaked seeds with lemon juice in a blender until whipped to a cream. Add filtered water, if needed, to prevent thickening. Texture should be smooth and not jelly-like. Add remaining ingredients and mix until blended. To make pâté, prepare ingredients and combine in a mixing bowl. Refrigerate to chill.

If you make this recipe for meals other than the Salmon Sushi recipe, you can serve the pâté with flax crackers or flat bread, wrapped in a romaine leaf or a Nori sheet.

Break-fast Salad

Yield: serves 8

This salad is a great way to add deliciously cleansing vegetables and fruits to your diet, including raisins, which rate extremely high in the ORAC scale—a measurement for the antioxidant levels in foods. Peaches, too, are high in antioxidants, which strengthen the immune system. The added fiber "topping" helps maintain a clean digestive system.

Dressing for the salad is not needed or missed because it satisfies every taste bud. The salad can be eaten any time during the day and can even replace a regular breakfast. Keep prepared ingredients refrigerated for easy assembly.

Ingredients

2 green leaf lettuce leaves, shredded

1 carrot, shredded

1 stalk celery, diced

1 peach or persimmon, diced

2 bananas, sliced

4 small radishes, diced

1 avocado, diced

1 slice red cabbage, shredded

1 tomato, diced

1 plum or pear, diced

¼ cup raisins

8 dates, diced

1 apple, shredded

½ cup walnuts, chopped

Directions

Layer ingredients in listed order. Arrange salad to include all the ingredients for a colorful display on a white dinner plate.

ALTs

Yield: serves 8

ALTs (avocado, lettuce, and tomatoes) are made with vegetable-based wraps and contain avocados—a rich source of monounsaturated fatty acids, including oleic acid, the carotenoid lutein, and significant quantities of the antioxidant vitamin E. The lettuce and tomatoes also add fiber and antioxidants.

Ingredients for Flaxnaise:

¼ cup golden flaxseeds, soaked

1 cup filtered water

2 tsp. ground mustard powder

¼ cup lemon juice

1 Tbsp. raw honey

½ tsp. Celtic sea salt

Filling:

2 avocados, sliced

1 cup alfalfa sprouts

Mrs. Dash seasoning, to taste

2 cups mixed greens

2 tomatoes, sliced

Equipment needed: Blender

Directions

Prepare filling ingredients. To make Flaxnaise, grind flaxseeds to a meal. Blend ingredients in a blender. Texture should be smooth and not a jelly-like texture. Add filtered water to prevent thickening. Fill wraps with filling and drizzle immediately with Flaxnaise. Serve wraps for a light meal.

ADDITIONAL ONLINE RESOURCES

The importance of shopping for locally grown organic fruits, vegetables, and dairy cannot be underestimated. Several websites are tremendous resources:

- **www.localharvest.org**
- **www.eatwild.com**
- **www.realmilk.com**

In addition, www.eatwellguide.org is an easy and comprehensive way to find wholesome, fresh, sustainable food in the U.S. and Canada. Find food in your neighborhood and when you travel that is healthful, humane, better for the environment, and that supports family farmers.

We also recommend **www.westonaprice.org**. The Weston A. Price Foundation is a nonprofit, tax-exempt charity founded in 1999 to disseminate the research of nutrition pioneer Dr. Weston Price, whose studies of isolated non-industrialized peoples established the parameters of human health and determined the optimum characteristics of human diets.

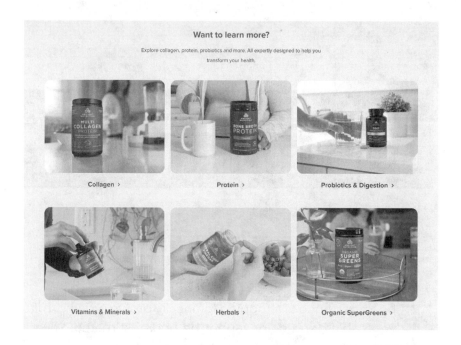

Want to learn more?

Explore collagen, protein, probiotics and more. All expertly designed to help you transform your health.

Collagen >

Protein >

Probiotics & Digestion >

Vitamins & Minerals >

Herbals >

Organic SuperGreens >

Finally, check out **www.ancientnutrition.com**. Ancient Nutrition provides supplements for digestive health, foundational nutrition, immunity support, optimal wellness, and weight management, as well as fitness and beauty supplements. This website not only discusses these products in detail but also contains our blog as well as scores of great recipes. Dr. Josh Axe and I co-founded Ancient Nutrition with an emphasis on gut health. For this reason, we believe our line of bone broth and collagen powders are among the best supplements for enhancing your gut health journey. We also love our SBO probiotic and watch it transform the lives of our customers when they use it along with the Probiotic Diet. Using our knowledge gained from years of studying health and wellness, we set out to create high-quality functional products, nutritional supplements, and educational resources to help you on your road to optimal health. Whether you use our products or other supplements, we are honored you trust us enough to pick up this book and to prioritize your gut health and feel well again!

NOTES

1. Free Probiotics

1. From the "John and Ken Show," KFI 640-AM radio in Los Angeles, from a show broadcast January 12, 2009.
2. "Facts About Antibiotic Resistance," an article on the U.S. Food and Drug Administration website and available at http://www.fda.gov/oc/opacom/hottopics/antiresist_facts.html and from "Overprescribing Antibiotics Creating 'Superbugs,'" *USA Today* newspaper, October 1, 1996, and available at http://findarticles.com/p/articles/mi_m1272?tag=content;col1
3. "Model Dies After Losing Hands, Feet to Urinary Tract Infection," FoxNews.com., January 24, 2009, and available at http://www.foxnews.com/story/0,2933,482548,00.html
4. "Milk: It Does a Body Good?" by Lori Lipinski, an article on the Weston A. Price Foundation website, and available at http://www.westonaprice.org/transition/dairy.html
5. "'Good' Germs May Fight Bad Ones in Hospital," Reuters, November 5, 2008.

2. "It's the Terrain"

1. René Dubos, *Louis Pasteur: Free Lance of Science* (New York, Charles Scribner's Sons, 1950, 1976), 8.
2. William Campbell Douglass II, M.D., *The Milk Book: The Milk of Human Kindness Is Not Pasteurized, 3rd ed.* (Panama, Republic of Panama: 2003), 42.

3. "The Post-Antibiotic Age: Germ Theory," by Tim O'Shea, which is available online at http://whale.to/vaccine/shea1.html

4. "Was the Man Behind Orthodox Medicine Louis Pasteur Wrong?" An article on the Expert Life Skills website, and available at http://expertlifeskills.com/was-the-man-behind-modern-medicine-louis-pasteur-wrong-what-are-the-implications-for-cancer-cure-if-he-was-wrong/

5. Joel Stein, "The Nuts Behind Kids' Allergies," *Los Angeles Times*, January 9, 2009.

6. "Claude Bernard: A Brief Biography," by Renato M.E. Sabbatini, Ph.D., an article on the cerebromente.org website at http://www.cerebromente.org.br/n06/historia/bernard_i.htm

7. "The Post-Antibiotic Age: Germ Theory," by Tim O'Shea, which is available online at http://whale.to/vaccine/shea1.html

8. Michael A. Schmidt, Lendon H. Smith, and Keith W. Sehnert, *Beyond Antibiotics: 50 (or so) Ways to Boost Immunity and Avoid Antibiotics* (Berkeley, California: North Atlantic Books, 1993), 14.

9. Jane G. Goldberg, *Deceits of the Mind and Their Effects on the Body* (Transaction Publishers, 1991), 56.

10. Ibid.

3. The Guts of the Matter

1. Rolf Benirschke, *Embracing Life: Great Comebacks from Ostomy Surgery* (Rolf Benirschke Enterprises, 2009), 53-54.

2. "Heartburn Fast Facts," by Sharon Gillson, columnist for the About.com website, and available at http://heartburn.about.com/od/understandingheartburn/a/hrtbrnfastfacts.htm

3. Jerry Lee Hutchens, *Simple Cleanse* (Book Publishing Company, 2005), 59.

4. "Auto-Intoxication: Death and Health Begin in the Colon," an article on the Light Party website at http://www.lightparty.com/Health/HealingRegeneration/html/Auto-Intoxication.html

5. T.S. Chen and P.S. Chen, "intestinal autointoxication: a medical leitmotif," *J Clin Gastroenterol.*, 1989, Aug;11(4):434-41, and available at http://www.ncbi.nlm.nih.gov/pubmed/2668399

6. Jennifer Ackerman, *Sex Sleep Eat Drink Dream* (Houghton Mifflin Harcourt, 2007), 60.

7. "Infants with Poor Intestinal Flora Often Develop Eczema," *ScienceDaily*, January 27, 2008, and available at http://www.sciencedaily.com/releases/2008/01/080123175324.htm

8. F. Guarner and J.R. Malagelada, 2003, Gut flora in health and disease, *The Lancet*, Volume 361, Issue 9356, 8 February 2003, pgs. 512-519.

9. Ackerman, *Sex Sleep Eat Drink Dream*, 60.

10. CNW Group press release, "The gut microflora and probiotics can impact stress and behaviour," November 25, 2008, and available at http://www.newswire.ca/en/releases/archive/November2008/25/c3874.html

4. Probiotics: The Good Germs

1. Some of the biographical material for Élie Metchnikoff was gleaned from the Nobel Prize Foundation website and from *Nobel Lectures, Physiology or Medicine 1901-1921* (Amsterdam: Elsevier Publishing Company, 1967).

2. John G. Simmons, *Doctors and Discoveries* (Houghton Mifflin Harcourt, 2002), 189.

3. Peter Cartwright, *Probiotics for Crohn's & Colitis* (Prentice Publishing, 2003), 21.

4. Frank Heynick, *Jews and Medicine* (KTAV Publishing House, Inc., 2002), 329.

5. "The Big Yogurt Binge," *Time* magazine, August 4, 1967.

6. Kingsley C. Anukam, Ph.D., and Gregor Reid, Ph.D., *Probiotics: 100 Years (1907-2007) After Élie Metchnikoff's Observation*, a scientific paper available online at http://www.formatex.org/microbio/pdf/Pages466-474.pdf

7. Ibid.

8. Jessica Siegel, "Asses' Milk and Melons," *The Record* newspaper, Bergen County, New Jersey, March 15, 1993.

9. Denise Dador, "Health Benefits of Probiotics," KABC-TV in Los Angeles, and available at http://abclocal.go.com/kabc/story?section=news/health&id=6274118

5. The True Probiotic Heroes

1. Dr. Mehmet Oz's PodCast on probiotics is available online at http://www .digestiveadvantage.com/transcript_understandingprobiotics.html

6. They Are What You Eat

1. Elaine Gottschall, *Breaking the Vicious Cycle* (Kirkton Press, 2004), 68.
2. Ibid., 80.

7. Probiotic Foods from Around the World

1. William Campbell Douglass, M.D., *The Milk Book* (Rhino Publishing, 1984, 1995 and 2003), 253.
2. Robert W. Hutkins, *Microbiology and Technology of Fermented Foods* (IFT Press, Blackwell Publishing, 2006), 3.
3. Ibid., 4.
4. John Roach, "'Antibiotic' Beer Gave Ancient Africans Health Buzz," National Geographic News, May 16, 2005, and available at http://news .nationalgeographic.com/news/pf/30891748.html
5. "Fermented Beverages of Pre- and Proto-History China, a research study available at http://www4.hmc.edu:8001/Chemistry/hvr/good%20ones/ Chinese%20Wine/Chinese%20Beer.pdf
6. Jim Ridley, "Kombucha: Anything That Tastes This Awful Must Be Good for You," Nashville Scene, February 4, 2009, and available at http://blogs .nashvillescene.com/bites/2009/02/kombucha_anything_that_tastes .php
7. Sally Fallon, *Nourishing Traditions* (Washington, DC: New Trends Publishing, Inc., 2001), 89.
8. Jill Neimark, "Cooking Culture: Tangy, Tasty, and Teeming with Health Benefits, Fermented Foods Are the New Stars of a Wholesome Diet," *Natural Health* magazine, April 2004, and available online at http:// findarticles.com/p/articles/mi_m0NAH/is_4_34/ai_114783531
9. Choe Sang-Hun, "*Kimchi* Goes to Space, Along with First Korean Astronaut," International Herald Tribune, February 22, 2008, and available at http://www.iht.com/articles/2008/02/22/asia/*kimchi*.php

10. Joel McConvey, "On *Kimchi*," found on the Walrus Blogs website at http://www.walrusmagazine.com/blogs/2008/05/13/korea-kimchi/ ?ref=2008.06-online-exclusive-korea-*kimchi*-joel-mcconvey-jeju -do&page=

8. Ladies and Germs

1. "Milton Berle," an obituary found on the Legacy.com website at http:// www.legacy.com/Obituaries.asp?Page=LifeStory&PersonID=272559

2. Vaginitis," an article on the MayoClinic.com website and available at http://www.mayoclinic.com/health/vaginitis/DS00255

3. Tracee Cornforth, "Bacterial Vaginosis/Vaginitis," on the About.com website, and available at http://womenshealth.about.com/cs/vaginosis/a/ bacterialvagin.htm

4. Larry Trivieri, Jr., editor, *Alternative Medicine: The Definitive Guide* (Celestial Arts, 2002), 967.

5. "Defensive Medicine Practice Leads to Dramatic Increase in Cesarean Section Rate," Chicago Community Midwives, November 19, 2005, and available at http://www.chicagocommunitymidwives.org/2005/11/19/ press-release-defensive-medicine-practice-leads-to-dramatic-increase -in-cesarean-section-rate/

9. Say Ah to Oral Probiotics

1. Chris Iliades, M.D., "The Mouthwash and Oral Cancer Connection," an article found on the EverydayHealth.com website at http://www .everydayhealth.com/oral-head-and-neck-cancer/mouthwash-and-oral -cancer.aspx

12. The Probiotic Diet Protocols

1. James Balch, M.D., *Prescription for Nutritional Cures* (Hoboken, NJ: John Wiley & Sons: 2004), 251.

2. "Antibiotics Linked to Asthma: Try Probiotics," an article posted on the ChicagoTribune.com website on June 13, 2007 at http://featuresblogs .chicagotribune.com/features_julieshealthclub/2007/06/antibiotics_up_ .html

3. *Encyclopedia of Natural Healing* (Burnaby, BC, Canada: Alive Publishing Group, Inc., 1997), 1037.

4. "How to Avoid—Gesundheit!—the Cold and Flu," by Amy Cox of cnn .com and available at http://www.cnn.com/2004/HEALTH/12/13/cold.flu .overview/

5. "Children's Illnesses: Top Four Causes of Missed School," an article on the MayoClinic.com website and available at http://www.mayoclinic.com/ health/childrens-conditions/CC00059

6. Tracee Cornforth, "Urinary Tract Infections," an article on the About.com website, May 13, 2008, and available at http://womenshealth.about.com/ cs/bladderhealth/a/UTI.htm

7. "High Blood Cholesterol," an article found on the MayoClinic.com website and available at http://www.mayoclinic.com/health/high-blood -cholesterol/DS00178

8. American Cancer Society's *Cancer Facts & Figures 2005* (Atlanta: American Cancer Society, 2005).

ABOUT THE AUTHORS

Jordan Rubin

JORDAN RUBIN is the *New York Times* bestselling author of *The Maker's Diet* and 29 additional titles. Jordan is the founder of Garden of Life, Beyond Organic, and Ancient Nutrition where he serves as CEO.

Josh Axe

JOSH AXE, DNM, DC, CNS, is the founder of DrAxe.com, one of the largest natural health websites in the world. Dr. Axe is the bestselling author of *Eat Dirt, Keto Diet, The Collagen Diet*, and *Ancient Remedies*. He is the co-founder of Ancient Nutrition.

Dr. Joseph Brasco

Specializing in the field of gastroenterology, DR. BRASCO offers customized treatment and management plans for patients suffering from issues of the gastrointestinal tract, also known as the digestive system. Treating conditions such as Crohn's disease, IBS or gastroesophageal reflux disease, Dr. Brasco is also competent in the effects of diet & nutrition, and their impact on your general well-being. Dr. Brasco is the co-author along with Jordan Rubin of *Restoring Your Digestive Health*.

YOUR Prophetic
COMMUNITY

Are you passionate about hearing God's voice, walking with Jesus, and experiencing the power of the Holy Spirit?

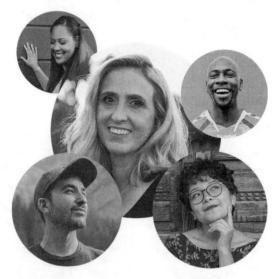

Destiny Image is a community of believers with a passion for equipping and encouraging you to live the prophetic, supernatural life you were created for!

We offer a fresh helping of practical articles, dynamic podcasts, and powerful videos from respected, Spirit-empowered, Christian leaders to fuel the holy fire within you.

Sign up now to get awesome content delivered to your inbox
destinyimage.com/sign-up

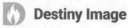 Destiny Image